Cardio-Oncology

Editor

MONIKA JACQUELINA LEJA

CARDIOLOGY CLINICS

www.cardiology.theclinics.com

November 2019 • Volume 37 • Number 4

ELSEVIER

1600 John F. Kennedy Boulevard • Suite 1800 • Philadelphia, Pennsylvania, 19103-2899

http://www.theclinics.com

CARDIOLOGY CLINICS Volume 37, Number 4
November 2019 ISSN 0733-8651, ISBN-13: 978-0-323-71186-9

Editor: Stacy Eastman
Developmental Editor: Laura Kavanaugh

Cardiology Clinics (ISSN 0733-8651) is published quarterly by Elsevier Inc., 360 Park Avenue South, New York, NY 10010-1710. Months of issue are February, May, August, and November. Business and Editorial Offices: 1600 John F. Kennedy Blvd., Ste. 1800, Philadelphia, PA 19103-2899. Customer Service Office: 3251 Riverport Lane, Maryland Heights, MO 63043. Periodicals post-age paid at New York, NY and additional mailing offices. Subscription prices are $349.00 per year for US individuals, $672.00 per year for US institutions, $100.00 per year for US students and residents, $432.00 per year for Canadian individuals, $843.00 per year for Canadian institutions, $466.00 per year for international individuals, $843.00 per year for international institutions and $220.00 per year for Canadian and international students/residents. To receive student/resident rate, orders must be accompanied by name of affiliated institution, data of term, and the *signature* of program/residency coordinator on institution letterhead. Orders will be billed at individual rate until proof of status is received. Foreign air speed delivery is included in all *Clinics* subscription prices. All prices are subject to change without notice. **POSTMASTER:** Send address changes to *Cardiology Clinics*, Elsevier Health Sciences Division, Subscription Customer Service, 3251 Riverport Lane, Maryland Heights, MO 63043. **Customer Service: 1-800-654-2452 (U.S. and Canada); 314-447-8871 (outside U.S. and Canada). Fax: 314-447-8029. E-mail: journalscustomerservice-usa@ elsevier.com (for print support); journalsonlinesupport-usa@elsevier.com (for online support).**

Reprints. For copies of 100 or more, of articles in this publication, please contact the Commercial Reprints Department, Elsevier Inc., 360 Park Avenue South, New York, NY 10010-1710. Tel.: 212-633-3874; Fax: 212-633-3820; E-mail: reprints@elsevier.com.

Cardiology Clinics is also published in Spanish by McGraw-Hill Interamericana Editores S. A., P.O. Box 5-237, 06500, Mexico D. F., Mexico; in Portuguese by Reichmann and Alfonso Editores Rio de Janeiro, Brazil; and in Greek by Dimitrios P. Lagos, 8 Pondon Street, GR115-28 Ilissia, Greece.

Cardiology Clinics is covered in *MEDLINE/PubMed (Index Medicus), Excerpta Medica, The Cumulative Index to Nursing and Allied Health Literature* (CINAHL).

Contributors

AUTHORS

KEVIN M. ALEXANDER, MD
Division of Cardiovascular Medicine, Stanford
Amyloid Center, Stanford University School of
Medicine, Stanford Cardiovascular Institute,
Stanford, California, USA; Instructor,
Advanced Heart Failure and Transplant
Cardiology, Stanford University School of
Medicine, Palo Alto, California, USA

JOSE ALVAREZ-CARDONA, MD
Division of Cardiovascular Medicine,
Fellow and Instructor, Cardio-Oncology
Center of Excellence, Washington University
in St. Louis, St Louis, Missouri,
USA

ANITA M. ARNOLD, DO, FACC, MBA
Assistant Professor of Medicine, Florida State
University School of Medicine, Director,
Cardio-Oncology, Lee Health, Ft Myers,
Florida, USA

AARTI ASNANI, MD
Director, Cardio-Oncology Program, Division
of Cardiovascular Medicine, CardioVascular
Institute, Beth Israel Deaconess Medical
Center, Boston, Massachusetts, USA

DINU VALENTIN BALANESCU, MD
Department of Cardiology, The University of
Texas MD Anderson Cancer Center, Houston,
Texas, USA

ANA BARAC, MD, PhD
Director, Cardio-Oncology Program, MedStar
Heart and Vascular Institute, Associate
Professor of Medicine and Oncology,
Georgetown University, Washington, DC, USA

TAREK BARBAR, MD
Department of Medicine, NewYork-
Presbyterian Hospital, Weill Cornell Medical
Center, New York, New York, USA

RACHEL BARISH, MSN, NP
Nurse Practitioner, MedStar Georgetown
Physicians Group, Division of Cardiology,
Washington, DC, USA

CATHLEEN BIGA, MSN, FACC
President/CEO, Cardiovascular
Management of Illinois, Woodridge, Illinois,
USA

PAULA HERNANDEZ BURGOS, MD
Department of Internal Medicine, Morsani
College of Medicine, University of South
Florida, Cardio-Oncology Program, Moffitt
Cancer Center, Tampa, Florida, USA

EDWARD Y. CHAN, MD
Department of Surgery, Houston
Methodist Hospital, Houston, Texas, USA

KONSTANTINOS CHARITAKIS, MD
Department of Cardiology, McGovern
Medical School, The University of Texas Health
Science Center at Houston, Houston, Texas,
USA

MEHMET CILINGIROGLU, MD
Department of Cardiology, Arkansas
Heart Hospital, Little Rock, Arkansas, USA

ROBERT J. CUSIMANO, MD
Division of Cardiac Surgery, Peter Munk
Cardiac Centre, Toronto General Hospital,
University of Toronto, Toronto, Ontario,
Canada

TEODORA DONISAN, MD
Department of Cardiology, The University of
Texas MD Anderson Cancer Center, Houston,
Texas, USA

ALESSANDRO EVANGELISTI, BS
Stanford Cardiovascular Institute,
Stanford University School of Medicine,
Stanford, California, USA; Research
Assistant, Stanford University School
of Medicine, Palo Alto, California, USA

MICHAEL G. FRADLEY, MD
Division of Cardiovascular Medicine,
Morsani College of Medicine, Associate
Professor of Medicine, University
of South Florida, Director, Cardio-Oncology
Program, Moffitt Cancer Center, Tampa,
Florida, USA

SARJU GANATRA, MD
Cardio-Oncology Program, Division of
Cardiovascular Medicine, Department of
Medicine, Lahey Hospital and Medical Center,
Burlington, Massachusetts, USA; Cardio-
Oncology and Adult Cancer Survivorship
Program, Dana-Farber Cancer Institute,
Division of Cardiovascular Medicine,
Department of Medicine, Brigham and
Women's Hospital, Boston, Massachusetts,
USA

EMILY GATES, MS
Research Assistant, MedStar Heart and
Vascular Institute, Georgetown University,
Washington, DC, USA

ANURADHA GODISHALA, MD
Division of Cardiovascular Medicine, Beth
Israel Deaconess Medical Center, Boston,
Massachusetts, USA

JUSTIN GODOWN, MD
Assistant Professor, Department of
Pediatrics, Division of Pediatric Cardiology,
Monroe Carell Jr. Children's Hospital
at Vanderbilt, Nashville, Tennessee,
USA

SALIM S. HAYEK, MD
Division of Cardiology, Department
of Medicine, University of Michigan,
University of Michigan Frankel
Cardiovascular Center, Ann Arbor,
Michigan, USA

JOERG HERRMANN, MD
Department of Cardiovascular Diseases,
Mayo Clinic, Rochester, Minnesota, USA

CHRISTOPHER W. HOEGER, MD
Department of Medicine, University
of Michigan, Ann Arbor, Michigan,
USA

WILLIAM GREGORY HUNDLEY, MD
Professor, Pauley Heart Center, Virginia
Commonwealth University Health Sciences,
Richmond, Virginia, USA

CEZAR ILIESCU, MD, FACC
Professor, Department of Cardiology,
The University of Texas MD Anderson
Cancer Center, Houston, Texas,
USA

JENNIFER HAWTHORNE JORDAN, PhD, MS
Assistant Professor, Department of
Biomedical Engineering, Virginia
Commonwealth University, Pauley
Heart Center, Virginia Commonwealth
University Health Sciences, Richmond,
Virginia, USA

JAYA KANDURI, MD
Department of Medicine, Beth Israel
Deaconess Medical Center, Boston,
Massachusetts, USA

YU KANG, MD, PhD
Division of Cardiovascular Diseases,
Department of Medicine, Hospital of the
University of Pennsylvania, Philadelphia,
Pennsylvania, USA

KAVEH KARIMZAD, MD
Department of Cardiology, The University of
Texas MD Anderson Cancer Center, Houston,
Texas, USA

PETER KIM, MD
Department of Cardiology, The University of
Texas MD Anderson Cancer Center, Houston,
Texas, USA

DANIEL J. LENIHAN, MD, FACC
Division of Cardiovascular Medicine, Professor
of Medicine, Director, Cardio-Oncology Center
of Excellence, Washington University in St.
Louis, St Louis, Missouri, USA

JENNIFER E. LIU, MD
Cardiology Service, Department of
Medicine, Memorial Sloan Kettering Cancer
Center, Department of Medicine, Weill
Cornell Medical College, New York, New York,
USA

JUAN LOPEZ-MATTEI, MD
Department of Cardiology, The University of
Texas MD Anderson Cancer Center, Houston,
Texas, USA

SYED S. MAHMOOD, MD, MPH
Cardiology Division, NewYork-Presbyterian
Hospital, Weill Cornell Medical Center, New
York, New York, USA

KONSTANTINOS MARMAGKIOLIS, MD
Florida Hospital, Pepin Heart Institute, Tampa,
Florida, USA

LUIS ALBERTO MORE, MD
CardioVascular Institute, Beth Israel
Deaconess Medical Center, Boston,
Massachusetts, USA

RAJARAM NAGARAJAN, MD, MS
Co-Director, Cardio-Oncology, Professor,
Department of Pediatrics, Division of
Oncology, Cancer and Blood Diseases
Institute, Cincinnati Children's Hospital
Medical Center, University of Cincinnati
College of Medicine, Cincinnati, Ohio, USA

TOMAS G. NEILAN, MD, MPH
Cardio-Oncology Program, Division of
Cardiology, Department of Medicine, Cardiac
MR/PET Program, Department of Radiology,
Division of Cardiology, Massachusetts General
Hospital, Boston, Massachusetts, USA

NICOLAS PALASKAS, MD
Department of Cardiology, The University of
Texas MD Anderson Cancer Center, Houston,
Texas, USA

ROHAN PARIKH, MD
Department of Medicine, Western Reserve
Health Education, Warren, Ohio, USA

DANIEL PERRY, MD
Division of Cardiology, Department of
Medicine, University of Michigan, Ann Arbor,
Michigan, USA

MICHAEL J. REARDON, MD
Department of Cardiovascular Surgery,
Houston Methodist DeBakey Heart & Vascular
Center, Houston Methodist Hospital, Houston,
Texas, USA

ISAAC RHEA, MD
Division of Cardiovascular Medicine,
Morsani College of Medicine, University
of South Florida, Cardio-Oncology Program,
Moffitt Cancer Center, Tampa, Florida,
USA

THOMAS D. RYAN, MD, PhD
Co-Director, Cardio-Oncology, Associate
Professor, Department of Pediatrics,
Division of Pediatric Cardiology, Heart
Institute, Cincinnati Children's Hospital
Medical Center, University of Cincinnati
College of Medicine, Cincinnati, Ohio,
USA

MARIELLE SCHERRER-CROSBIE, MD, PhD
Division of Cardiovascular Diseases,
Department of Medicine, Hospital of the
University of Pennsylvania, Philadelphia,
Pennsylvania, USA

SANA SHOUKAT, MD
The University of Texas Health Science Center
at Houston, Houston, Texas, USA

RONALD M. WITTELES, MD
Associate Professor, Division of
Cardiovascular Medicine, Co-Director,
Stanford Amyloid Center, Stanford University
School of Medicine, Stanford, California, USA

BOBBY YANAGAWA, MD, PhD
Division of Cardiac Surgery, Department
of Surgery, St Michael's Hospital,
University of Toronto, Toronto, Ontario,
Canada

SYED WAMIQUE YUSUF, MD
The University of Texas MD Anderson
Cancer Center, Houston, Texas,
USA

DANYI ZHENG, MD
The University of Texas Health Science
Center at Houston, Houston, Texas,
USA

Contents

underlying cause. Prospective studies are needed to develop evidence-based approaches to cardioprotection in patients receiving fluoropyrimidines.

Trastuzumab-Induced Cardiomyopathy

Rachel Barish, Emily Gates, and Ana Barac

Trastuzumab targets the human epidermal growth factor receptor 2 (HER2). Its overexpression occurs in 25% of breast cancers and is associated with aggressive tumor characteristics and poor prognosis in absence of targeted therapy. Trastuzumab dramatically improves HER2-positive breast cancer outcomes; however, its clinical use is associated with left ventricular dysfunction and heart failure. Patients receiving trastuzumab or other HER2-targeted therapies undergo routine cardiac function assessment. Holding and/or stopping trastuzumab treatment in the setting of left ventricular dysfunction is recommended. This article summarizes the role of trastuzumab in cancer treatment, the mechanisms of trastuzumab-induced cardiotoxicity, recent clinical investigations, and current controversies.

Echocardiography Imaging of Cardiotoxicity

Yu Kang and Marielle Scherrer-Crosbie

Heart disease is the most important cause of non-cancer death for patients with cancer. Addressing the cardiotoxic effects of anticancer therapies to prevent increased cardiovascular risk in this population is crucial. Echocardiography plays a big role in monitoring cardiotoxicity induced by cancer treatment. Many emerging modalities, including tissue Doppler imaging measures, speckle tracking imaging, and three-dimensional echocardiography, may provide improved sensitivity and specificity to detect cancer treatment-induced cardiotoxicity. Additional research is critical to define the value of both conventional and novel indices in guiding the clinical management of cancer treatment-induced cardiotoxicity.

MRI of Cardiotoxicity

Jennifer Hawthorne Jordan and William Gregory Hundley

Cardiovascular magnetic resonance (CMR) imaging is useful to identify systolic dysfunction, particularly when echocardiographic imaging is not acceptable because of poor acoustic windows or when left ventricular ejection fraction (LVEF) is inconclusive by other modalities and an accurate LVEF measurement is needed. Of particular advantage in cardio-oncology is CMR's capability to perform tissue characterization to noninvasively identify changes in pathologic conditions related to cancer therapy or to discriminate causes of disease that may confound presentation in cardio-oncology patients. For these reasons, there is an increasing use of CMR in the screening and surveillance of cardio-oncology patients.

Cardiomyopathy Prevention in Cancer Patients

Tarek Barbar, Syed S. Mahmood, and Jennifer E. Liu

Left ventricular systolic dysfunction (LVSD) and overt heart failure are well known manifestations of chemotherapy-induced cardiotoxicity. The development of LVSD is clinically significant because it can impact the delivery of lifesaving chemotherapy and increase the risk of developing heart failure, compromising quality of life and survival years after cure of the cancer. Cancer treatment–related cardiomyopathy is most commonly associated with anthracyclines and trastuzumab. Several interventions have been identified to prevent cancer-induced cardiomyopathy. Anthracyclines is a major culprit, and prevention strategies with limiting cumulative dose, continuous infusion, dexrazoxane, and liposomal formulation have been shown to decrease the risk of cardiotoxicity.

With increasing survival from cancer, the incidence of cardiovascular diseases is increasing as a chronic side effect of radiation therapy. Prevention, early recognition, and prompt intervention should be the major focus in the care of these patients.

Multiple cancer therapies are associated with cardiac arrhythmias through a variety of pathophysiologic mechanisms. Atrial fibrillation and atrial flutter are common during cancer therapy but should rarely limit continued delivery of therapy. Ventricular arrhythmias are not common during cancer therapy and are more often secondary to other cardiac pathologies. QT interval monitoring is recommended for some agents, although it is often not a reliable predictor of ventricular arrhythmias. Bradyarrhythmias are common and rarely require intervention, but special attention must be paid to heart block in checkpoint inhibitor therapy.

Comorbidities specific to the cardio-oncology population contribute to the challenges in the interventional management of patients with cancer and cardiovascular disease (CVD). Patients with cancer have generally been excluded from cardiovascular randomized clinical trials. Endovascular procedures may represent a valid option in patients with cancer with a range of CVDs because of their minimally invasive nature. Patients with cancer are less likely to be treated according to societal guidelines because of perceived high risk. This article presents the specific challenges that interventional cardiologists face when caring for patients with cancer and the modern tools to optimize care.

Light chain amyloidosis is a deadly disease in which a monoclonal plasma cell dyscrasia produces misfolded immunoglobulin light chains (AL) that aggregate and form rigid amyloid fibrils. The amyloid deposits infiltrate one or more organs, leading to injury and severe dysfunction. The degree of cardiac involvement is a major driver of morbidity and mortality. Early diagnosis and treatment are crucial to prevent irreversible end-organ damage and improve overall survival. Treatment of AL cardiac amyloidosis involves eliminating the underlying plasma cell dyscrasia with chemotherapy and pursuing supportive heart failure management.

Video content accompanies this article at http://www.cardiology.theclinics.com.

Carcinoid heart disease is the collective term for all cardiac manifestations that develop in patients with carcinoid. The cardiac manifestations of carcinoid tumors are attributed to the paraneoplastic effects of vasoactive substances released by the malignant cells. The clinical manifestations of carcinoid heart disease include valvular destruction leading to valvular regurgitation and stenosis, right-sided heart failure, and metastatic carcinoid disease. A combination of biomarkers and cardiac imaging is used in screening and diagnosis of carcinoid heart disease in patients with carcinoid syndrome. The management of carcinoid heart disease involves medical and surgical treatment and requires a multidisciplinary approach for optimized care.

Cardiovascular effects of cancer therapies are of concern. Prediction, diagnosis, and management of cardiotoxicity is a challenge. Cardiovascular biomarkers are being studied in relationship to cancer therapy, showing promise in detection and prevention of cardiotoxicity. We summarize the use of biomarkers in cardio-oncology and presents recommendations for their use. Troponins and natriuretic peptides are the most commonly used biomarkers. High-quality evidence supporting their use is lacking. Biomarkers can be incorporated into a detection strategy for cardiotoxicity. Large, well-powered studies are needed to delineate care strategies using biomarkers in the prediction and management of the cardiovascular effects of cancer therapy.

Cardiac tumors are rare. Most surgeons will encounter few primary cardiac tumors outside of myxomas. This article offers the authors' approach to simple and complex primary and secondary cardiac tumors. Symptoms of primary cardiac tumors are primarily determined by tumor size and anatomic location. Most simple primary tumors and some complex primary tumors are best managed by surgical resection. Secondary tumors are 30 times more frequent than primary cardiac tumors. Surgical resection of secondary tumors is rational in a few highly selected patients. For complex primary and secondary tumors, the authors recommend referral to an experienced multidisciplinary cardiac tumor team.

Advances in cancer therapies have significantly improved patient outcomes. However, with improvements in survival, the toxicities associated with cancer therapy have become of paramount importance and oncologists are faced with the challenge of establishing therapeutic efficacy while minimizing toxicity. Cardiovascular disease represents a significant risk to survivors of childhood cancer and is a major cause of morbidity and mortality. This article outlines the current state of knowledge regarding cardiotoxicity in children undergoing cancer therapies, including the impact of specific oncologic therapies, recommendations for cardiovascular screening, the management of established cardiac disease, and the evolving field of pediatric cardio-oncology.

Implementing a Cardio-oncology Center of Excellence: Nuts and Bolts, Including Coding and Billing

Anita M. Arnold and Cathleen Biga

Cardio-oncology is rapidly expanding as part of cancer therapy in both the acute phase and later stages after treatment. The shifting paradigm of cancer becoming a chronic disease requires long-term follow-up for ongoing cardiac toxicity. As more cancer patients enter the survivorship phase, there needs to be identification of those at risk and strategies for how best to monitor long-term cancer therapy–related cardiac disease. This article serves as a template decide if a cardio-oncology program should be started and expanded as a center of excellence for the discipline as well as to help in implementing and financially sustaining a program.

CARDIOLOGY CLINICS

SERIES OF RELATED INTEREST

Cardiac Electrophysiology Clinics
Heart Failure Clinics
Interventional Cardiology Clinics

THE CLINICS ARE AVAILABLE ONLINE!
Access your subscription at:
www.theclinics.com

Anthracycline Cardiotoxicity
It Is Possible to Teach an Old Dog Some New Tricks

Jose Alvarez-Cardona, MD, Daniel J. Lenihan, MD*

KEYWORDS

- Anthracycline cardiotoxicity • Chemotherapeutic agents • Left ventricular ejection fraction (LVEF)
- Cardioprotection

KEY POINTS

- Anthracyclines have proved to be one of the most effective chemotherapeutic agents in the treatment of numerous solid tumors and hematologic malignancies in both adult and pediatric patients.
- Their clinical benefit, however, is sometimes hampered by the development of cardiotoxicity, a process that still remains elusive despite decades of investigation.
- Detection of cardiac damage is best performed with a multimodality approach including biomarkers.
- Early involvement with a cardio-oncologist can enhance cardioprotective strategies.

HISTORICAL SIGNIFICANCE

Anthracyclines have proved to be one of the most effective chemotherapeutic agents in the treatment of numerous solid tumors and hematologic malignancies in both adult and pediatric patients. Their clinical benefit, however, is sometimes hampered by the development of cardiotoxicity, a process that still remains elusive despite decades of investigation. It has been postulated that anthracycline-induced cardiotoxicity is mediated in part by reactive oxygen species (ROS) and redox cycling. In addition, DNA topoisomerase-IIβ has been identified as an important mediator in doxorubicin-induced DNA changes responsible for mitochondrial dysfunction and generation of ROS.[1] The severity of cardiotoxicity and myocardial damage is proportional to the cumulative dose received, dosing modality (continuous infusion vs bolus), and the additive or synergistic effects from other chemotherapeutic agents.[2]

Anthracycline-induced cardiotoxicity has previously been classified as acute (within 2 weeks after the end of treatment), early-onset chronic (within 1 year after the end of treatment), and late-onset chronic (more than a year after the end of treatment). The definition of cardiotoxicity has focused on a reduced left ventricular (LV) ejection fraction (EF), usually assessed in symptomatic patients and, thus, excluding those with asymptomatic LV dysfunction. This issue is important because cellular changes are evident as early as 4 hours after the first dose of doxorubicin, and the early detection of any degree of LV dysfunction would allow initiation of cardioprotective therapy in a timely manner.[3] This study is further supported by the findings of Cardinale and colleagues[4]

Disclosure: None.
Division of Cardiovascular Medicine, Cardio-Oncology Center of Excellence, Washington University in St Louis, 660 South Euclid Avenue, Campus Box 8086, St Louis, MO 63110-1093, USA
* Corresponding author.
E-mail address: djlenihan@wustl.edu

Cardiol Clin 37 (2019) 355–363
https://doi.org/10.1016/j.ccl.2019.08.001
0733-8651/19/© 2019 Elsevier Inc. All rights reserved.

showing that cardiotoxicity (defined as a reduction in LVEF >10% points from baseline and <50%) usually occurs within the first year of treatment, and initiation of cardioprotective therapy influences recovery of cardiac function.

The development of advanced imaging modalities (eg, strain imaging and cardiac MRI) and cardiac biomarkers (eg, troponin and natriuretic peptides) now allows identification of patients with subclinical LV dysfunction. In fact, the American Society of Echocardiography considers global longitudinal strain (GLS) as the optimal parameter of deformation for the early detection of subclinical LV dysfunction.[5] This has led to a paradigm shift in patients treated with anthracycline-based chemotherapy. Further research is needed to understand the implications of different subtypes of cardiotoxicity, such as the presence of elevated biomarkers or abnormal cardiac imaging in asymptomatic patients (**Fig. 1**, **Table 1**).

EPIDEMIOLOGY

It is well established that anthracycline cardiotoxicity is a dose-dependent and cumulative process of variable onset that may present with subclinical LV dysfunction or overt clinical symptoms. Historically, cardiotoxicity has been defined based on LVEF, which may result in underestimation of the true incidence. Cardiotoxicity is a broad term that encompasses asymptomatic detectable structural changes on the heart, which can

manifest by the onset of arrhythmias, elevation in cardiac biomarkers related to stress and myocardial injury, and LV dysfunction (systolic and diastolic) without symptoms of heart failure. As shown in **Table 2**, the risk for LV dysfunction and heart failure varies by anthracycline and its cumulative dose. In addition, such risk may be even higher in patients exposed to other cardiotoxic chemotherapeutic agents and in those with pre-existing cardiovascular conditions. Using LVEF as the sole marker for cardiotoxicity is also problematic because there is interobserver and intraobserver variability even among expert echocardiographers (see **Table 2**).

CURRENT DETECTION STRATEGIES

Early recognition of subclinical LV dysfunction plays a major role in the treatment of patients with cancer, thus allowing clinicians to incorporate cardioprotective therapy before there is evidence of a decline in LVEF, which may or may not be reversible. The goal is to decrease the risk for interruptions in cancer therapy, which could otherwise affect a patient's survival. It is therefore reasonable to broaden the definition of cardiotoxicity to include different subtypes of subclinical LV dysfunction as defined by an elevation in cardiac biomarkers (eg, troponin, N-terminal pro-B-type natriuretic peptide [NT-proBNP]) and abnormalities in cardiac imaging.

Troponin

Cardiac troponin elevation is a marker of myocardial injury and provides prognostic information in patients with acute coronary syndrome. Different studies have validated its use to detect cardiotoxicity after chemotherapy. Minimal elevation in troponin level is associated with a higher risk for cardiac events, including a decline in LVEF after completing high-dose chemotherapy.[6,7] It is important, however, to obtain a baseline troponin level before starting chemotherapy, since it could be elevated owing to the burden of disease.[8,9] This is particularly important in patients with leukemia because of the increased risk for thrombosis secondary to leukocytosis and leukostasis.[10–12] It is certainly reasonable to consider initiation of carvedilol and/or an angiotensin-converting enzyme (ACE) inhibitor or angiotensin-receptor blocker (ARB) in patients with elevated troponin after anthracycline therapy.

N-Terminal pro-B-Type Natriuretic Peptide

Elevation of NT-proBNP or BNP is considered a useful screening tool for the early detection

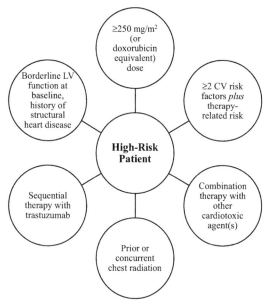

Fig. 1. Patient with increased risk for developing cardiac dysfunction.

Table 1
Cardiotoxicity assessment for patients receiving anthracycline-containing chemotherapy

Therapy	Patient
Establishing the risk for cardiotoxicity	

• High-dose anthracycline monotherapy
  ○ A higher cumulative dose carries a higher risk for cardiotoxicity.
• Combination with other potentially cardiotoxic agents
  ○ High-dose cyclophosphamide
  ○ Trastuzumab
  ○ Trastuzumab + pertuzumab
• Concurrent chest radiation
	• Age <15 or >65 y
	• Female
	• Obesity
	• Known cardiomyopathy or heart failure
	• Coronary artery disease
	• Peripheral vascular disease
	• Diabetes mellitus
	• Hypertension
	• Hyperlipidemia
	• Chronic kidney disease
	• Prior anthracycline therapy (eg, doxorubicin $\geq$250 mg/m^2, epirubicin $\geq$600 mg/m^2)
	• Prior chest radiation ($\geq$30 Gy)
	• Tobacco use

Screening cardiovascular tests	

• Ventricular function assessment
  ○ 2D or 3D echo with strain imaging
  ○ Cardiac MRI with late gadolinium enhancement $\pm$ strain imaging
• ECG to detect any conduction or rhythm abnormality, ischemia, infarction
• Chest imaging (eg, radiograph, CT scan)
• Troponin I or T
• NT-proBNP or BNP
• High-sensitivity C-reactive protein
	ANY ABNORMALITY...
	Consider referral to a cardio-oncologist

Table 2
Incidence of left ventricular dysfunction and heart failure with different anthracyclines

Anthracycline and Cumulative Dose (mg/m^2)	Incidence of LV Systolic Dysfunction (%)	Incidence of Heart Failure (%)
Doxorubicin		
100	0.5	0
150	7	0.2
300	16	0.6
400	32	3–5
550	65	7–26
700	86	18–48
Idarubicin (>90)	NA	5–18
Epirubicin (>900)	NA	0.9–11.4
Mitoxantrone (>120)	NA	2.6
Liposomal anthracyclines (>900)	NA	2

Abbreviation: NA, not applicable.

Data from Swain SM, Whaley FS, Ewer MS. Congestive heart failure in patients treated with doxorubicin: a retrospective analysis of three trials. Cancer 2003;97:2869-79; and Zamorano JL, Lancellotti P, Rodriguez Munoz D et al. 2016 ESC Position Paper on cancer treatments and cardiovascular toxicity developed under the auspices of the ESC Committee for Practice Guidelines: The Task Force for cancer treatments and cardiovascular toxicity of the European Society of Cardiology (ESC). Eur Heart J 2016;37:2768-2801.

of subclinical LV dysfunction during anthracycline chemotherapy. It has been demonstrated that BNP elevation preceded cardiac events in patients receiving anthracycline therapy.[13] Thus, a baseline NT-proBNP or BNP should be checked before starting treatment and possibly after each cycle, or on discovering clinical symptoms that would suggest heart failure.

Imaging Techniques

Different imaging techniques are available to assess LV function, including 2-dimensional and 3-dimensional (2D and 3D) echocardiography, radionuclide ventriculography (multiple-gated acquisition [MUGA]), and cardiac MRI. Each has its own advantages and disadvantages, so a multimodality approach is sometimes warranted (**Table 3**).[5] MUGA is not recommended at this time mainly because of expense, radiation exposure, and lack of additional data beyond LVEF (see **Table 3**).

PREVENTION STRATEGIES

Various cardioprotective strategies have been explored over the last decades, including the use of cardioselective β-blockers, renin-angiotensin-system antagonists, dexrazoxane, and modified formulations and dosing of anthracyclines (**Fig. 2**). These have shown mixed clinical results, and larger studies are needed to validate their findings.

The OVERCOME trial (preventiOn of left Ventricular dysfunction with Enalapril and caRvedilol in patients submitted to intensive ChemOtherapy for the treatment of Malignant hEmopathies) showed that combined treatment with enalapril and carvedilol may prevent LV systolic dysfunction in patients with malignant hemopathies treated with high-dose chemotherapy. Patients in the intervention group had a lower incidence of the combined event of death or heart failure (6.7% vs 22%, $P = .036$) and of death, heart failure, or a final LVEF less than 45% (6.7% vs 24.4%, $P = .02$).[14] In the PRADA trial (Prevention of cardiac dysfunction

Table 3
Imaging modalities for detection of anthracycline-associated cardiotoxicity

Technique	Diagnostic Information	Advantages	Limitations

Echocardiography
• 2D
• 3D
	• Cardiotoxicity:
	  ○ Decline in LVEF >10% to a value ≤50%
	  ○ Change in GLS >15%
	• Tissue Doppler imaging: measurement of mitral and tricuspid annular plane systolic excursion; RVs
		• Widely available
		• Lack of radiation
		• Provides additional information: hemodynamic assessment, valvular disease, and other cardiac structures
			• Interobserver variability
			• GLS: vendor and software specific
			• Image quality affects interpretation

Radionuclide ventriculography (MUGA)	• Cardiotoxicity: ○ Decline in LVEF by ≥10% from baseline to a value ≤50%	• High reproducibility • Low intra- and interobserver variability • Widely available	• Radiation exposure • Lack of information regarding pericardial and valvular heart disease and RV function
Cardiac MRI	• Reference standard for LV and RV volumes and function	• Reproducibility • Gadolinium-based contrast and T1 mapping • Assessment for myocardial fibrosis, pericardial and valvular heart disease	• Limited availability • Electromagnetic interference

Abbreviations: GLS, global longitudinal strain; LV, left ventricular; LVEF, left ventricular ejection fraction; MUGA, multiple-gated acquisition; RV, right ventricle.

Data from Plana JC, Galderisi M, Barac A et al. Expert consensus for multimodality imaging evaluation of adult patients during and after cancer therapy: a report from the American Society of Echocardiography and the European Association of Cardiovascular Imaging. Journal of the American Society of Echocardiography: official publication of the American Society of Echocardiography 2014;27:911-39.

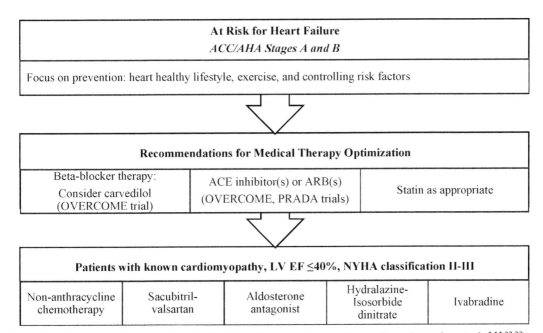

Fig. 2. Modification of anthracycline chemotherapy to reduce cardiotoxicity risk. (*Data from* Refs.[25–31])

during adjuvant breast cancer therapy), 130 adult women with early-stage breast cancer and no serious comorbidities receiving adjuvant anthracycline-containing regimens with or without trastuzumab were randomized to candesartan, metoprolol succinate, or matching placebos. Candesartan was shown to confer protection against early decline in LVEF when compared with metoprolol succinate and placebo.[15] More recently, the CECCY (Carvedilol Effect in preventing Chemotherapy-induced CardiotoxicitY) trial evaluated the role of carvedilol in preventing cardiotoxicity under contemporary anthracycline dosage in 200 patients with HER2-negative breast cancer. The study showed a 13.5% to 14.5% overall incidence of cardiotoxicity with no impact on the incidence of early onset of LVEF reduction with carvedilol. It did, however, show a significant reduction

in troponin levels and diastolic dysfunction in patients treated with carvedilol.[16]

In a group of patients with metastatic breast cancer and stage-III or stage-IV ovarian cancer, a 6-h infusion regimen of doxorubicin versus rapid infusion over 15 to 20 minutes was associated with a lower decline in LVEF.[17] However, in a study conducted by Lipshultz and colleagues,[9] no significant difference was noted regarding LV systolic dysfunction, LV dilation, LV wall thickness, and LV mass at 8 years in children receiving doxorubicin by either continuous (over 48 hours) or bolus infusion.

Dexrazoxane is currently approved in patients with metastatic breast cancer who have already received more than 300 mg/m^2 of doxorubicin.[18,19] A meta-analysis showed that dexrazoxane reduced the rate of heart failure but did not improve survival in patients receiving anthracyclines.[20] The limited use of dexrazoxane is due to suspicion for the occurrence of secondary malignancies, although such a suspicion is unfounded.[21]

The effect of uninterrupted statin therapy over 2.55 ± 1.68 years was assessed in 628 women with newly diagnosed breast cancer treated with anthracycline-containing chemotherapy. This observational clinical cohort study demonstrated that statin use was associated with a lower risk for incident heart failure (hazard ratio 0.3, 95% confidence interval 0.1–0.9; $P = .03$).[22] Although this result is consistent with prior animal studies, a prospective randomized clinical trial is warranted to validate this finding.

At Risk for Heart Failure				
ACC/AHA Stages A and B				
Focus on prevention: heart healthy lifestyle, exercise, and controlling risk factors				

Recommendations for Medical Therapy Optimization				
Beta-blocker therapy: Consider carvedilol (OVERCOME trial)	ACE inhibitor(s) or ARB(s) (OVERCOME, PRADA trials)		Statin as appropriate	

Patients with known cardiomyopathy, LV EF ≤40%, NYHA classification II-III				
Non-anthracycline chemotherapy	Sacubitril-valsartan	Aldosterone antagonist	Hydralazine-Isosorbide dinitrate	Ivabradine

Fig. 3. Stepwise approach to cardioprotection in patients receiving anthracyclines. (*Data from* Refs.[4,14,23,32])

In patients with pre-existing cardiovascular conditions, it is reasonable to optimize their medical therapy by incorporating an ACE inhibitor or ARB and carvedilol before receiving anthracycline-containing chemotherapy (**Fig. 3**). Statins should be recommended based on the patient's cardiovascular risk. Those with pre-existing cardiomyopathy and heart failure with reduced EF should be treated with guideline-based medical therapy[23] (see **Figs. 2** and **3**).

CARDIOVASCULAR CARE AFTER ANTHRACYCLINE-BASED CHEMOTHERAPY

Over the last decade there has been significant improvement in cancer treatment, and this has translated into a growing number of cancer survivors among different age groups. Classifying patients based on their risk for anthracycline-induced cardiotoxicity has allowed the early implementation of preventive strategies such as the use of renin-angiotensin-system antagonists, β-blockers, and statins. For some patients this is recommended before starting treatment, whereas for others this is done on treatment completion. Although ultrastructural changes in myocytes have been noticed within hours of doxorubicin treatment, it is unclear why some patients experience progression to clinical heart failure while others only have subclinical manifestations. It is therefore important to establish survivorship programs that focus on the cardiovascular care of the oncology patient.

The American Society of Clinical Oncology developed clinical practice guideline recommendations focusing on 5 important aspects of the cardio-oncology patient, including the identification of patients with increased risk for developing cardiac dysfunction, preventive strategies before, during, and after treatment, and surveillance and monitoring approaches during and after treatment.[24] Recommendations about surveillance and monitoring approaches after treatment in patients at risk for cardiac dysfunction are summarized in **Box 1**.

We present 3 cases involving patients of different age groups treated with anthracycline-containing chemotherapy. These cases highlight important issues regarding the diagnosis and management of LV systolic dysfunction in this population.

CASE 1

A 60-year-old woman diagnosed with invasive lobular carcinoma of the left breast in 2001 and treated with a left modified radical mastectomy followed by adjuvant chemotherapy (FAC—fluorouracil, doxorubicin, cyclophosphamide—for 6 cycles, followed by paclitaxel for 4 cycles) and no adjuvant radiation or endocrine therapy initially was diagnosed with recurrent, metastatic lobular breast cancer (ER/PR$^+$, HER2$^+$) in 2015. She was treated with different chemotherapy regimens because of disease progression and occasional intolerance to treatment. These regimens included docetaxel, trastuzumab (held 3 times because of depressed LV systolic function), pertuzumab, denosumab, palbociclib, paclitaxel (nanoparticle albumin-bound), T-DM1, capecitabine, and lapatinib. The patient had been experiencing depressed LV systolic function since 2017 with the lowest EF (20%–25%) in 2019. She had not been able to tolerate guideline-directed medical therapy for heart failure because of low blood pressure and was only on low-dose carvedilol (6.25 mg twice daily) and eplerenone (25 mg daily). The patient has evidence of a left bundle branch block and is being evaluated for cardiac resynchronization therapy with a biventricular pacemaker.

Key points about this case:

- Surveillance for late-onset heart failure is warranted in patients treated with an anthracycline.
- The significance of exposure to trastuzumab and pertuzumab more than a decade after treatment with an anthracycline suggests that there is a major risk for developing heart failure.
- Optimizing heart-failure therapy in patients with cancer can be challenging.

CASE 2

A 72-year-old African American man was diagnosed in July 2018 with diffuse large B-cell lymphoma (stage IVA) and received R-CHOP plus C-122 (a lenalidomide analog) between August and November 2018. Before initiating treatment, an MUGA showed a normal LV systolic function with an EF of 61% (normal >50%). The patient was able to complete treatment without any major complications. MUGA was repeated about 2 months after treatment, whereby LVEF was still within normal range but mildly depressed (EF 52%) when compared with baseline. The patient, who has hypertension and significant calcification of the native coronary arteries (based on staging PET), was referred to the cardio-oncology clinic where he was found to have New York Heart Association (NYHA) class I symptoms. The patient was already on lisinopril 10 mg daily, which

Box 1
Recommendations for surveillance after treatment in patients at risk for cardiac dysfunction

History and physical examination

- At least annually by a cardiologist or health care provider with cardio-oncology expertise
- Address any pre-existing or new cardiovascular risk factors
- Emphasize the importance of a heart-healthy lifestyle including diet and exercise

Individuals with clinical signs or symptoms concerning for LV dysfunction

- 2D or 3D echocardiogram with strain imaging and contrast as needed
- Cardiac MRI (with gadolinium contrast) if echocardiogram is not available or technically feasible
- Serum cardiac biomarkers: troponin I or T, NT-proBNP or BNP
- Referral to a cardio-oncologist based on findings

Asymptomatic patients at increased risk for LV dysfunction

- 2D or 3D echocardiogram with strain imaging and contrast as needed between 6 and 12 months after completion of cardiotoxic treatment
- Cardiac MRI (with gadolinium contrast) if echocardiogram is not available or technically feasible
- Consider periodic assessment of serum cardiac biomarkers (troponin I or T, NT-proBNP or BNP) at the time of each echocardiogram
- Referral to a cardio-oncologist if asymptomatic LV dysfunction is detected

Asymptomatic patients at increased risk for LV dysfunction but without evidence on 6- to 12-month post-treatment echocardiogram

- American Society of Clinical Oncology clinical guideline cannot provide recommendations for these patients because of insufficient evidence
- Consider the combination of an imaging diagnostic test and serum cardiac biomarkers (troponin I or T, NT-proBNP or BNP) if risk of cardiac dysfunction or heart failure is considered high
- 2D or 3D echocardiogram with strain imaging and contrast as needed every 5 years after treatment completion

Data from Armenian SH, Lacchetti C, Barac A et al. Prevention and Monitoring of Cardiac Dysfunction in Survivors of Adult Cancers: American Society of Clinical Oncology Clinical Practice Guideline. J Clin Oncol 2017;35:893-911; and Armenian SH, Hudson MM, Mulder RL et al. Recommendations for cardiomyopathy surveillance for survivors of childhood cancer: a report from the International Late Effects of Childhood Cancer Guideline Harmonization Group. Lancet Oncol 2015;16:e123-36.

was increased to 20 mg daily. A cardiac MRI was performed about 3 months after treatment, which showed LVEF 37%, LV end-diastolic volume (EDV) 222 mL, right ventricular (RV) EF 39%, RVEDV 142 mL, no evidence of late gadolinium enhancement, and no hemodynamically significant valvular abnormality. He also had evidence of worsening cardiac biomarkers troponin I and NT-proBNP (**Fig. 4**). At this point, carvedilol was added and he was continued on lisinopril. He still had NYHA class I symptoms. About 9 months after chemotherapy, the patient was complaining of shortness of breath and dyspnea on exertion. A transthoracic echocardiogram showed severe LV systolic dysfunction with EF 13%, LVEDV 172 mL, and restrictive physiology by tissue Doppler imaging.

Key points about this case:

- Although there was no evidence of prior infarction or scarring on the cardiac MRI, one cannot conclusively state that this is

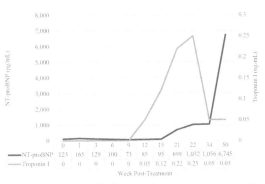

Fig. 4. Depiction of changes in troponin I and NT-proBNP over time.

solely due to anthracycline cardiotoxicity without definitively excluding coronary artery disease.

- The patient showed worsening heart failure despite treatment with carvedilol and lisinopril. Further optimization of heart-failure therapy is appropriate.
- Troponin I elevation preceded NT-proBNP elevation, supporting the use of these cardiac biomarkers during and after treatment. This timeline of events is expected because anthracyclines cause ultrastructural changes at the myocyte level, and troponin is an early marker of myocardial injury.
- Troponin I was the highest around the time when LVEF began to decline.
- GLS may have been helpful in identifying subclinical LV systolic dysfunction.

CASE 3

A 24-year-old woman was diagnosed with classical Hodgkin lymphoma in August 2018 and was immediately started on ABVD (doxorubicin, bleomycin, vincristine, and dacarbazine). After completing the first cycle, the patient developed chest pain and troponin elevation. Left heart catheterization showed no evidence of obstructive coronary artery disease. Transthoracic echocardiogram showed a newly depressed LV systolic function with estimated LVEF 30% to 40%. The patient was started on low-dose carvedilol 3.125 mg twice daily and referred to our cardio-oncology clinic. Dexrazoxane was added to ABVD for the remaining cycles. A repeat transthoracic echocardiogram about 2 months after the initial diagnosis of heart failure demonstrated an EF of 40%. The patient had continued to experience episodes of shortness of breath and palpitations. She was found to be having episodes of nonsustained ventricular tachycardia. She did not tolerate a higher dose of carvedilol because of low-normal blood pressure. A cardiac MRI was performed about 4 months after the initial decline in LV function, which showed an LVEF of 41% and LVEDV of 126 mL. Nonspecific patchy and extensive late gadolinium enhancement in a nonvascular pattern was detected. As the patient continued to experience NYHA class II symptoms, she was referred for cardiac rehabilitation. Her symptoms have improved. Reassessment of LVEF is pending.

Key points about this case:

- Anthracycline-induced cardiotoxicity can present acutely within days to weeks after first exposure.

- Other causes of acute heart failure should be assessed. Perhaps evaluation for acute myocarditis would have been justified.
- No evidence of worsening LV dysfunction was detected after adding dexrazoxane to the chemotherapy regimen and initiating carvedilol. This highlights the importance of early detection and initiation of cardioprotective therapy.
- Long-term surveillance will be warranted for this patient.

REFERENCES

1. Zhang S, Liu X, Bawa-Khalfe T, et al. Identification of the molecular basis of doxorubicin-induced cardiotoxicity. Nat Med 2012;18:1639–42.
2. van Dalen EC, van der Pal HJ, Caron HN, et al. Different dosage schedules for reducing cardiotoxicity in cancer patients receiving anthracycline chemotherapy. Cochrane Database Syst Rev 2009;(4):CD005008. https://doi.org/10.1002/14651858.CD005008.pub3.
3. Unverferth BJ, Magorien RD, Balcerzak SP, et al. Early changes in human myocardial nuclei after doxorubicin. Cancer 1983;52:215–21.
4. Cardinale D, Colombo A, Bacchiani G, et al. Early detection of anthracycline cardiotoxicity and improvement with heart failure therapy. Circulation 2015;131:1981–8.
5. Plana JC, Galderisi M, Barac A, et al. Expert consensus for multimodality imaging evaluation of adult patients during and after cancer therapy: a report from the American Society of Echocardiography and the European Association of Cardiovascular Imaging. J Am Soc Echocardiogr 2014;27:911–39.
6. Cardinale D, Sandri MT, Colombo A, et al. Prognostic value of troponin I in cardiac risk stratification of cancer patients undergoing high-dose chemotherapy. Circulation 2004;109:2749–54.
7. Sandri MT, Cardinale D, Zorzino L, et al. Minor increases in plasma troponin I predict decreased left ventricular ejection fraction after high-dose chemotherapy. Clin Chem 2003;49:248–52.
8. Auner HW, Tinchon C, Linkesch W, et al. Prolonged monitoring of troponin T for the detection of anthracycline cardiotoxicity in adults with hematological malignancies. Ann Hematol 2003;82:218–22.
9. Lipshultz SE, Rifai N, Dalton VM, et al. The effect of dexrazoxane on myocardial injury in doxorubicin-treated children with acute lymphoblastic leukemia. N Engl J Med 2004;351:145–53.
10. Colovic N, Bogdanovic A, Virijevic M, et al. Acute myocardial infarction during induction chemotherapy for acute MLL t(4;11) leukemia with lineage switch and extreme leukocytosis. Srp Arh Celok Lek 2015;143:734–8.

11. Landolfi R, Di Gennaro L, Barbui T, et al. Leukocytosis as a major thrombotic risk factor in patients with polycythemia vera. Blood 2007;109:2446–52.

12. Schmid-Schonbein GW. The damaging potential of leukocyte activation in the microcirculation. Angiology 1993;44:45–56.

13. Lenihan DJ, Stevens PL, Massey M, et al. The utility of point-of-care biomarkers to detect cardiotoxicity during anthracycline chemotherapy: a feasibility study. J Card Fail 2016;22:433–8.

14. Bosch X, Rovira M, Sitges M, et al. Enalapril and carvedilol for preventing chemotherapy-induced left ventricular systolic dysfunction in patients with malignant hemopathies: the OVERCOME trial (prevention of left Ventricular dysfunction with Enalapril and caRvedilol in patients submitted to intensive ChemOtherapy for the treatment of Malignant hEmopathies). J Am Coll Cardiol 2013;61:2355–62.

15. Gulati G, Heck SL, Ree AH, et al. Prevention of cardiac dysfunction during adjuvant breast cancer therapy (PRADA): a 2 x 2 factorial, randomized, placebo-controlled, double-blind clinical trial of candesartan and metoprolol. Eur Heart J 2016;37:1671–80.

16. Avila MS, Ayub-Ferreira SM, de Barros Wanderley MR Jr, et al. Carvedilol for prevention of chemotherapy-related cardiotoxicity: the CECCY trial. J Am Coll Cardiol 2018;71:2281–90.

17. Shapira J, Gotfried M, Lishner M, et al. Reduced cardiotoxicity of doxorubicin by a 6-hour infusion regimen. A prospective randomized evaluation. Cancer 1990;65:870–3.

18. Hensley ML, Hagerty KL, Kewalramani T, et al. American Society of Clinical Oncology 2008 clinical practice guideline update: use of chemotherapy and radiation therapy protectants. J Clin Oncol 2009;27:127–45.

19. Swain SM, Whaley FS, Gerber MC, et al. Delayed administration of dexrazoxane provides cardioprotection for patients with advanced breast cancer treated with doxorubicin-containing therapy. J Clin Oncol 1997;15:1333–40.

20. van Dalen EC, Caron HN, Dickinson HO, et al. Cardioprotective interventions for cancer patients receiving anthracyclines. Cochrane Database Syst Rev 2011;(6):CD003917. https://doi.org/10.1002/14651858.CD003917.pub3.

21. Asselin BL, Devidas M, Chen L, et al. Cardioprotection and safety of dexrazoxane in patients treated for newly diagnosed T-cell acute lymphoblastic leukemia or advanced-stage lymphoblastic non-Hodgkin lymphoma: a report of the Children's Oncology Group Randomized Trial Pediatric Oncology Group 9404. J Clin Oncol 2016;34:854–62.

22. Seicean S, Seicean A, Plana JC, et al. Effect of statin therapy on the risk for incident heart failure in patients with breast cancer receiving anthracycline chemotherapy: an observational clinical cohort study. J Am Coll Cardiol 2012;60:2384–90.

23. Yancy CW, Jessup M, Bozkurt B, et al. 2017 ACC/AHA/HFSA focused update of the 2013 ACCF/AHA guideline for the management of heart failure: a report of the American College of Cardiology/American Heart Association Task Force on Clinical Practice Guidelines and the Heart Failure Society of America. Circulation 2017;136:e137–61.

24. Armenian SH, Lacchetti C, Barac A, et al. Prevention and monitoring of cardiac dysfunction in survivors of adult cancers: American Society of Clinical Oncology Clinical practice guideline. J Clin Oncol 2017;35:893–911.

25. Batist G. Cardiac safety of liposomal anthracyclines. Cardiovasc Toxicol 2007;7:72–4.

26. Cortes J, Di Cosimo S, Climent MA, et al. Nonpegylated liposomal doxorubicin (TLC-D99), paclitaxel, and trastuzumab in HER-2-overexpressing breast cancer: a multicenter phase I/II study. Clin Cancer Res 2009;15:307–14.

27. Hortobagyi GN, Frye D, Buzdar AU, et al. Decreased cardiac toxicity of doxorubicin administered by continuous intravenous infusion in combination chemotherapy for metastatic breast carcinoma. Cancer 1989;63:37–45.

28. Legha SS, Benjamin RS, Mackay B, et al. Adriamycin therapy by continuous intravenous infusion in patients with metastatic breast cancer. Cancer 1982;49:1762–6.

29. Rayson D, Suter TM, Jackisch C, et al. Cardiac safety of adjuvant pegylated liposomal doxorubicin with concurrent trastuzumab: a randomized phase II trial. Ann Oncol 2012;23:1780–8.

30. Swain SM, Whaley FS, Gerber MC, et al. Cardioprotection with dexrazoxane for doxorubicin-containing therapy in advanced breast cancer. J Clin Oncol 1997;15:1318–32.

31. van Dalen EC, van der Pal HJ, Kremer LC. Different dosage schedules for reducing cardiotoxicity in people with cancer receiving anthracycline chemotherapy. Cochrane Database Syst Rev 2016;(3):CD005008.

32. Yancy CW, Jessup M, Bozkurt B, et al. 2013 ACCF/AHA guideline for the management of heart failure: executive summary: a report of the American College of Cardiology Foundation/American Heart Association Task Force on practice guidelines. Circulation 2013;128:1810–52.

Common Vascular Toxicities of Cancer Therapies

Joerg Herrmann, MD

KEYWORDS

- Atherosclerosis • Cancer • Myocardial infarction • Peripheral arterial disease • Stroke
- Thrombosis • Vasospasm

KEY POINTS

- A broad spectrum of vascular toxicities has been recognized in the patient who has cancer and even more so since the introduction of targeted therapies.
- Vascular toxicities of cancer therapies can involve all vascular territories, can be functional or structural in nature, and can be of lasting or only temporary duration.
- The management of cancer therapy–related vascular toxicities is directed toward the underlying pathologic mechanism: thrombosis, abnormal vasoreactivity, or structural alteration (remodeling).

Historically, venous thromboembolism (VTE) has been the main and, very often the only, vascular disease entity noted in patients who have cancer. Furthermore, the risk of VTE has been considered to be present in these patients irrespective of cancer therapy. Thus, in the past, there has not been much concern for vascular toxicities as a consequence of cancer therapy, with the exception of 5-fluorouracil (5-FU) and radiation therapy. However, the introduction of targeted therapies, especially those that inhibit the vascular endothelial growth factor (VEGF) signaling pathway, has changed this view and has drawn more attention to the topic of vascular toxicities with cancer therapies.

As outlined in **Fig. 1**, the vascular disease spectrum that can be seen in patients who have cancer is very broad. It can affect all vascular territories, can involve both the venous and the arterial circulation, can be functional or structural in nature, and can be of lasting or only temporary duration. For this reason, it is difficult to devise a uniform classification system of vascular toxicities of cancer therapies. For practical purposes, an approach by type of presentation might be preferred and is the structure for this article. The focus is on clinical aspects and less so on basic and translational science.

CEREBROVASCULAR EVENTS

Cerebrovascular events (CVAs), including transient ischemic attack and stroke, have been only rarely reported with the classic chemotherapeutics of the past. This changed with the introduction of VEGF inhibitors, including the monoclonal antibody bevacizumab and several tyrosine kinase inhibitors (TKIs) that target the VEGF receptor II (eg, sunitinib, sorafenib). VEGF inhibitors increase the risk of ischemic and hemorrhagic strokes. The relative risk of either type of stroke is increased 3-fold in patients on bevacizumab, with an absolute incidence of ischemic and hemorrhagic strokes of 0.5% and 0.3%, respectively.[1] A higher relative risk of CVAs was noted in patients who have colorectal cancer (6.4-fold increased risk), and the highest absolute incidence of CVAs was reported in patients with mesothelioma (1.9%).[1] The risk of any CVA doubled with doubling of the dose of bevacizumab; that is, CVA incidence 2%

Conflict of Interest: None related to this content.
Department of Cardiovascular Diseases, Mayo Clinic, 200 First Street SW, Rochester, MN 55902, USA
E-mail address: herrmann.joerg@mayo.edu

Cardiol Clin 37 (2019) 365–384
https://doi.org/10.1016/j.ccl.2019.07.003

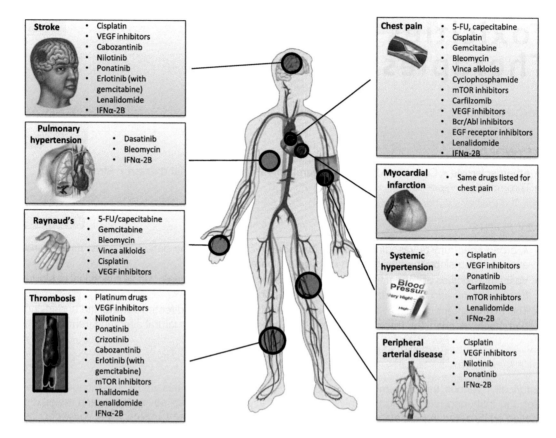

Fig. 1. The spectrum of common vascular toxicities and related cancer therapeutics. IFN, interferon; mTOR, mammalian target of rapamycin.

and 4% with 2.5 and 5 mg/kg/wk bevacizumab dose regimen, respectively.[1] Hemorrhagic strokes tend to occur earlier (median time 2.6 months), often in the setting of tumor progression with a poor prognosis (owing [50% mortality] to tumor progression and 50% mortality of intracranial bleeding events).[2] On the contrary, ischemic strokes tend to be seen later on in the course of therapy (median 16.2 months) and do not associate with a rapidly fatal outcome in most cases. Key risk factors for intracranial bleeding are use of additional medications that increase the risk for bleeding and thrombocytopenia but not, importantly, central nervous system tumors or metastases.[3,4] In regard to ischemic stroke, vascular risk factors apply as in the general population.

The most common type of stroke in patients who have cancer is thromboembolic in nature, and the rate of cryptogenic strokes is nearly twice as high (50% vs 30% in the general population).[5] The risk of arterial thromboembolic events emerges within 6 months before and peaks within a 1 month window before and after cancer diagnosis (**Fig. 2**).[5–7] The risk is highest in patients with gastrointestinal

tract, lung cancers, and non-Hodgkin lymphoma. It is also seen more commonly with advanced stages (stage III and IV).[5–7] These dynamics and clear similarities with VTE suggest that general thrombophilia in patients who have cancer is an important determining factor.[8] A nidus for thrombus in the heart can be the valves (marantic endocarditis), the left atrium or left atrial appendage (atrial fibrillation), or the venous circulation with or without indwelling central venous catheters in the setting of a patent foramen oval. Other sources for emboli to the brain in patients who have cancer include septic emboli and tumor emboli. Platinum drugs, next to VEGF inhibitors, are the main cancer drugs that associate with thromboembolic events.[9]

The second group to consider (after thromboembolism) in patients who have cancer with ischemic stroke are those with vasculopathy. This is mainly atherosclerosis of the carotid arteries though the intracranial vasculature can be affected as well. Again, against the premise that targeted therapies would be more specific and associated with less toxicity, progressive atherosclerosis has been reported with the Bcr-Abl inhibitors nilotinib and

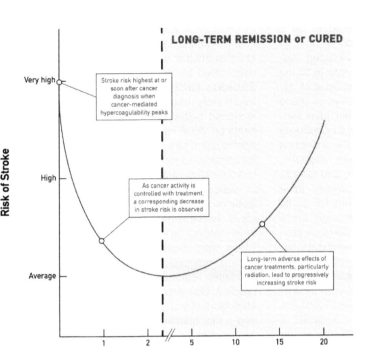

Fig. 2. The risk of stroke relative to the time of cancer diagnosis. (*From* Navi BB, Iadecola C. Ischemic stroke in cancer patients: A review of an underappreciated pathology. *Ann Neurol.* 2018;83(5):873-883; with permission.)

ponatinib.[10–12] These drugs can cause acute CVAs with evidence of carotid artery disease or an intracranial vascular pathology condition similar to Moya Moya disease.[13,14] Although these drugs cause injury to the endothelium, this does not seem to provide a full explanation.[15] For instance, other drugs, such as cisplatin, also bestow endothelial toxicity but have been associated more with thrombotic events rather than atherosclerosis.[16,17] Other factors are therefore likely playing an important role in determining the outcome of endothelial injury with cancer therapeutics.

Abnormal vasoreactivity is less likely to be a prominent contributing factor for stroke in patients who have cancer even though stroke cases have been described in patients on 5-FU and capecitabine, which are known to affect vascular reactivity, most of the time without an identifiable cause. In fact, the term chemotherapy-induced stroke mimic has been used[18] Another stroke mimic in patients who have cancer is posterior reversible encephalopathy syndrome, which can present as an acute cerebral event with headache, confusion, visual symptoms, and seizures. Posterior cerebral white matter edema on neuroimaging is the pathognomic sign, related to impaired autoregulation of the cerebral vasculature, often in the setting of severe hypertension. Numerous cases have been reported with a broad range of cancer therapeutics, especially those that can cause endothelial or vascular injury, such as

VEGF signaling pathway inhibitors, but also immune checkpoint inhibitors.[19–21]

Finally, stroke presentations in patients who have cancer can be the consequence of cerebral artery dissections or compression of vessels by tumors.[22] Both, venous compression or thrombosis are additional possibilities.

From a management standpoint, each patient should undergo a standard workup within the guideline recommended time metrics for stroke evaluation.[23] This includes a timely head computed tomography (CT with read out completed within 45 minutes of arrival), which is key evaluation step in patients who have cancer and is important to identify hemorrhage and/or central nervous system masses. If these are not seen, an ischemic cause is to be assumed and further workup should include evaluation for carotid artery disease and cardioembolic causes, as well as dissections and venous thrombosis.

CHEST PAIN

Various chemotherapeutic agents have been associated with a broad spectrum of chest pain presentations, including typical effort angina and atypical variant and microvascular angina.[24] The classic example is 5-FU and its oral prodrug capecitabine, which can cause coronary vasospasm and related symptoms.[25] Cardiac injury seen with the use of these drugs is considered to be a consequence of myocardial ischemia (though direct cardiotoxic effects have also been discussed).[26] Cardiac dysfunction can evolve to the point of cardiogenic shock.[27] Takotsubo is of differential diagnostic consideration, even in these cases.[28] The latter and various chest pain syndromes can also be encountered with paclitaxel and docetaxel, similarly related to the induction of abnormal vasoreactivity.[25] Finally, cisplatin, often in combination with bleomycin, can lead to presentations of chest pain, commonly in a manner that should increase concern for acute coronary syndrome (ACS).[29-31] Although these drugs lead to endothelial injury and can thus provoke signs and symptoms of endothelial dysfunction, platinum drugs are especially well-known to induce thrombotic events. Abnormal vasoreactivity, arterial thrombosis, and progressive atherosclerosis have all been noted with VEGF inhibitor therapy.[32,33] For the VEGF inhibitor sunitinib, it has furthermore been shown that it alters coronary microcirculatory structure with a reduction in coronary flow reserve (CFR).[34] This effect is due to inhibition of platelet-derived growth factor beta signaling with impairment of pericyte viability.[34]

The possibility of preexisting coronary artery disease should not be forgotten in patients who have cancer and needs to be entertained in the evaluation of these patients. Of importance, patients with a history of ischemic heart disease, especially myocardial infarction (MI), have an 8-fold increased risk of developing cardiotoxicity with the use of 5-FU. Other etiologic factors of ischemic chest pain in patients who have cancer to consider include coronary artery compression by cardiac and noncardiac tumors.[35-37] True invasion in the coronary arteries should increase suspicion for angiosarcoma. On the other hand, nonobstructive encasement of the right coronary artery in the right ventricular grove by diffuse large B-cell lymphoma or thymoma has become known as the floating artery sign.[38] Last, but not least, other causes of chest pain need to be entertained in patients who have cancer, just as they are in the general population, including aortopathies, pericardial diseases (even aortic stenosis), costochondritis, and gastrointestinal and pulmonary etiologic factors.

From a management perspective, most patients can be started empirically on vasodilator therapy with sublingual nitroglycerin, long-acting nitroglycerin, or the long-acting calcium channel blocker amlodipine, unless hypotension poses concerns. In patients with vasospastic disease, this intervention is curative (and thereby diagnostic). In individuals with endothelial dysfunction or microvascular

disease, these vasodilators may remain insufficient in ameliorating symptom burden. Other calcium channel blocker such as nifedipine and felodipine might need to be used, or diltiazem or verapamil if cardiac function is normal. Beta-blocker have traditionally been used to maintain the cardiac workload below the ischemic threshold. For patients on VEGF inhibitors or other endothelial toxic agents, such as cisplatin, various interventions can be considered to improve vascular health (**Fig. 3**). Vasoreactivity testing can be used as a parameter of vascular health and can be assessed, for instance, with an Endo-PAT (Itamar Medical, Caesarea, Israel). Additional evaluation steps include stress testing, as in the general population. In those cases with microvascular dysfunction, with expected reduced CFR, quantitative PET, which measures regional myocardial blood flow, would be ideal. However, in view of the multiple possible etiologic factors, several of them being structural, and a key question being the need for structural intervention, an anatomic imaging approach, possibly combined with functional assessment, might be recommendable. Coronary CT angiography with virtual fractional flow reserve and myocardial perfusion imaging provides such a tool. Triple rule-out chest CTs address the concerns related to aortic and pulmonary disease processes and pulmonary embolism, as well as coronary artery disease. For patients with coronary artery disease not controlled by medications or signs of severe extent (including any left main coronary artery disease), an invasive coronary angiogram should be performed to define the next best step in terms of revascularization. Anemia and thrombocytopenia are important considerations in patients who have cancer and need to be carefully weighted into the decision-making. Estimates of the duration of cytopenias are important, as well as the overall prognosis of the patient. However, a case can be made for percutaneous coronary intervention as a palliative measure to improve quality of life not accomplished by medical therapy alone.

ACUTE CORONARY SYNDROME

All cancer therapeutics associated with chest pain can also cause ACS; in fact, unstable angina may be considered not infrequently in those with resting chest pain secondary to abnormal vasoreactivity of the epicardial and/or microvascular circulation. Furthermore, profound coronary vasospasm as seen with 5-FU, particularly with continuous infusion (less so with bolus infusion of 5-FU and capecitabine), can lead to ST segment elevation and, if prolonged, to MI, ventricular arrhythmias, such as

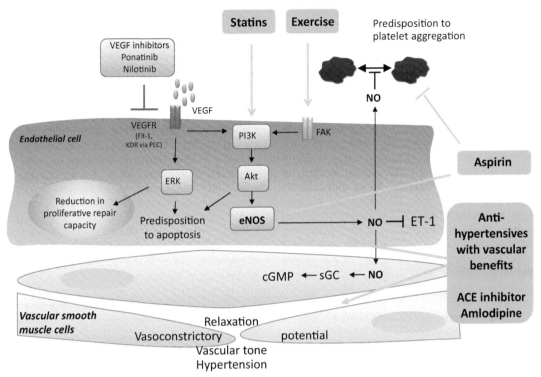

Fig. 3. Therapeutic intervention to improve vascular health, especially in patients on cancer therapeutics with an inhibitory effect on the VEGF signaling pathway. ACE, angiotensin-converting enzyme; eNOS, endothelial nitric oxide synthase; VEGFR, VEGF receptor. (*From* Touyz RM, Herrmann SMS, Herrmann J. Vascular toxicities with VEGF inhibitor therapies-focus on hypertension and arterial thrombotic events. *J Am Soc Hypertens.* 2018;12(6):409-425; with permission.)

ventricular tachycardia and fibrillation, and even sudden cardiac death.[39–41] Profound and prolonged vasospasm is considered to also underlie ACS presentations with paclitaxel, gemcitabine, rituximab, and sorafenib.[42–47]

The level of suspicion for an acute thrombotic event should be high in patients who present with chest pain while on cisplatin (and especially in those on concomitant therapy with additional endothelial toxic drugs, such as vinca alkaloids, bleomycin, or gemcitabine).[48,49] Intravascular evaluations in patients presenting with such a constellation indicated plaque erosion as the underlying pathologic condition.[50] Plaque hemorrhage can destabilize plaques in patients receiving treatment with vascular disrupting agents.[51] Even if not acutely, plaque hemorrhage fosters the growth and vulnerability of atherosclerotic plaques.[52] VEGF inhibitors would be expected to elicit an antiangiogenic response and thereby plaque stabilization rather than plaque destabilization.[53,54] Any increased risk in thromboembolic events may, therefore, be more due to impairment in the viability of surface-lining endothelial cells. VEGF inhibitors also suppress endothelial repair to injury, and this combined effect

may ultimately be a key factor (similar to cisplatin in this regard).[55] Conceivably, immune checkpoint inhibitors may increase plaque inflammation and thereby predispose to classic plaque rupture. However, this has not yet been proven. Alternative etiologic factors of thrombotic coronary artery occlusions and related ACS that need to be entertained in patients who have cancer (similar to stroke) are embolic events via a patent foramen ovale, from the cardiac chambers, and/or even tumor embolization.[56,57] Another consideration is spontaneous coronary artery dissection, possibly as a consequence of the effects of cancer therapy on vascular remodeling.[58–60]

As outlined in a recent study on ACS in subjects with active hematological malignancies, type II MIs were adjudicated in two-thirds of the MI subjects who underwent coronary angiography.[61,62] Other than altered vasoreactivity, tachycardia, hypotension, hypoxia, and anemia may predispose to demand–supply mismatch in those with significant coronary artery disease or, potentially, with pathoanatomical variants, such as (severe) myocardial bridging.[62] Of note, severe coronary artery disease (3-vessel and left main coronary artery disease) was seen in half of the subjects with active hematological malignancies and ACS who underwent coronary angiography.[61]

Another very important observation pertains to the impact of guideline-recommended therapies on mortality outcomes.[61] Aspirin, beta-blocker, and angiotensin-converting enzyme (ACE) inhibitor or angiotensin receptor blocker reduced mortality, whereas heparin use and an invasive approach did not.[61] The latter might be because type I MIs constituted only the minority and medical management sufficed in most subjects. Other studies support these observations in broader cohorts of subjects, including those with solid tumors. The Society for Cardiovascular Angiography and Interventions (SCAI)-based algorithm advises on an approach based on a modified Thrombolysis in Myocardial Infarction (TIMI) risk score and takes the platelet count of the patient into consideration (**Fig. 4**).[63] Revascularization strategies should follow practice guidelines (taking into account regional differences).[64–67] If stenting is performed, the European Society of Cardiology guidelines recommend a drug-eluting stent (DES) regardless of (patient and lesion) presentation type.[67] This is because improvements in DES design has reduced their thrombotic risk so much that it may be lower than with a bare-metal stent (BMS).[68,69] In the LEADERS FREE trial in subjects at high bleeding risk (including 15% with anemia, 15% with

anticipated surgery in the next year, and 10% with malignancy), for instance, a polymer-free biolimus A9-coated DES in combination with just 1 month of dual antiplatelet therapy (DAPT) was superior to BMS in terms of safety (stent thrombosis, death, and MI) and efficacy (repeat revascularization).[70] It is important to point out that most reports on acute stent thrombosis in patients who have cancer have been in the setting of BMS, often shortly after discontinuation of DAPT.[71] This, however, does not exclude the possibility of this event after DES. In fact, malignancy has been listed as a key risk factor for early stent thrombosis and the most important patient-related risk factor for late stent thrombosis.[72] For patients with ACS, DAPT duration should be for a minimum of 1 year, regardless of coronary management strategy; that is, even when medical therapy alone or surgery is chosen. This recommendation may even apply more so to patients who have cancer; however, the bleeding risk of these patients (especially with anticipated thrombocytopenia) needs to be taken in consideration. At this point, it is not known if a prediction score for thrombosis and bleeding risk, such as the DAPT score or the Predicting Bleeding Complications in Patients Undergoing Stent Implantation and Subsequent Dual Antiplatelet Therapy (PRECISE-DAPT) score, serve equally well in patients who have cancer.[73,74]

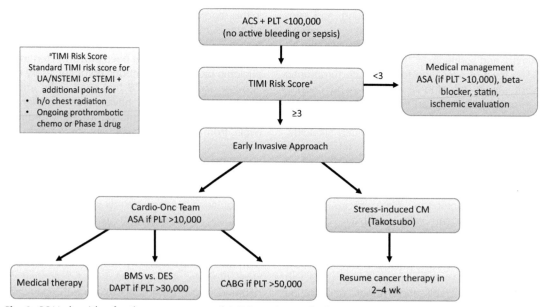

Fig. 4. SCAI algorithm for the management of ACS in patients who have cancer. (*Adapted from* Iliescu CA, Grines CL, Herrmann J, et al. SCAI Expert consensus statement: Evaluation, management, and special considerations of cardio-oncology patients in the cardiac catheterization laboratory (endorsed by the Cardiological Society of India, and Sociedad Latino Americana de Cardiologia Intervencionista). *Catheter Cardiovasc Interv.* 2016;87(5):E202-223; with permission.)

CLAUDICATION OR ACUTE LIMB ISCHEMIA

Other than in patients with preexisting peripheral arterial disease, signs and symptoms of chronic limb ischemia are very rarely seen as a consequence of cancer therapy, other than, for example, radiation therapy. This, however, changed with the introduction of TKIs targeting the *Bcr-Abl* oncogenic fusion gene product, namely nilotinib and ponatinib.[12,75] These drugs were found to cause what has been termed progressive peripheral arterial occlusion disease, characterized by diffuse stenosis of the lower arterial circulation, vascular occlusions and formation of collateral circulation.[10] The dynamics of these changes were perceived to be out of proportion to the risk factor profile. Indeed, in a carefully conducted matched-control study, chronic myeloid leukemia (CML) patients on nilotinib experienced a significantly higher rate of arterial occlusive events, 80% and 20% involving the peripheral and coronary circulation, respectively.[15] Furthermore, atherosclerotic cardiovascular disease risk factors models, such as the EURO score, were still predictive of risk.[15] Collectively, these findings support the view that nilotinib plays a causal role and that the disease process is consistent with accelerated atherosclerosis rather than a different disease process. The same seems to hold true for ponatinib.[12,25,76] Although the underlying pathophysiology is not fully defined, recent experimental studies indicate that nilotinib downregulates VEGF receptor II and thereby shares inhibitory VEGF signaling properties with ponatinib.[15,77] Both drugs have a profoundly negative impact on endothelial cell viability, even in a therapeutic dose spectrum.[78,79] In an animal model, nilotinib, and ponatinib were found to shift the balance more toward vascular instability, including both the solid and the fluid phase.[80] Plaque rupture with acute thrombosis is a conceivable mechanism of acute events in patients undergoing therapy with these drugs but they have not necessarily been confirmed in all cases. Rather, it seems that, at least in some patients, events of acute ischemia are due to rapid progression to the point of occlusion with insufficient collateral formation.[81]

In patients who have cancer at large, however, thromboembolism likely remains the more common mechanism of acute limb ischemia.[82] Similar to acute thrombotic events in other vascular territories, the source of embolism can be anywhere proximal to the occlusion point in the peripheral arteries, aorta, the valves, the left ventricle, the left atrium or appendage, or even on the venous side with paradoxic emboli. Patients with acute promyelocytic leukemia are particularly prone to acute arterial thrombosis in all vascular territories.[83]

Management of patients who have cancer with suspected peripheral arterial disease is as recommended by the American Heart Association and American College of Cardiology (AHA/ACC) guidelines.[84] Pulse status on physical examination is the first step followed by assessment of the ankle-brachial index (ABI), which takes center stage. Patients with noncompressible vessels should have an assessment of the toe-brachial index (TBI), whereas those with symptoms of claudication and normal or borderline normal ABI should have an exercise ABI. Those with any abnormal findings should be started on guideline-directed medical therapy, including aspirin or clopidogrel, statin, and optimal blood pressure control, considering an ACE inhibitor or angiotensin II receptor blocker. If symptoms persist, anatomic assessment of the lower extremity vascular is to be pursued, including (Duplex) ultrasound, CT angiography, or magnetic resonance angiography. For patients with suspected chronic limb ischemia; that is, physical examination suggestive of peripheral artery disease (PAD) with rest pain, nonhealing wound, or gangrene, any abnormality on ABI testing is to be followed in by additional perfusion assessment, including TBI with waveforms, transcutaneous oxygen pressure, and skin perfusion pressure; and, if any of these are abnormal, by anatomic assessment, as previously noted, or by invasive angiography. Patients presenting with acute limb ischemia need to be immediately recognized (acutely cold and painful leg) with motor and sensory assessment, and ultrasound for arterial and venous Doppler signals. The differentiation then is between a viable limb, a marginally or immediately threatened limb, or a nonviable limb. Amputation is indicated for the latter scenario, whereas all other cases should undergo emergent revascularization and anticoagulation, unless contraindicated.

At present, it is unknown how to best assess patients to be started on nilotinib or ponatinib at baseline and during follow-up (**Table 1**).[77,85] Various recommendations have been provided, including alteration of dose and overall treatment regimens.[11,12] In principle, for PAD and other atherosclerotic diseases with these drugs, the intensity for screening and preventive efforts should increase and the threshold for intervention and cessation of therapy should decrease with increasing risk category. As previously outlined, the EURO score may be a unique tool to tailor screening efforts. The SCAI vascular surveillance algorithm takes into account the duration of risk, as well the impact of radiation therapy (**Fig. 5**).

Table 1
Recommendation for vascular assessment of patients on Bcr/Abl therapy, namely nilotinib and ponatinib

Symptoms	Peripheral Pulse Status	Risk Factors	Vascular Tests	F/u
None	Normal	None	None	Every 12 mo
None	Reduced +/−	None or present	ABI	If ABI ≥0.9: 12 mo f/u If ABI <0.9: additional tests[a] and 6 mo f/u
Present +/−	Reduced +/−	None or present	ABI	Vascular specialist 3–6 mo f/u If ABI <0.7: stop

Abbreviations: CTA, computed tomography angiography; F/u, follow-up; IMT, intima-media thickness; U/S, ultrasound.
   [a] Exercise ABI, duplex U/S, and lower extremity CT angiography, as well as evaluation of carotid IMT and coronary CTA or stress test.
   Data from Breccia M, Arboscello E, Bellodi A, et al. Proposal for a tailored stratification at baseline and monitoring of cardiovascular effects during follow-up in chronic phase chronic myeloid leukemia patients treated with nilotinib frontline. *Crit Rev Oncol Hematol.* 2016;107:190-198.

Raynaud

Raynaud is a clinical diagnosis with a distinction between primary or secondary Raynaud. Abnormal vasoconstriction or vasospasm of digital arteries and cutaneous arterioles is thought to be the underlying mechanism, which, in its most severe form, can lead to ischemic fingertip necrosis. In a number of patients who have cancer, an underlying cause can be identified, especially medications. Raynaud has been reported with bleomycin, vinca

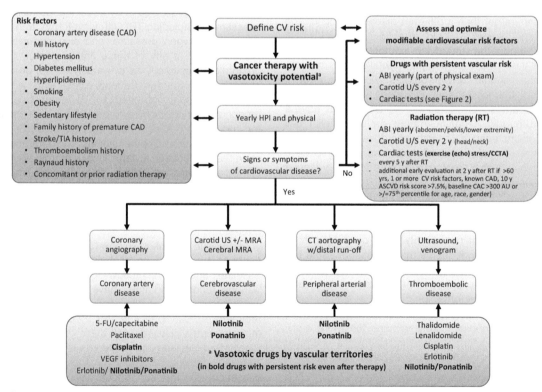

Fig. 5. SCAI algorithm for the surveillance of vascular toxicities with cancer therapies. PAH, pulmonary arterial hypertension; TIA, transient ischemic attack. (*Adapted from* Iliescu CA, Grines CL, Herrmann J, et al. SCAI Expert consensus statement: Evaluation, management, and special considerations of cardio-oncology patients in the cardiac catheterization laboratory (endorsed by the Cardiological Society of India, and Sociedad Latino Americana de Cardiologia Intervencionista). *Catheter Cardiovasc Interv.* 2016;87(5):E202-223; with permission.)

alkaloids, cisplatin, carboplatin, gemcitabine, and interferon (IFN)-alpha, even as early as after the first dose.[86–91] Endothelial injury has been a leading consideration; however, evolving endothelial dysfunction may not suffice to explain this phenomenon. For IFN-alpha, for instance, immune-mediated vasculitis has been discussed in addition to thrombus formation and vasospasm.[92] Raynaud can also occur as a paraneoplastic phenomenon, even before the diagnosis of malignancy is made.[93]

Usually, no additional testing is performed and vasodilator therapy is the treatment of choice. Calcium channel blockers are the preferred agents, whereas beta-blocker should be avoided (or switched to carvedilol if absolutely needed due to its additional alpha-blocking properties, which may ease peripheral vasoconstriction, but there is no guarantee that patients will benefit or tolerate this beta-blocker either). As with all vascular toxicities the risks and benefits of continuing versus discontinuing any culprit cancer therapeutic need to be carefully weighed.

Venous Thromboembolic Disease

Because patients who have cancer face a higher risk of VTE in general, it has been challenging to assign a high-risk potential for VTE to any given specific cancer therapeutic.[94] However, a few drugs do seem to increase the risk beyond what would be expected in the population. These include cisplatin, bevacizumab, and TKIs targeting the VEGF signaling pathway and others; mammalian target of rapamycin (mTOR) inhibitors; immunomodulatory agents, including thalidomide and lenalidomide; and possibly even immune checkpoint inhibitors and antihormonal agents such as tamoxifen. The PROTECHT (PROphylaxis of ThromboEmbolism during CHemoTherapy) risk prediction score for VTE in patients who have cancer takes platinum-based and gemcitabine chemotherapy into consideration and may perform better than other risk prediction scores, including the extensively validated Khorana risk score.[95] Despite the promise of such risk scores and promising results in clinical trials, generalized risk score–guided VTE prophylaxis is not recommended in outpatients who have cancer. In fact, primary prophylaxis is recommended only for patients with multiple myeloma: aspirin, if no additional risk factors, or low-molecular-weight heparin (LMWH) or warfarin, if additional risk factors are present, including the use of immunomodulators with steroids.[96]

In patients who have cancer with VTE, guideline recommendations for treatment vary by the society (**Table 2**). Importantly, the most recent 2019 National Comprehensive Cancer Network (NCCN) guideline now lists rivaroxaban as a viable option for monotherapy aside from dalteparin, as well as apixaban for patients who cannot or will not take LMWH (eg, due to HIT [heparin-induced thrombocytopenia]). Furthermore, LMWH or unfractionated heparin for 5 to 10 days followed by edoxaban (or dabigatran) is another viable option. For many years LMWHs had been the preferred choice over warfarin given its greater efficacy in preventing recurrent VTE. However, there are many obstacles to LMWH, including administration and costs. direct oral anticoagulants (DOACs) have been found to be as effective as LMWH but with a higher bleeding risk potential, especially upper gastrointestinal bleeding (and possibly genitourinary bleeding).[97] The International Society of Thrombosis and Haemostasis Guidance Statement, therefore, suggests the use of specific DOACs (edoxaban and rivaroxaban) only for patients who have cancer with an acute diagnosis of VTE and a low risk of bleeding and no drug–drug interactions with current systemic therapy.[98] They continue to recommend LMWHs for patients who have cancer with an acute diagnosis of VTE and a high risk of bleeding, including patients with luminal gastrointestinal cancers with an intact primary; patients with cancers at risk of bleeding from the genitourinary tract, bladder, or nephrostomy tubes; or patients with active gastrointestinal mucosal abnormalities, such as duodenal ulcers, gastritis, esophagitis, or colitis.

It is recommended to use the same anticoagulant for 3 months and to continue as long as the cancer is active, under active treatment, or risk factors for recurrence persist. In case of recurrent VTE on anticoagulation, patients should be switched to LMWH if not on it already; otherwise, the dose of LMWH should be increased by 25% (anti-Xa levels and HIT should be considered). For patients with thrombocytopenia, the NCCN guidelines have listed enoxaparin as the only agent at full dose, half-dose, or no dose in combination with platelet transfusion in cases of platelet counts of greater than 50,000, 25,000 to 50,000, or less than 25,000. Cost considerations are an important aspect because different insurance plans may not cover all anticoagulant (but only one or the other).

PULMONARY HYPERTENSION

Pulmonary hypertension is another example of a vascular toxicity that received a new level of attention with the introduction of targeted therapy. A cluster of 9 subjects on dasatinib therapy, a TKI of Bcr-Abl, used in subjects with Philadelphia chromosome-positive (Ph+) leukemias, was noted in the French Pulmonary Hypertension Registry.

Table 2
Treatment of cancer-related venous thrombosis

2016 ITAC-CME Consensus Recommendations	2015 International Society of Thrombosis and Haemostasis Guidance Statements on Diagnosis and Treatment of the Incidental Venous Thrombosis in Cancer Patients	2019 NCCN Guidelines on Cancer-Associated Venous Thromboembolic Disease	2016 ACCP Guidelines
Initial treatment of established VTE: first 10 d of anticoagulation 1. LMWH is recommended for the initial treatment of established VTE in patients with cancer (grade 1B). 2. Fondaparinux and unfractionated heparin can also be used for the initial treatment of established VTE in patients with cancer (grade 2D). 3. Thrombolysis in patients with cancer with established VTE should only be considered on a case-by-case basis, with specific attention paid to contraindications, especially bleeding risk (eg, specifically if brain metastasis), guidance based on evidence of very low quality, and the high bleeding risk of thrombolytic therapy. 4. In the initial treatment of VTE, inferior vena cava (IVA) filters can be considered in the case of contraindication for anticoagulant treatment or in the case of pulmonary embolism recurrence under optimal anticoagulation. Periodic reassessment of contraindications for anticoagulation is	• In patients who have cancer with a diagnosis of incidental VTE, the author recommends a careful review of the history to exclude symptomatic VTE. • In patients with incidental PE involving the main, lobar, segmental, or multiple subsegmental pulmonary arteries, the author suggests that no further testing is required to confirm the diagnosis. • In patients with isolated SSPE, the author recommends careful review of the images by radiologists, and suggest that compression ultrasonography of the lower limbs be performed to detect concomitant incidental DVT. • In patients with incidental ileofemoral DVT on CT of the abdomen and pelvis, the author suggests confirming the diagnosis with Doppler ultrasonography of the pelvis and compression ultrasonography of the lower limbs. • In patients who have cancer with incidental VTE, the author recommends standard anticoagulation with LMWH in those with symptoms compatible with VTE.	Monotherapy • LMWH: dalteparin 200 U/kg SC daily for 30 d, then 150 U/kg once daily for 2–6 mo (category 1), enoxaparin (category 2A) • Rivaroxaban 15 mg bid for 21 d, then 20 mg daily (category 2A) • Fondaparinux 5, 75, 10 mg (<50, 50–100, and >100 kg) (category 2A) • UFH (category 2B) • UFH IV, then SC (category 2A) • UFH SC (category 2A) • For patients who refuse or have compelling reasons to avoid LMWH: apixaban (category 2A) Combination therapy with edoxaban • LMWH (dalteparin 200 U/kg SC daily or enoxaparin 1 mg/kg SC bid) (category 1) or UFH IV or SC for 5–10 d, then edoxaban 60 mg daily (or 30 mg if CrCl 30–50 mL or <60 kg weight or concomitant p-glycoprotein inhibitors or inducers) for at least 6 mo Combination therapy with warfarin • LMWH (see previous), fondaparinux, or UFH IV or SC for 5–10 d, then warfarin with INR 2–3 for at least 6 mo	• In patients with DVT of the leg or PE and cancer (cancer-associated thrombosis), as long-term (first 3 mo) anticoagulant therapy, the author suggests LMWH over VKA therapy (grade 2B), dabigatran (grade 2C), rivaroxaban (grade 2C), apixaban (grade 2C), or edoxaban (grade 2C). • In patients with DVT of the leg or PE who receive extended therapy, the author suggests that there is no need to change the choice of anticoagulant after the first 3 mo (grade 2C). • In patients with DVT of the leg or PE and active cancer (cancer-associated thrombosis) and who (1) do not have a high bleeding risk, the author recommends extended anticoagulant therapy (no scheduled stop date) over 3 mo of therapy (grade 1B); or (2) have a high bleeding risk, the author suggests extended anticoagulant therapy (no scheduled stop date) over 3 mo of therapy (grade 2B). • In patients with an unprovoked proximal DVT or PE who are stopping anticoagulant therapy and do

recommended, and anticoagulation should be resumed when safe.

Early maintenance (10 d to 3 mo) and long-term (beyond 3 mo)

1. LMWHs are preferred over vitamin K antagonists (VKAs) for the treatment of VTE in patients with cancer (grade 1A).
2. LMWH should be used for a minimum of 3 mo to treat established VTE in patients with cancer (grade 1A).
3. Direct oral anticoagulants can be considered for VTE treatment of patients with stable cancer not receiving systemic anticancer therapy, and in cases in which VKA is an acceptable but not an available treatment choice (guidance).
4. After 3–6 mo, termination or continuation of anticoagulation (LMWH, VKA, or direct oral anticoagulants) should be based on individual assessment of the benefit-to-risk ratio, tolerability, drug availability, patient preference, and cancer activity (guidance, in the absence of data).

Treatment of VTE recurrence in patients with cancer given anticoagulant treatment:

1. Increase in LMWH dose (by 20%–25%) in patients treated with LMWH
2. Switch from VKA to LMWH in patients treated with VKA; and 3. IVA filter insertion, with

- In patients with incidental proximal DVT, or PE of the main, lobar, segmental, or multiple subsegmental pulmonary arteries, the author recommends therapeutic anticoagulation for at least 6 mo.
- In patients with isolated SSPE with proximal DVT, the author recommends therapeutic anticoagulation for at least 6 mo.
- In patients with isolated SSPE with distal DVT or without DVT, the author suggests that the decision to provide anticoagulation be made on a case-by-case basis, considering the risk of bleeding, the presence of risk factors for recurrent thrombosis, the performance status of the patient, and patient preference. If the decision is not to anticoagulate, the author suggests clinical monitoring and serial bilateral compression ultrasonography after 1 wk in those with distal DVT, to detect thrombus extension.
- In patients with incidental splanchnic vein thrombosis, the author suggests anticoagulant therapy in patients with thrombosis that seems to be acute, or that shows progression or extension over time, and in those who are neither actively bleeding nor have a very high risk of bleeding.
- In patients who have cancer with evidence of disease or ongoing systemic or locoregional therapy,

- Combination therapy with dabigatran
- LMWH (dalteparin 200 U/kg SC daily or enoxaparin 1 mg/kg SC bid) (category 1) or UFH IV or SC for 5–10 d, then dabigatran 150 mg bid (as long as CrCl >30 mL/min) for at least 6 mo

Duration:

- Minimum of 3 mo
- For noncatheter-associated DVT/PE indefinite while cancer is active, under treatment, or risk factors for recurrence persist
- For catheter-associated thrombosis, anticoagulation as long as catheter is in place, recommended at least 3 mo

not have a contraindication to aspirin, the author suggests aspirin over no aspirin to prevent recurrent VTE (grade 2B).

- In patients with acute DVT or PE who are treated with anticoagulants, the author recommends against the use of an IVC filter (grade 1B).
- In patients with acute DVT of the leg, the author suggests not using compression stockings routinely to prevent PTS (grade 2B).

(continued on next page)

Table 2
(continued)

2016 ITAC-CME Consensus Recommendations	2015 International Society of Thrombosis and Haemostasis Guidance Statements on Diagnosis and Treatment of the Incidental Venous Thrombosis in Cancer Patients	2019 NCCN Guidelines on Cancer-Associated Venous Thromboembolic Disease	2016 ACCP Guidelines
continued anticoagulant therapy, unless contraindicated. Treatment of established catheter-related thrombosis 1. For the treatment of symptomatic catheter-related thrombosis in patients with cancer, anticoagulant treatment is recommended for a minimum of 3 mo; in this setting, LMWHs are suggested. Direct comparisons between LMWHs and VKAs have not been made in this setting. 2. The central venous catheter can be kept in place if it is functional, well positioned, and noninfected with good resolution of symptoms under close surveillance; irrespective of whether the central venous catheter is kept or removed, no standard approach in terms of duration of anticoagulation is established (guidance)	the author suggests periodic re-evaluation of the risks of bleeding and VTE recurrence, as well as patient preferences, to guide the decision of whether to extend LMWH beyond 6 mo.		

Abbreviations: ACCP, American College of Chest Physicians; CrCl, creatinine clearance; ITAC-CME, international initiative on thrombosis and cancer; IV, intravenous; PE, pulmonary embolism; PTS, post-thrombotic syndrome; SC, subcutaneous; SSPE, subsegmental PE; UFH, unfractionated heparin.

Common to all subjects, pulmonary capillary wedge pressure was normal and all but one subject had no response to vasodilator therapy. Mean pulmonary artery pressure was 46 mm Hg and the average right ventricular systolic pressure was 65 mm Hg.[99] In a larger follow-up study of 21 subjects, pulmonary vascular resistance and arterial pressure dropped on discontinuation of dasatinib but remained elevated in one-third of the subjects over an average follow-up period of 24 months. Whether 1 treatment strategy (eg, endothelin receptor antagonists) is better than another is unknown at present. Universal screening has not been endorsed but patients developing dyspnea or signs and symptoms of right heart failure on dasatinib therapy need to be evaluated by echocardiography and additional right heart catheterization if found to have pulmonary hypertension (Fig. 6).[100,101] As many as 1 in 10 patients on dasatinib may develop pulmonary hypertension.[99,102] Pathomechanistically, dasatinib leads to endothelial injury and increases the susceptibility to experimental pulmonary hypertension; for example, by chronic hypoxia, with structural alterations of the pulmonary arteries.[103] In addition, immune mechanisms have been discussed to contribute to dasatinib-induced pulmonary hypertension based on the frequently concomitant exudative pleural and pericardial effusions with lymphocytic accumulations.[104]

The combination of a VEGF receptor 2 inhibitor with chronic hypoxia likewise results in reproducible pulmonary hypertension in experimental models.[105] Furthermore, VEGF receptor 2 deficiency, even if confined to the endothelial cells only, impairs vascularization and resolution of intrapulmonary artery thrombi, which may contribute to chronic thromboembolic pulmonary hypertension.[106] In addition to structural alteration, Rho kinase-mediated vasoconstriction is a contributing factor to severe occlusive pulmonary hypertension under the outlined conditions.[107] Other newer agents that have been implicated in pulmonary hypertension include nilotinib, ponatinib, carfilzomib, and ruxolitinib, but causality is not confirmed, especially in view of contradictory

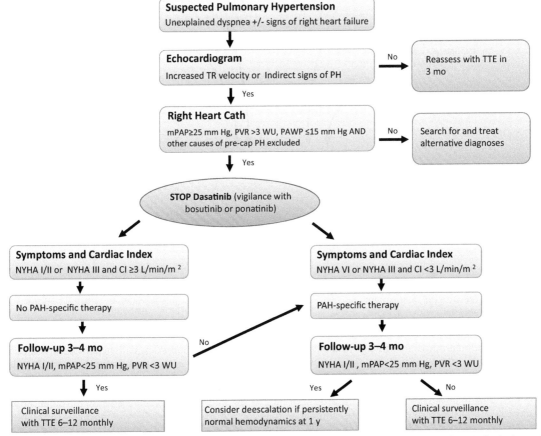

Fig. 6. Suggested algorithm for the evaluation for pulmonary hypertension in patients on dasatinib. (*Adapted from* Weatherald J, Chaumais MC, Savale L, et al. Long-term outcomes of dasatinib-induced pulmonary arterial hypertension: a population-based study. *Eur Respir J.* 2017;50(1); with permission.)

findings.[108] Trastuzumab emtansine, rituximab, and bevacizumab have been implicated in isolated case reports of pulmonary hypertension.[108]

Another chemotherapeutic that historically has been associated with pulmonary hypertension is bleomycin. Approximately 1 in 10 patients treated are affected, and the risk emerges gradually over the course of therapy and even years later.[109] The underlying pathologic condition is pulmonary fibrosis as a consequence of the stimulation and transformation of fibroblasts into collagen-producing myofibroblasts by activated alveolar macrophages and epithelial cells in a response-to-injury pattern to inflammation.[109] Statins have been shown to ameliorate bleomycin-induced lung injury as have Rho kinase inhibition, endothelin receptor antagonism, arginase inhibition, and provision of inhaled or even dietary nitric oxide (NO), and sildenafil.[110–117]

Finally, IFN alpha can induce pulmonary vasculitis and pulmonary hypertension for unknown reasons.[90] Immune mechanisms, among others, are discussed similar to the discussion on the effects of IFN alpha on the peripheral arterial vasculature.

SYSTEMIC HYPERTENSION

Increase in systemic blood pressure is a notorious characteristic of agents designed to target the VEGF signaling pathway. On average, systolic and diastolic blood pressure increase by 10 to 20 mm Hg and 5 to 15 mm Hg, respectively. Absolute numbers, as well as the reported incidence rates, of hypertension, however, are influenced by the monitoring techniques and definitions used. Ambulatory blood pressure monitoring has the advantage of detecting early and mild forms of hypertension. Chemotherapy-related systemic

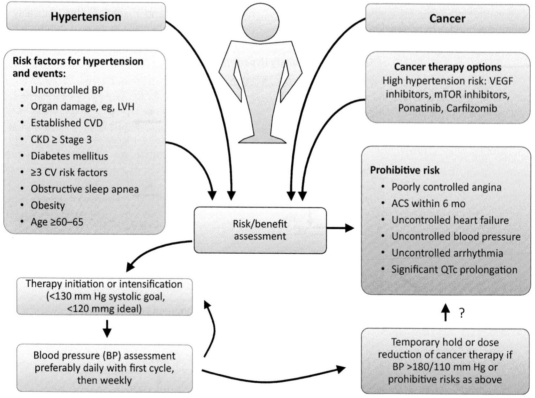

Fig. 7. Evaluation proposal for patients who have cancer undergoing chemotherapy with hypertension risk, such as those targeting the VEGF pathway. Baseline evaluation should take into account risk factors for cardiovascular (CV) events, including uncontrolled blood pressure (BP), left ventricular hypertrophy (LVH), CV disease (CVD), chronic kidney disease (CKD), and diabetes. Ideally, patients should be optimized before starting chemotherapy and should be followed more closely early after starting therapy. In case of severe BP elevation or complications related or aggravated by it, cessation of therapy should be considered. A BP goal for patients on VEGF inhibitor therapy that is less than 130 mm Hg systolic (2017 hypertension guideline) and less than 120 mm Hg systolic ideally (SPRINT [Systolic Blood Pressure Intervention] trial target) is proposed. (*From* Touyz RM, Herrmann SMS, Herrmann J. Vascular toxicities with VEGF inhibitor therapies-focus on hypertension and arterial thrombotic events. *J Am Soc Hypertens.* 2018;12(6):409-425; with permission.)

hypertension occurs over the course of the first few cycles of therapy; in fact, as early as within hours of therapy initiation, especially with TKIs.[118] Reported incidences of hypertension also tend to be as much as 2 times higher with TKIs than with bevacizumab (up to 70% for all-grade and up to nearly 20% for high-grade; life-threatening hypertensive crisis is still uncommon at <5%).[25,119,120] Patients with preexisting hypertension are at greater risk of developing worsening blood pressure control.[121,122] Age from 60 to 65 years, smoking, hypercholesterolemia, and obesity may further increase the risk, but these factors have not been universally confirmed as predictors. Ethnicity may play a role, as does cancer type (higher in Asians and patients who have renal cell carcinoma).[123]

The mechanisms by which VEGF inhibitors increase blood pressure remain debated.[124] Changes in systemic vascular resistance, secondary to endothelial dysfunction and capillary rarefication, are potential mechanisms of systemic hypertension with VEGF signaling pathway inhibitors.[118] This is in keeping with the well-documented effects of VEGF in angiogenesis and NO production by endothelial NO synthase (eNOS), with NO being crucial for normal endothelial function, vascular homeostasis, and angiogenesis.[124] In addition, inhibition of renal NO signaling leads to a rightward shift of the renal pressure-natriuresis curve with impaired sodium excretion, fluid retention, and salt-dependent hypertension.[125]

The other class of chemotherapeutics that have been associated with hypertension are the mTOR inhibitors. Everolimus carries a higher risk (up to 30%, hypertensive crisis 1%) than temsirolimus (overall <10%). The mechanisms of mTOR inhibitor-induced hypertension are not well-defined. The same holds true for carfilzomib; hypertension is seen in more than 40% of patients treated with this proteasome inhibitor. Hypertensive crisis and emergency are rare but can occur.

In view of the potential worsening of systemic blood pressures to the point of life-threatening levels, it is generally recommended to control

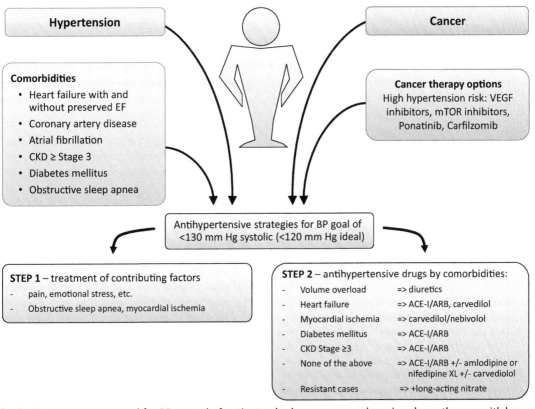

Fig. 8. Management proposal for BP control of patients who have cancer undergoing chemotherapy with hypertension risk. As outlined in the article, the author proposes that patients on VEGF inhibitor therapy should be treated toward a goal of less than 130 mm Hg systolic (2017 hypertension guideline) and less than 120 mm Hg systolic ideally (SPRINT trial target). Two steps toward reaching this goal are to be pursued: (1) treatment of contributing and aggravating factors and (2) antihypertensive therapy by comorbidity. (*From* Touyz RM, Herrmann SMS, Herrmann J. Vascular toxicities with VEGF inhibitor therapies-focus on hypertension and arterial thrombotic events. *J Am Soc Hypertens.* 2018;12(6):409-425; with permission.)

blood pressure before initiation of therapy and to follow closely, especially early in the course of therapy (**Figs. 7** and **8**). In view of the higher cardiovascular event risk in patients on VEGF inhibitor therapy, an argument for more intensive blood pressure targets can be made.[125] No antihypertensive has been shown to be superior per se, but some studies suggest more favorable survival outcomes with ACE inhibitors, though this has not been universally confirmed.[126–129] Nondihydropyridines should be avoided because they inhibit cytochrome P450 3A4 and can result in higher levels of VEGF inhibitors.[124] Fluid volume management is an important factor in patients on carfilzomib. In severe, resistant hypertension, cancer therapy should be interrupted, which promptly and effectively decreases blood pressures.

ACKNOWLEDGMENTS

Funding was received from the National Institutes of Health (HL116952 and CA233610).

REFERENCES

1. Zuo PY, Chen XL, Liu YW, et al. Increased risk of cerebrovascular events in patients with cancer treated with bevacizumab: a meta-analysis. PLoS One 2014;9(7):e102484.
2. Letarte N, Bressler LR, Villano JL. Bevacizumab and central nervous system (CNS) hemorrhage. Cancer Chemother Pharmacol 2013;71(6):1561–5.
3. Sandler A, Hirsh V, Reck M, et al. An evidence-based review of the incidence of CNS bleeding with anti-VEGF therapy in non-small cell lung cancer patients with brain metastases. Lung Cancer 2012;78(1):1–7.
4. Khasraw M, Holodny A, Goldlust SA, et al. Intracranial hemorrhage in patients with cancer treated with bevacizumab: the Memorial Sloan-Kettering experience. Ann Oncol 2012;23(2):458–63.
5. Navi BB, Iadecola C. Ischemic stroke in cancer patients: a review of an underappreciated pathology. Ann Neurol 2018;83(5):873–83.
6. Navi BB, Reiner AS, Kamel H, et al. Risk of arterial thromboembolism in patients with cancer. J Am Coll Cardiol 2017;70(8):926–38.
7. Navi BB, Reiner AS, Kamel H, et al. Arterial thromboembolic events preceding the diagnosis of cancer in older persons. Blood 2019;133(8):781–9.
8. Oren O, Herrmann J. Arterial events in cancer patients-the case of acute coronary thrombosis. J Thorac Dis 2018;10(Suppl 35):S4367–85.
9. El Amrani M, Heinzlef O, Debroucker T, et al. Brain infarction following 5-fluorouracil and cisplatin therapy. Neurology 1998;51(3):899–901.
10. Aichberger KJ, Herndlhofer S, Schernthaner GH, et al. Progressive peripheral arterial occlusive disease and other vascular events during nilotinib therapy in CML. Am J Hematol 2011;86(7):533–9.
11. Valent P, Hadzijusufovic E, Hoermann G, et al. Risk factors and mechanisms contributing to TKI-induced vascular events in patients with CML. Leuk Res 2017;59:47–54.
12. Valent P, Hadzijusufovic E, Schernthaner GH, et al. Vascular safety issues in CML patients treated with BCR/ABL1 kinase inhibitors. Blood 2015;125(6):901–6.
13. Coon EA, Zalewski NL, Hoffman EM, et al. Nilotinib treatment-associated cerebrovascular disease and stroke. Am J Hematol 2013;88(6):534–5.
14. Mayer K, Gielen GH, Willinek W, et al. Fatal progressive cerebral ischemia in CML under third-line treatment with ponatinib. Leukemia 2014;28(4):976–7.
15. Hadzijusufovic E, Albrecht-Schgoer K, Huber K, et al. Nilotinib-induced vasculopathy: identification of vascular endothelial cells as a primary target site. Leukemia 2017;31(11):2388–97.
16. Dieckmann KP, Struss WJ, Budde U. Evidence for acute vascular toxicity of cisplatin-based chemotherapy in patients with germ cell tumour. Anticancer Res 2011;31(12):4501–5.
17. Dursun B, He Z, Somerset H, et al. Caspases and calpain are independent mediators of cisplatin-induced endothelial cell necrosis. Am J Physiol Renal Physiol 2006;291(3):F578–87.
18. Nguyen MT, Stoianovici R, Brunetti L. Chemotherapy induced stroke mimic: 5-Fluorouracil encephalopathy fulfilling criteria for tissue plasminogen activator therapy. Am J Emerg Med 2017;35(9):1389–90.
19. Baytan B, Ozdemir O, Demirkaya M, et al. Reversible posterior leukoencephalopathy induced by cancer chemotherapy. Pediatr Neurol 2010;43(3):197–201.
20. Hottinger AF. Neurologic complications of immune checkpoint inhibitors. Curr Opin Neurol 2016;29(6):806–12.
21. How J, Blattner M, Fowler S, et al. Chemotherapy-associated posterior reversible encephalopathy syndrome: a case report and review of the literature. Neurologist 2016;21(6):112–7.
22. Nguyen T, DeAngelis LM. Stroke in cancer patients. Curr Neurol Neurosci Rep 2006;6(3):187–92.
23. Powers WJ, Rabinstein AA, Ackerson T, et al. 2018 guidelines for the early management of patients with acute ischemic stroke: a guideline for healthcare professionals from the American Heart Association/American Stroke Association. Stroke 2018;49(3):e46–110.
24. Sestito A, Sgueglia GA, Pozzo C, et al. Coronary artery spasm induced by capecitabine. J Cardiovasc Med (Hagerstown) 2006;7(2):136–8.

25. Herrmann J, Yang EH, Iliescu CA, et al. Vascular toxicities of cancer therapies: the old and the new–an evolving avenue. Circulation 2016; 133(13):1272–89.

26. Sara JD, Kaur J, Khodadadi R, et al. 5-fluorouracil and cardiotoxicity: a review. Ther Adv Med Oncol 2018;10. 1758835918780140.

27. Kobayashi N, Hata N, Yokoyama S, et al. A case of Takotsubo cardiomyopathy during 5-fluorouracil treatment for rectal adenocarcinoma. J Nippon Med Sch 2009;76(1):27–33.

28. Y-Hassan S, Tornvall P, Tornerud M, et al. Capecitabine caused cardiogenic shock through induction of global Takotsubo syndrome. Cardiovasc Revasc Med 2013;14(1):57–61.

29. Dixon A, Nakamura JM, Oishi N, et al. Angina pectoris and therapy with cisplatin, vincristine, and bleomycin. Ann Intern Med 1989;111(4):342–3.

30. Rodriguez J, Collazos J, Gallardo M, et al. Angina pectoris following cisplatin, etoposide, and bleomycin in a patient with advanced testicular cancer. Ann Pharmacother 1995;29(2):138–9.

31. Fukuda M, Oka M, Itoh N, et al. Vasospastic angina likely related to cisplatin-containing chemotherapy and thoracic irradiation for lung cancer. Intern Med 1999;38(5):436–8.

32. Pantaleo MA, Mandrioli A, Saponara M, et al. Development of coronary artery stenosis in a patient with metastatic renal cell carcinoma treated with sorafenib. BMC Cancer 2012;12:231.

33. Winnik S, Lohmann C, Siciliani G, et al. Systemic VEGF inhibition accelerates experimental atherosclerosis and disrupts endothelial homeostasis–implications for cardiovascular safety. Int J Cardiol 2013;168(3):2453–61.

34. Chintalgattu V, Rees ML, Culver JC, et al. Coronary microvascular pericytes are the cellular target of sunitinib malate-induced cardiotoxicity. Sci Transl Med 2013;5(187):187ra169.

35. Weinberg BA, Conces DJ Jr, Waller BF. Cardiac manifestations of noncardiac tumors. Part I: direct effects. Clin Cardiol 1989;12(5):289–96.

36. Zeymer U, Hirschmann WD, Neuhaus KL. Left main coronary stenosis by a mediastinal lymphoma. Clin investigator 1992;70(11):1024–6.

37. Orban M, Tousek P, Becker I, et al. Cardiac malignant tumor as a rare cause of acute myocardial infarction. Int J Cardiovasc Imaging 2004;20(1): 47–51.

38. Juan YH, Chatzizisis YS, Saboo SS, et al. Tumor encasement of the right coronary artery: role of anatomic and functional imaging in diagnosis and therapeutic management. Open Cardiovasc Med J 2014;8:110–2.

39. Lu JI, Carhart RL, Graziano SL, et al. Acute coronary syndrome secondary to fluorouracil infusion. J Clin Oncol 2006;24(18):2959–60.

40. Cardinale D, Colombo A, Colombo N. Acute coronary syndrome induced by oral capecitabine. Can J Cardiol 2006;22(3):251–3.

41. Frickhofen N, Beck FJ, Jung B, et al. Capecitabine can induce acute coronary syndrome similar to 5-fluorouracil. Ann Oncol 2002;13(5):797–801.

42. Schrader C, Keussen C, Bewig B, et al. Symptoms and signs of an acute myocardial ischemia caused by chemotherapy with Paclitaxel (Taxol) in a patient with metastatic ovarian carcinoma. Eur J Med Res 2005;10(11):498–501.

43. Shah K, Gupta S, Ghosh J, et al. Acute non-ST elevation myocardial infarction following paclitaxel administration for ovarian carcinoma: a case report and review of literature. J Cancer Res Ther 2012; 8(3):442–4.

44. Gemici G, Cincin A, Degertekin M, et al. Paclitaxel-induced ST-segment elevations. Clin Cardiol 2009; 32(6):E94–6.

45. Ozturk B, Tacoy G, Coskun U, et al. Gemcitabine-induced acute coronary syndrome: a case report. Med Princ Pract 2009;18(1):76–80.

46. Armitage JD, Montero C, Benner A, et al. Acute coronary syndromes complicating the first infusion of rituximab. Clin Lymphoma Myeloma 2008;8(4):253–5.

47. Arima Y, Oshima S, Noda K, et al. Sorafenib-induced acute myocardial infarction due to coronary artery spasm. J Cardiol 2009;54(3):512–5.

48. Jafri M, Protheroe A. Cisplatin-associated thrombosis. Anticancer Drugs 2008;19(9):927–9.

49. Karabay KO, Yildiz O, Aytekin V. Multiple coronary thrombi with cisplatin. J Invasive Cardiol 2014; 26(2):E18–20.

50. Ito D, Shiraishi J, Nakamura T, et al. Primary percutaneous coronary intervention and intravascular ultrasound imaging for coronary thrombosis after cisplatin-based chemotherapy. Heart Vessels 2012;27(6):634–8.

51. Michel JB, Martin-Ventura JL, Nicoletti A, et al. Pathology of human plaque vulnerability: mechanisms and consequences of intraplaque haemorrhages. Atherosclerosis 2014;234(2):311–9.

52. Michel JB, Virmani R, Arbustini E, et al. Intraplaque haemorrhages as the trigger of plaque vulnerability. Eur Heart J 2011;32(16):1977–85, 1985a, 1985b, 1985c.

53. Jain RK, Finn AV, Kolodgie FD, et al. Antiangiogenic therapy for normalization of atherosclerotic plaque vasculature: a potential strategy for plaque stabilization. Nat Clin Pract Cardiovasc Med 2007; 4(9):491–502.

54. Kolodgie FD, Narula J, Yuan C, et al. Elimination of neoangiogenesis for plaque stabilization: is there a role for local drug therapy? J Am Coll Cardiol 2007; 49(21):2093–101.

55. Ramcharan KS, Lip GY, Stonelake PS, et al. Effect of standard chemotherapy and antiangiogenic

therapy on plasma markers and endothelial cells in colorectal cancer. Br J Cancer 2014;111(9):1742–9.

56. Kushiyama S, Ikura Y, Iwai Y. Acute myocardial infarction caused by coronary tumour embolism. Eur Heart J 2013;34(48):3690.

57. Diaz Castro O, Bueno H, Nebreda LA. Acute myocardial infarction caused by paradoxical tumorous embolism as a manifestation of hepato-carcinoma. Heart 2004;90(5):e29.

58. Mir MA, Patnaik MM, Herrmann J. Spontaneous coronary artery dissection during hematopoietic stem cell infusion. Blood 2013;122(19):3388–9.

59. Ghosh N, Chow CM, Korley V, et al. An unusual case of chronic coronary artery dissection: did cisplatin play a role? Can J Cardiol 2008;24(10):795–7.

60. Abbott JD, Curtis JP, Murad K, et al. Spontaneous coronary artery dissection in a woman receiving 5-fluoro-uracil–a case report. Angiology 2003;54(6):721–4.

61. Park JY, Guo W, Al-Hijji M, et al. Acute coronary syndromes in patients with active hematologic malignancies - incidence, management, and outcomes. Int J Cardiol 2019;275:6–12.

62. Thygesen K, Alpert JS, Jaffe AS, et al. Fourth universal definition of myocardial infarction (2018). J Am Coll Cardiol 2018;72(18):2231–64.

63. Iliescu CA, Grines CL, Herrmann J, et al. SCAI expert consensus statement: evaluation, management, and special considerations of cardio-oncology patients in the cardiac catheterization laboratory (endorsed by the Cardiological Society of India, and Sociedad Latino Americana de Cardiologia Intervencionista). Catheter Cardiovasc Interv 2016;87(5):E202–23.

64. Rodriguez F, Mahaffey KW. Management of patients with NSTE-ACS: a comparison of the recent AHA/ACC and ESC guidelines. J Am Coll Cardiol 2016;68(3):313–21.

65. Amsterdam EA, Wenger NK, Brindis RG, et al. 2014 AHA/ACC guideline for the management of patients with non-ST-elevation acute coronary syndromes: a report of the American College of Cardiology/American Heart Association Task Force on Practice Guidelines. Circulation 2014;130(25):e344–426.

66. Roffi M, Patrono C, Collet JP, et al. 2015 ESC guidelines for the management of acute coronary syndromes in patients presenting without persistent ST-segment elevation: task force for the management of acute coronary syndromes in patients presenting without persistent ST-segment elevation of the European Society of Cardiology (ESC). Eur Heart J 2016;37(3):267–315.

67. Neumann FJ, Sousa-Uva M, Ahlsson A, et al. 2018 ESC/EACTS guidelines on myocardial revascularization. Eur Heart J 2019;40(2):87–165.

68. Gogas BD, McDaniel M, Samady H, et al. Novel drug-eluting stents for coronary revascularization. Trends Cardiovasc Med 2014;24(7):305–13.

69. Palmerini T, Biondi-Zoccai G, Della Riva D, et al. Stent thrombosis with drug-eluting and bare-metal stents: evidence from a comprehensive network meta-analysis. Lancet 2012;379(9824):1393–402.

70. Urban P, Meredith IT, Abizaid A, et al. Polymer-free drug-coated coronary stents in patients at high bleeding risk. N Engl J Med 2015;373(21):2038–47.

71. Smith SC, Winters KJ, Lasala JM. Stent thrombosis in a patient receiving chemotherapy. Cathet Cardiovasc Diagn 1997;40(4):383–6.

72. Gori T, Polimeni A, Indolfi C, et al. Predictors of stent thrombosis and their implications for clinical practice. Nat Rev Cardiol 2019;16(4):243–56.

73. Yeh RW, Secemsky EA, Kereiakes DJ, et al. Development and validation of a prediction rule for benefit and harm of dual antiplatelet therapy beyond 1 year after percutaneous coronary intervention. JAMA 2016;315(16):1735–49.

74. Costa F, van Klaveren D, James S, et al. Derivation and validation of the predicting bleeding complications in patients undergoing stent implantation and subsequent dual antiplatelet therapy (PRECISE-DAPT) score: a pooled analysis of individual-patient datasets from clinical trials. Lancet 2017;389(10073):1025–34.

75. Herrmann J, Lerman A. An update on cardio-oncology. Trends Cardiovasc Med 2014;24(7):285–95.

76. Herrmann J. Tyrosine kinase inhibitors and vascular toxicity: impetus for a classification system? Curr Oncol Rep 2016;18(6):33.

77. Moslehi JJ, Deininger M. Tyrosine kinase inhibitor-associated cardiovascular toxicity in chronic myeloid leukemia. J Clin Oncol 2015;33(35):4210–8.

78. Gover-Proaktor A, Granot G, Pasmanik-Chor M, et al. Bosutinib, dasatinib, imatinib, nilotinib, and ponatinib differentially affect the vascular molecular pathways and functionality of human endothelial cells. Leuk Lymphoma 2019;60(1):189–99.

79. Gover-Proaktor A, Granot G, Shapira S, et al. Ponatinib reduces viability, migration, and functionality of human endothelial cells. Leuk Lymphoma 2017;58(6):1455–67.

80. Pouwer MG, Pieterman EJ, Verschuren L, et al. The BCR-ABL1 inhibitors imatinib and ponatinib decrease plasma cholesterol and atherosclerosis, and nilotinib and ponatinib activate coagulation in a translational mouse model. Front Cardiovasc Med 2018;5:55.

81. Herrmann J, Bell MR, Warren RL, et al. Complicated and advanced atherosclerosis in a young woman with Philadelphia chromosome-positive acute lymphoblastic leukemia: success and challenges of BCR/ABL1-Targeted cancer therapy. Mayo Clin Proc 2015;90(8):1167–8.

82. Tsang JS, Naughton PA, O'Donnell J, et al. Acute limb ischemia in cancer patients: should we surgically intervene? Ann Vasc Surg 2011;25(7):954–60.

83. Kalk E, Goede A, Rose P. Acute arterial thrombosis in acute promyelocytic leukaemia. Clin Lab Haematol 2003;25(4):267–70.

84. Gerhard-Herman MD, Gornik HL, Barrett C, et al. 2016 AHA/ACC guideline on the management of patients with lower extremity peripheral artery disease: a report of the American College of Cardiology/American Heart Association task force on clinical practice guidelines. J Am Coll Cardiol 2017;69(11):e71–126.

85. Breccia M, Arboscello E, Bellodi A, et al. Proposal for a tailored stratification at baseline and monitoring of cardiovascular effects during follow-up in chronic phase chronic myeloid leukemia patients treated with nilotinib frontline. Crit Rev Oncol Hematol 2016;107:190–8.

86. Staff S, Lagerstedt E, Seppanen J, et al. Acute digital ischemia complicating gemcitabine and carboplatin combination chemotherapy for ovarian cancer. Acta Obstet Gynecol Scand 2011;90(11): 1296–7.

87. Vogelzang NJ, Bosl GJ, Johnson K, et al. Raynaud's phenomenon: a common toxicity after combination chemotherapy for testicular cancer. Ann Intern Med 1981;95(3):288–92.

88. Kuhar CG, Mesti T, Zakotnik B. Digital ischemic events related to gemcitabine: report of two cases and a systematic review. Radiol Oncol 2010;44(4): 257–61.

89. Zeidman A, Dicker D, Mittelman M. Interferon-induced vasospasm in chronic myeloid leukaemia. Acta Haematol 1998;100(2):94–6.

90. Al-Zahrani H, Gupta V, Minden MD, et al. Vascular events associated with alpha interferon therapy. Leuk Lymphoma 2003;44(3):471–5.

91. McGrath SE, Webb A, Walker-Bone K. Bleomycin-induced Raynaud's phenomenon after single-dose exposure: risk factors and treatment with intravenous iloprost infusion. J Clin Oncol 2013; 31(4):e51–2.

92. Raanani P, Ben-Bassat I. Immune-mediated complications during interferon therapy in hematological patients. Acta Haematol 2002;107(3):133–44.

93. Madabhavi I, Revannasiddaiah S, Rastogi M, et al. Paraneoplastic Raynaud's phenomenon manifesting before the diagnosis of lung cancer. BMJ Case Rep 2012;2012 [pii:bcr0320125985].

94. Timp JF, Braekkan SK, Versteeg HH, et al. Epidemiology of cancer-associated venous thrombosis. Blood 2013;122(10):1712–23.

95. van Es N, Di Nisio M, Cesarman G, et al. Comparison of risk prediction scores for venous thromboembolism in cancer patients: a prospective cohort study. Haematologica 2017;102(9):1494–501.

96. Lyman GH, Bohlke K, Khorana AA, et al. Venous thromboembolism prophylaxis and treatment in patients with cancer: American Society of Clinical Oncology clinical practice guideline update 2014. J Clin Oncol 2015;33(6):654–6.

97. Raskob GE, van Es N, Verhamme P, et al. Edoxaban for the treatment of cancer-associated venous thromboembolism. N Engl J Med 2018;378(7): 615–24.

98. Khorana AA, Noble S, Lee AYY, et al. Role of direct oral anticoagulants in the treatment of cancer-associated venous thromboembolism: guidance from the SSC of the ISTH. J Thromb Haemost 2018;16(9):1891–4.

99. Montani D, Bergot E, Gunther S, et al. Pulmonary arterial hypertension in patients treated by dasatinib. Circulation 2012;125(17):2128–37.

100. Weatherald J, Chaumais MC, Montani D. Pulmonary arterial hypertension induced by tyrosine kinase inhibitors. Curr Opin Pulm Med 2017;23(5): 392–7.

101. Weatherald J, Chaumais MC, Savale L, et al. Long-term outcomes of dasatinib-induced pulmonary arterial hypertension: a population-based study. Eur Respir J 2017;50(1) [pii:1700217].

102. Jeon Y-W, Lee S-E, Kim S-H, et al. Six-year follow-up of dasatinib-related pulmonary arterial hypertension (PAH) for chronic myeloid leukemia in single center. Blood 2013;122(21):4017.

103. Guignabert C, Phan C, Seferian A, et al. Dasatinib induces lung vascular toxicity and predisposes to pulmonary hypertension. J Clin Invest 2016; 126(9):3207–18.

104. Bergeron A, Rea D, Levy V, et al. Lung abnormalities after dasatinib treatment for chronic myeloid leukemia: a case series. Am J Respir Crit Care Med 2007;176(8):814–8.

105. Sakao S, Tatsumi K. The effects of antiangiogenic compound SU5416 in a rat model of pulmonary arterial hypertension. Respiration 2011;81(3): 253–61.

106. Alias S, Redwan B, Panzenbock A, et al. Defective angiogenesis delays thrombus resolution: a potential pathogenetic mechanism underlying chronic thromboembolic pulmonary hypertension. Arterioscler Thromb Vasc Biol 2014;34(4):810–9.

107. Oka M, Homma N, Taraseviciene-Stewart L, et al. Rho kinase-mediated vasoconstriction is important in severe occlusive pulmonary arterial hypertension in rats. Circ Res 2007;100(6):923–9.

108. McGee M, Whitehead N, Martin J, et al. Drug-associated pulmonary arterial hypertension. Clin Toxicol (Phila) 2018;56(9):801–9.

109. Reinert T, Baldotto CSdR, Nunes FAP, et al. Bleomycin-induced lung injury. J Cancer Res 2013; 2013:9.

110. Lee AH, Dhaliwal R, Kantores C, et al. Rho-kinase inhibitor prevents bleomycin-induced injury in neonatal rats independent of effects on lung inflammation. Am J Respir Cell Mol Biol 2014;50(1):61–73.

111. Bei Y, Hua-Huy T, Duong-Quy S, et al. Long-term treatment with fasudil improves bleomycin-induced pulmonary fibrosis and pulmonary hypertension via inhibition of Smad2/3 phosphorylation. Pulm Pharmacol Ther 2013;26(6):635–43.

112. Schroll S, Lange TJ, Arzt M, et al. Effects of simvastatin on pulmonary fibrosis, pulmonary hypertension and exercise capacity in bleomycin-treated rats. Acta Physiol (Oxf) 2013;208(2):191–201.

113. Baliga RS, Milsom AB, Ghosh SM, et al. Dietary nitrate ameliorates pulmonary hypertension: cytoprotective role for endothelial nitric oxide synthase and xanthine oxidoreductase. Circulation 2012;125(23):2922–32.

114. Van Rheen Z, Fattman C, Domarski S, et al. Lung extracellular superoxide dismutase overexpression lessens bleomycin-induced pulmonary hypertension and vascular remodeling. Am J Respir Cell Mol Biol 2011;44(4):500–8.

115. Schroll S, Arzt M, Sebah D, et al. Improvement of bleomycin-induced pulmonary hypertension and pulmonary fibrosis by the endothelin receptor antagonist Bosentan. Respir Physiol Neurobiol 2010;170(1):32–6.

116. Hemnes AR, Zaiman A, Champion HC. PDE5A inhibition attenuates bleomycin-induced pulmonary fibrosis and pulmonary hypertension through inhibition of ROS generation and RhoA/Rho kinase activation. Am J Physiol Lung Cell Mol Physiol 2008;294(1):L24–33.

117. Grasemann H, Dhaliwal R, Ivanovska J, et al. Arginase inhibition prevents bleomycin-induced pulmonary hypertension, vascular remodeling, and collagen deposition in neonatal rat lungs. Am J Physiol Lung Cell Mol Physiol 2015;308(6):L503–10.

118. Izzedine H, Ederhy S, Goldwasser F, et al. Management of hypertension in angiogenesis inhibitor-treated patients. Ann Oncol 2009;20(5):807–15.

119. Qi WX, He AN, Shen Z, et al. Incidence and risk of hypertension with a novel multi-targeted kinase inhibitor axitinib in cancer patients: a systematic review and meta-analysis. Br J Clin Pharmacol 2013;76(3):348–57.

120. Qi WX, Lin F, Sun YJ, et al. Incidence and risk of hypertension with pazopanib in patients with cancer: a meta-analysis. Cancer Chemother Pharmacol 2013;71(2):431–9.

121. Wicki A, Hermann F, Pretre V, et al. Pre-existing antihypertensive treatment predicts early increase in blood pressure during bevacizumab therapy: the prospective AVALUE cohort study. Oncol Res Treat 2014;37(5):230–6.

122. Hamnvik OP, Choueiri TK, Turchin A, et al. Clinical risk factors for the development of hypertension in patients treated with inhibitors of the VEGF signaling pathway. Cancer 2015;121(2):311–9.

123. Tomita Y, Uemura H, Fujimoto H, et al. Key predictive factors of axitinib (AG-013736)-induced proteinuria and efficacy: a phase II study in Japanese patients with cytokine-refractory metastatic renal cell Carcinoma. Eur J Cancer 2011;47(17):2592–602.

124. Small HY, Montezano AC, Rios FJ, et al. Hypertension due to antiangiogenic cancer therapy with vascular endothelial growth factor inhibitors: understanding and managing a new syndrome. Can J Cardiol 2014;30(5):534–43.

125. Touyz RM, Herrmann SMS, Herrmann J. Vascular toxicities with VEGF inhibitor therapies-focus on hypertension and arterial thrombotic events. J Am Soc Hypertens 2018;12(6):409–25.

126. Keizman D, Huang P, Eisenberger MA, et al. Angiotensin system inhibitors and outcome of sunitinib treatment in patients with metastatic renal cell carcinoma: a retrospective examination. Eur J Cancer 2011;47(13):1955–61.

127. Mc Menamin UC, Murray LJ, Cantwell MM, et al. Angiotensin-converting enzyme inhibitors and angiotensin receptor blockers in cancer progression and survival: a systematic review. Cancer Causes Control 2012;23(2):221–30.

128. Izzedine H, Derosa L, Le Teuff G, et al. Hypertension and angiotensin system inhibitors: impact on outcome in sunitinib-treated patients for metastatic renal cell carcinoma. Ann Oncol 2015;26(6):1128–33.

129. Sorich MJ, Kichenadasse G, Rowland A, et al. Angiotensin system inhibitors and survival in patients with metastatic renal cell carcinoma treated with VEGF-targeted therapy: a pooled secondary analysis of clinical trials. Int J Cancer 2016;138(9):2293–9.

Cardiotoxicity of Immune Therapy

Sarju Ganatra, MD[a,b,c,*], Rohan Parikh, MD[d], Tomas G. Neilan, MD, MPH[e,f]

KEYWORDS

- Immunotherapy • Immune checkpoint inhibitor • Cardiotoxicity • Myocarditis
- Chimeric antigen receptor • CAR T- cell therapy • Cytokine release syndrome

KEY POINTS

- Immunotherapy, in the form of immune checkpoint inhibitors and chimeric antigen receptor T-cell therapy, has dramatically improved outcomes for wide variety of cancers with an otherwise poor prognosis.
- However, both these therapies are associated with therapy-limiting and potentially life-threatening cardiovascular adverse effects.
- Immune checkpoint inhibitors can cause myocarditis, which usually occurs early after initiation, and prompt treatment with high-dose corticosteroids is crucial.
- Chimeric antigen receptor T-cell therapy can cause cytokine release syndrome, which may result in circulatory collapse. Supportive treatment as well as tocilizumab, an anti–interleukin-6 receptor antibody, are cornerstones of treatment.
- As immunotherapy uses expands, cardio-oncologists will be required to play a fundamental role in the comprehensive care of these patients.

INTRODUCTION

Harnessing the power of the immune system to target cancer cells has been the subject of research for more than a decade. In 1891, Dr William Coley injected beta-hemolytic *Streptococcus* into a patient with an inoperable osteosarcoma, causing the tumor to shrink, likely by upregulation and priming the immune system against the tumor, albeit nonspecifically.[1] Almost 100 years later, immunotherapies such as interleukin (IL)-2, interferon, and bacillus Calmette-Guérin vaccine became available.[2]

The first immune checkpoint inhibitor (ICI) was approved in 2011. ICIs work by releasing restrained antitumor immune responses.[3,4] These agents have changed the landscape of available cancer treatment by improving overall survival of various cancers with an otherwise dismal prognosis and their use is expected to grow substantially in coming years. However, high-grade immune-related adverse events (irAEs) can occur, particularly with combination immunotherapy.[5] Although most irAEs are manageable with temporary cessation of ICI therapy and immunosuppression, cardiotoxicity

[a] Cardio-Oncology Program, Division of Cardiovascular Medicine, Department of Medicine, Lahey Hospital and Medical Center, 41 Mall road, Burlington, MA 01805, USA; [b] Cardio-Oncology and Adult Cancer Survivorship Program, Dana Farber Cancer Institute, 450 Brookline Avenue, Boston, MA 02215, USA; [c] Division of Cardiovascular Medicine, Department of Medicine, Brigham and Women's Hospital, 75 Francis Street, Boston, MA 02115, USA; [d] Department of Medicine, Western Reserve Health Education, 1350 East Market St, Warren, OH 44482, USA; [e] Cardio-Oncology Program, Division of Cardiology, Department of Medicine, Massachusetts General Hospital, 55 Fruit Street, Boston, MA 02114, USA; [f] Cardiac MR/PET Program, Department of Radiology, Division of Cardiology, Massachusetts General Hospital, 55 Fruit Street, Boston, MA 02114, USA
* Corresponding author. Cardio-Oncology Program, Department of Cardiovascular Medicine, Lahey Hospital and Medical Center, 41 Mall Road, Burlington, MA 01805.
E-mail address: sarju.ganatra@lahey.org

Cardiol Clin 37 (2019) 385–397
https://doi.org/10.1016/j.ccl.2019.07.008
0733-8651/19/© 2019 Elsevier Inc. All rights reserved.

cardiology.theclinics.com

in the form of myocarditis is emerging as a potential therapy-limiting adverse event with a high rate of associated major morbidity and mortality.[6,7]

Adaptive cell transfer therapy was approved in late 2017 in the form of chimeric antigen receptor (CAR) T-cell therapy, after its successful application in advanced B-cell leukemia and lymphoma.[8] CAR T-cell therapy can cause a unique set of cardiotoxicities, the foremost of which is caused by on-target toxic effect leading to release of cytokines (cytokine release syndrome [CRS]) which may lead to systematic hemodynamic compromise and cardiovascular (CV) collapse.[9] Fatal cardiotoxicity caused by off-target cross reactivity against titin, a protein expressed only during contraction and expansion of cardiac tissue, has also been reported.[10,11]

This article reviews cardiotoxicity associated with ICI and CAR T-cell therapy and discusses the management strategies.

IMMUNE CHECKPOINT INHIBITORS

ICIs are a new class of anticancer therapies that amplify T cell–mediated immune responses against cancer cells. They work by blocking intrinsic immune downregulators, such as cytotoxic T-lymphocyte antigen 4 (CTLA-4) and programmed cell death 1 (PD-1) or its ligand, programmed cell death ligand 1 (PD-L1).[3,4] So far, 7 agents (1 CTLA-4–blocking antibody [ipilimumab]; 3 PD-1– blocking antibodies [nivolumab, pembrolizumab, and cemiplimab]; and 3 PD-L1–blocking antibodies [atezolizumab, avelumab, and durvalumab]) have been approved for 12 different cancers (**Table 1**) by the US Food and Drug Administration (FDA), and their efficacy is being evaluated in a variety of other cancers.[5]

Cardiotoxicity

Because ICIs unrestrain the innate immune system, irAEs were anticipated.[12] Although gastrointestinal tract, endocrine glands, skin, and liver are most commonly involved, any organ system can be affected by irAEs.[5,12] Myocarditis has emerged as a potentially life-threatening and therapy-limiting cardiotoxicity.[13] Although myocarditis has received the most attention given associated major morbidity and high mortality, other forms of cardiotoxicity, such as cardiomyopathy, arrhythmia, and vasculitis, have also been reported.[6,14–16] As the clinical use of ICI therapy increases rapidly, understanding, recognizing, and managing irAEs is becoming extremely important.[7]

Table 1
US Food and Drug Administration–approved immune checkpoint inhibitors and indications

Drug	Target	Indications
Ipilimumab	CTLA-4	Melanoma
Nivolumab	PD-1	Melanoma, NSCLC, RCC, HCC, HL, SCC of H&N, urothelial carcinoma, colorectal carcinoma
Pembrolizumab	PD-1	Melanoma, NSCLC, HL, SCC of H&N, urothelial carcinoma, gastric tumors, solid tumors with high microsatellite instability or mismatch repair deficiency
Atezolizumab	PD-L1	NSCLC, urothelial carcinoma
Avelumab	PD-L1	Merkel cell carcinoma, urothelial carcinoma
Durvalumab	PD-L1	Urothelial carcinoma

Abbreviations: HL, Hodgkin lymphoma; NSCLC, non–small cell lung cancer; RCC, renal cell carcinoma; SCC of H&N, squamous cell carcinoma of head and neck.

Mechanism of Toxicity

Although the exact mechanism of irAEs is not understood, presence of common high-frequency T-cell receptor sequences in tumor and cardiac muscle raises the possibility of a shared antigen target.[13,17] Both CTLA-4 and PD-1 have shown cardioprotective effects against immune-mediated damage after stress in animal models.[18–20] Genetic manipulation of this axis has provided some insight. Specifically, rapidly fatal autoimmune myocarditis mediated by CD8 T cells[18] was noted in CTLA-4 knockout mice. Deletion of PD-1 in mice showed development of spontaneous myocarditis and dilated cardiomyopathy likely secondary to anti–cardiac troponin (cTn) autoantibody–mediated myocardial injury.[19,20] PD-L1 upregulation in myocardium is noted in mouse models examining T cell–mediated myocarditis. This upregulation likely represents a cytokine-induced cardioprotective mechanism, which is crucial for limiting immune-mediated myocardial injury and may be abrogated by anti–PD-L1 antibody.[21]

Incidence and Risk Factors of Immune Checkpoint Inhibitor–Associated Myocarditis

The incidence of ICI-associated myocarditis is unclear. Initial clinical trials did not report any myocarditis, likely because of misclassification of adverse events. A pooled analysis of 448 patients from phase I to III clinical trials, treated with nivolumab and ipilimumab combination therapy, did not report any incidence of myocarditis.[22] In contrast, a pharmacovigilance study shows that myocarditis was noted in 0.27% of patients receiving combination therapy and 0.09% of patients on a single ICI.[13] A cohort study of patients from a multicenter registry reported a prevalence of 1.14%, which increased to as high as 2.4% for combination therapy with anti–PD-1/anti–CTLA-4.[6] The true incidence of myocarditis is likely somewhere in between. A small study noted that, for patients undergoing nivolumab therapy, troponin level was increased in 10% of patients without clear cause.[23]

The risk factors for ICI-associated myocarditis are not well understood. An international registry produced data showing that combination therapy, diabetes, obesity, and anti–CTLA-4 therapy were independent risk factors. The prevalence of ICI-related myocarditis was 0.5% with anti–PD-1 alone compared with 2.4% with combined anti–PD-1 and anti–CTLA-4 therapy.[6] The prevalence of myocarditis was lowest with anti–PD-1 agent (0.5%), whereas it was noted to be higher with anti–PD-L1 (2.4%) and anti–CTLA-4 monotherapy (3.3%).[6] In general, noncardiac irAEs are more frequently reported in patients with preexisting autoimmune disease.[5,13,24] However, with myocarditis, no association with preexisting autoimmune disease has been established. The type of cancer and preexisting cardiac disease have also not been shown to have any influence on the occurrence of myocarditis.[6]

Timing of Cardiotoxicity

Consistent data have shown that ICI-associated myocarditis usually occurs early after initiation of therapy. The reported median time is 2 months with most of the cases occurring within 3 months.[6,13] Although myocarditis is reported more frequently in the early phase of the treatment, it can occur at any time.[15] The early occurrence of myocarditis after initiation of ICI suggests that there may exist some preexisting immunologic risk factors that make some patients more prone to develop myocarditis.[7]

Clinical Presentation

The presenting symptoms vary widely. They range from mild, nonspecific symptoms such as fatigue and myalgia, chest pain, and shortness of breath, to syncope and sudden cardiac death.[13–16] Patients may present with a tachyarrhythmia (atrial or ventricular) or heart block or may develop these during the course of illness.[6,13]

Outcomes

It might be an overestimation caused by detection and reporting bias but ICI-associated myocarditis is reportedly associated with very high mortality ranging from 38% to 46% and nonfatal major adverse CV events (MACE) in nearly one-half of all myocarditis cases, including heart failure, cardiogenic shock, cardiac arrest, ventricular arrhythmia, and complete heart block.[6,25] Although fulminant myocarditis with arrhythmias has been more commonly reported, subclinical or smoldering myocarditis with minimal signs and symptoms may also occur and is likely underreported.[7,26]

Diagnosis

Understanding of the application of standard cardiac testing to the diagnosis of ICI myocarditis is rapidly evolving. This article discusses various diagnostic tests, their utility in diagnosis, as well as prognostication and their limitations.

- Electrocardiogram (ECG). It may show nonspecific findings such as sinus tachycardia, QRS/QT prolongation, conduction abnormalities, diffuse T-wave inversion, abnormal Q wave, ventricular arrhythmia, and local or diffuse ST elevation.[27,28] International registry data showed that ECG was abnormal in 89% of patients with myocarditis.[6] Although ECG abnormalities can be found in most patients with myocarditis at initial presentation, a normal ECG does not rule out myocarditis.[29] In a retrospective case control study, increase in QRS duration was observed with ICI-associated myocarditis compared with controls receiving ICI but without myocarditis. QRS prolongation was also associated with increased risk of MACE.
- cTn. Retrospective registry data show that troponin was the most sensitive test, with increased troponin level noted in 94% of patients with myocarditis.[6] However, an increased troponin level is not specific for myocarditis, and a normal troponin level, especially in cases that appear late after initiation of ICIs, does not exclude ICI-associated

myocarditis.[6] Troponin level has also been shown to have prognostic value in patients with ICI myocarditis, with a higher troponin level associated with worse CV outcomes.[6]

- Brain natriuretic peptide (BNP)/N-terminal pro-BNP. These peptides are markers of myocardial stretch and levels may be increased in patients with volume overload/heart failure, but they may also be normal.[30,31]
- Echocardiogram. Given its widespread availability and ease of performance, it is usually the first-line test for the assessment of patients with suspected ICI-associated myocarditis. However, the left ventricular ejection fraction (LVEF) may be normal even in fulminant myocarditis, and a normal LVEF does not exclude the occurrence of a major adverse cardiac event. In a retrospective international registry, 51% of patients with myocarditis had normal LVEF.[6] In addition, of the patients who experienced MACE, 38% occurred in patients with a normal LVEF.[6] Although LVEF has not been a reliable marker for either diagnosis or prognosis, emerging data show that global longitudinal strain (GLS) may help with both. A retrospective study of 101 patients with ICI-associated myocarditis shows that GLS was noted to be lower in patients with myocarditis compared with controls, for patients with both a preserved and a reduced ejection fraction. A lower GLS in this retrospective registry was strongly associated with subsequent adverse cardiac events among patients with myocarditis regardless of whether they had preserved or reduced ejection fraction.[32]
- Cardiac MRI (CMR). CMR is the gold standard noninvasive test for the diagnosis of myocarditis because of its excellent spatial resolution and additive ability to provide tissue characterization.[33] Increased capillary permeability associated with myocarditis leads to increased myocardial water content and cellular necrosis, which can be detected by CMR on T1-weighted and T2-weighted images.[34] CMR has sensitivity of 76% and specificity of 96% for diagnosing myocarditis of other causes.[35,36] However, recent data from an international registry show that more than half of patients with myocarditis had normal LVEF on CMR and only 46% had late gadolinium enhancement (LGE), making current CMR diagnostic criteria unreliable and a less sensitive tool for diagnosis of ICI-associated myocarditis.[37] Although LGE on CMR has been shown to be an effective tool for risk stratification and prognostication for

myocarditis of other causes, for ICI-associated myocarditis, LGE was not associated with MACE.[37–39] These data suggest caution in using an LGE-only approach to diagnose ICI-associated myocarditis, especially among patients with a normal LVEF. In addition, given its limited availability and the difficulty in obtaining this lengthy test in severely ill patients, its widespread use in every patient with suspected myocarditis is restricted.

- Endomyocardial biopsy (EMB). EMB is considered the gold standard for the diagnosis of myocarditis.[40] Although it is highly specific for diagnosis, the myocardial involvement with ICI-associated myocarditis is usually patchy, which makes EMB less sensitive. In addition, because of its invasive nature and the risk of cardiac perforation, with limited sensitivity, it is not performed as a first-line test.[7] When it is obtained from the affected area, histologic examination may show inflammatory infiltrates (usually T cell–predominant lymphocytic infiltrate) in the myocardium. Immune-mediated myocarditis usually shows the presence of cell-specific markers such as T lymphocytes (cluster of differentiation [CD] 3), macrophages (CD68), or human leukocyte antigens.[41]

A high level of vigilance is required given that immune-mediated myocarditis may present with nonspecific symptoms and potentially has a fulminant progression. There is no single test with high enough sensitivity to rule out ICI-associated myocarditis and hence it is important to consider multiple tests to increase the likelihood of accurate diagnosis.

It is also important to consider broad differential diagnosis, such as immune-mediated pneumonitis, acute coronary syndrome, and other causes of heart failure, especially for patients with prior exposure to cardiotoxic antineoplastic therapy. Several cases of sarcoidosis with immunotherapy have been reported, which may affect the heart and present in a manner similar to ICI-associated myocarditis with heart block, and heart failure in turn should also be considered in the differential.[42]

Treatment

The treatment algorithm for ICI-associated myocarditis is largely based on early clinical experience rather than large prospective trials. Cessation of ICI therapy and immunosuppression are the cornerstones of treatment. **Table 2** describe the current, albeit early, knowledge of the salient clinical features, diagnosis, and treatment strategies.

Table 2
Salient features of immune checkpoint inhibitor–associated myocarditis

What is ICI-associated myocarditis?	It is an immune-mediated inflammatory condition that affects the myocardium (heart muscle)
What are the symptoms?	Fatigue, myalgia, chest pain, shortness of breath, orthopnea, leg swelling, palpitation lightheadedness/dizziness, syncope, change in mental status
What is the differential diagnosis?	Acute coronary syndromes, pneumonitis, viral myocarditis, other causes of cardiomyopathy and heart failure, endocrinopathy, cardiac sarcoidosis and so forth
When does it occur?	Early in the course (median reported time is 17–65 d after the first dose of ICI therapy)
Who is most likely to develop?	Patients receiving combination ICI therapy are at highest risk. Other risk factors, such as prior autoimmune disease, have not been established
Why does it happen?	The precise mechanisms are unclear. Limited evidence suggests that autoreactive T cells infiltrate the myocardium. Given that similar T-cell clones were found in the tumor, it is plausible that myocardium and tumor may have shared antigen
How to diagnose	There are no universally accepted criteria. If myocarditis is suspected, cardiology consult, ECG, cTn, echocardiogram, CMR and EMB may be considered
ECG	Nonspecific findings, such as sinus tachycardia, QRS/QT prolongation, conduction abnormalities, diffuse T-wave inversion, abnormal Q wave, ventricular arrhythmia, and local or diffuse ST elevation, can be seen
cTn	cTn can be used as diagnostic and prognostic tool. Increase of cTn level is noted in most reported cases. However, a normal cTn level does not rule out myocarditis
Echocardiogram	Useful tool for assessing cardiac function and to rule out some other CV disease. However, it does not provide tissue characterization and lacks the ability to detect subtle myocardial abnormalities
CMR	CMR is highly sensitive and specific and can be used as the primary imaging tool for diagnosis in suspected cases of myocarditis, if available. Acute inflammation and cellular necrosis caused by myocarditis can be detected by T1-weighted and T2-weighted images as well as LGE sequence
EMB	EMB is considered gold standard for diagnosis but can be falsely negative because of patchy distribution of the lesion. Given its invasive nature and associated potential complications, it is not considered a first-line investigation and can be reserved for cases with high suspicion and otherwise negative work-up. A T cell–predominant lymphocytic infiltrate is the most common histologic finding
How to treat?	There are no prospective studies evaluating various treatment regimens but several clinical experience–based algorithms provide detailed practical guidance for management. Cessation of ICI therapy and immunosuppression are the cornerstones of treatment
Corticosteroids	High-dose corticosteroids (methylprednisolone 1000 mg/d for first 3 d followed by oral prednisone 1 mg/kg) is usually the first line of therapy in the acute phase
Immunosuppressive therapy	For unstable patients: ATG or IVIg and plasma exchange need to be considered For stable patients: tacrolimus or mycophenolate mofetil or infliximab may be considered with evidence of high-grade myocarditis on biopsy, in patients who fail to respond to corticosteroid therapy, or as a steroid-sparing agent Note: infliximab is contraindicated in presence of moderate to severe heart failure
When to start the treatment?	As soon as myocarditis is suspected, high-dose corticosteroids should be started promptly without any delay for confirmatory tests

(continued on next page)

Table 2
(continued)

How long to treat?	Unclear, but it is reasonable to continue the treatment until resolution of symptoms and normalization of cTn, LVEF, and conduction abnormalities
What is the prognosis?	Although most reported cases have a fulminant course with electrical instability and a fatal outcome, there may be a spectrum of the severity of myocarditis, and complete recovery is possible with prompt recognition and initiation of immunosuppressive therapy (as described in clinical vignette here)
What are the predictors of outcome?	Increased cTn level and presence of conduction abnormalities are predictors of worse outcomes/MACE
Pre-ICI LVEF	Retrospective data from the registry does not show any correlation between baseline LVEF and MACE
GLS	Subnormal GLS is shown to be a prognosticator for future adverse cardiac events in patients with ICI-associated myocarditis with preserved or low LVEF
cTn	Higher level of cTn is shown to be associated with MACE, heart failure, and arrhythmia
Electrical conduction abnormality	Electrical conduction abnormalities may suggest underlying severe myocarditis and have been reportedly associated with fulminant outcomes
Is it safe to restart ICI after myocarditis?	There may be a risk of recurrence. There are no prospective data to guide this complex decision, which needs to be individualized with multidisciplinary discussion considering the cancer status, response to immunotherapy, availability of alternative effective therapy, severity of cardiotoxicity, regression of toxicity with immunosuppressive therapy, and patient preference after weighing risks and benefits
Which agent to use if there is a need to restart immunotherapy?	Retrospective study has observed lower incidence of cardiotoxicity with anti–PD-1 monotherapy. Another retrospective study also shows the safety of anti–PD-1 therapy in patients who needed to restart ICI therapy after discontinuation of anti–CTLA-4 agent secondary to ir-AE requiring immunosuppression. It is unclear what to do if original cardiotoxicity was noted with anti–PD-1 agent

Abbreviations: ATG, antithymocyte globulin; IVIg, intravenous immunoglobulin.

- Corticosteroids. A high dosage of corticosteroids (ie, methylprednisolone 1000 mg/d for 3 days followed by prednisone 1 mg/kg) is considered the first-line therapy.[7] Along with dosing, timing of the therapy is also important. Prompt initiation of high-dose steroids has been shown to be beneficial for recovery of left ventricular (LV) systolic function as well as for reducing the burden of MACE.[6,15]
- Other immunosuppressive therapy. There is very little experience with using immunosuppressive agents beyond steroids. For stable patients with immune-mediated myocarditis, tacrolimus, mycophenolate mofetil, infliximab may be considered if there is an evidence of high-grade myocarditis on biopsy, for those who fail to respond to corticosteroid therapy, or as a steroid-sparing agent.[7] However, efficacy data with infliximab are mixed, and the use of infliximab has been associated with the development of heart failure among patients with rheumatoid arthritis.[43] In turn, infliximab is contraindicated in the presence of moderate to severe heart failure. Although tacrolimus and mycophenolate mofetil can be used, there is no evidence of their safety and efficacy in patients with ICI-associated myocarditis; their use is based on their proven efficacy in cardiac allograft rejection.[44]

If the patient is unstable, antithymocyte globulin, intravenous (IV) immunoglobulin, and plasma exchange should be considered.[45,46]

- Neurohormonal therapy. Concomitant standard heart failure management should also be initiated, especially if the LVEF is reduced.[7]

The optimal length of treatment with immunosuppressive agents is not clear; however, it is reasonable to continue until resolution of symptoms and normalization of LVEF, biomarker, and conduction abnormality.

Screening and Surveillance

Although the overall incidence of ICI-mediated myocarditis is likely low, it is associated with a high incidence (up to 46%) of MACE.[6,25] Delayed initiation and lower doses of initial steroid therapy may lead to higher rates of MACE, suggesting that prompt recognition of this entity is crucial.[6] Surveillance for cardiotoxicity in patients receiving ICI can be helpful for prompt recognition and risk stratification, particularly for high-risk patients such as those with preexisting autoimmune disease, diabetes, or CV conditions; for patients receiving combination ICI regimens; and coadministration or history of exposure to other agents with established CV toxicities.[7] However, currently, there are no guidelines regarding screening and surveillance of ICI-related cardiotoxicity in asymptomatic patients.

High-sensitivity cTn (hs-cTn) and ECG have shown the highest sensitivity for diagnosing ICI-associated myocarditis.[6] Because the median onset of myocarditis is early, checking cTn levels at baseline and at each cycle may therefore be of value. Retrospective registry data show that 70% of patients who developed myocarditis on ICI therapy had a normal pre-ICI LVEF and, hence, measurement of LVEF before ICI therapy may not provide utility.[6] However, recently a lower GLS has shown utility as a predictor of subsequent adverse cardiac events among patients with myocarditis regardless of LVEF.[32] Although not established yet, this novel imaging technique might be a helpful cardiotoxicity surveillance tool as well.

The utility of novel biomarkers such as soluble ST2 (sST2), a member of the IL-1 receptor family that is a biomarker of cardiac mechanical stress/fibrosis, and IL-10, a marker of inflammation, has been explored for variety of CV (CV) conditions, including myocardial infarction, heart failure, and myocarditis of other causes,[47–50] and they may also have a meaningful role in ICI-associated myocarditis. Eventually, detailed CV review of systems along with ECG, multibiomarker panel, and novel imaging techniques, may help build an effective surveillance strategy.

CHIMERIC ANTIGEN RECEPTOR T-CELL THERAPY

CARs are engineered receptors that graft a defined specificity onto T cells and augment T-cell function.[51] In this immunotherapy, the patient's own T cells are extracted, genetically engineered to express target tumor–associated antigens, multiplied, and infused back into the patient's body where they continue to multiply, recognize, and destroy cancer. CAR T cells engraft and undergo extensive proliferation once infused into the patient. Each CAR T cell can kill many tumor cells, and also provide ongoing immune surveillance to prevent tumor recurrence through antigen release, by assisting tumor-infiltrating lymphocytes to attack tumors, or by their own persistence. CAR T-cell therapy has revolutionized cancer treatment through significant improvement of survival for patients with otherwise deadly cancer.

Approved Agents and Indications

The FDA have approved 2 agents in 2017 that express CD19 on the surface: tisagenlecleucel and axicabtagene ciloleucel.[8,52–54] These agents are currently approved and used for refractory or relapsed acute lymphocytic leukemia (ALL) and diffuse large B-cell lymphoma. However, preliminary results from several phase I clinical trials of CAR T cells targeting B-cell maturation antigen have shown highly encouraging results in relapsed/refractory multiple myeloma.[55,56] Moreover, there is growing enthusiasm to explore the utility of genetically engineered T cells in the treatment of autoimmune disease, infection, inflammation, and fibrosis.[57]

Cardiovascular Effects of Chimeric Antigen Receptor T-cell Therapy

Mechanism

Most CV effects have been reported in the context of CRS. CRS occurs as a result of on-target toxicity, which clinically manifests because of excessive release of inflammatory cytokines by the activated CAR T cells or other immune cells.[58,59] Although cytokine release is an expected effect caused by immune activation by CAR T cells and is mostly mild, some patients develop life-threatening complications caused by systematic circulatory collapse.[60] A wide variety of cytokines are attributed to the occurrence of CRS; however, IL-6 is considered to be a key mediator of the systemic adverse effects.[61] Rarely, off-target cross reactivity against titin, a protein expressed only during contraction and expansion of cardiac tissue, may also occur, which may lead to cardiogenic shock, and 2 deaths have been attributed to this cause.[11]

Incidence and risk factors

The exact incidence of CRS-associated CV adverse outcomes is unknown. Although CRS is reported to occur fairly frequently (70%–90%), the toxic effects mediated by the cytokine release are most often mild. However, 20% to 50% of patients with CRS develop life-threatening complications such as vascular leak syndrome with circulatory collapse and multiorgan failure.[60]

Several patient-related and therapy-related predictors of CRS development during treatment have been identified (**Box 1**). The severity of CRS toxicity correlates with disease burden at the time of treatment and higher infused CAR T-cell dose.[62,63] A single study on patients with ALL has shown that preexisting systolic or diastolic dysfunction, ECG abnormalities, and presence of greater than 25% blasts in bone marrow were predictors for hypotension requiring inotropic support.[64]

Clinical manifestations and timing

The systemic inflammatory response during CRS causes fever and could be associated with hypotension and hypoxia. It varies in severity from mild to severe with life-threatening condition and can cause capillary leak syndrome, cardiac dysfunction, adult respiratory distress syndrome, neurologic toxicity, coagulopathy, and liver and renal failure.[9]

The understanding of CV impacts related to CAR T-cell therapy–induced CRS is limited and is based on early clinical trials and reported cases.[65] Clinical CV manifestations of CRS include a spectrum of adverse effects ranging from tachycardia, which often occurs with fever, to more severe CRS resulting in hypotension, troponin level increase, reduced LVEF, and distributive shock requiring vasopressor inotropic support. In a pediatric population undergoing CAR T-cell therapy, up to one-quarter of patients experienced LV systolic dysfunction as well as shock requiring ionotropic support.[64]

Symptom onset can occur within minutes to hours or days after infusion begins, coinciding with maximal T-cell expansion. Median time to development of CRS after CAR T-cell infusion is 2.2 days. The highest risk is in the first 2 weeks after infusion but theoretically it could occur as long as CAR T cells persist in the circulation, which could be years. The delay for CRS development after CAR T-cell infusion is usually inversely related to the severity of CRS.[66]

Pre–Chimeric Antigen Receptor T Cardiovascular Work-up

Despite of enrollment of highly selective patients without any significant active CV issues in clinical trials, serious CV events were observed. The clinical significance of CAR T-cell therapy–related cardiotoxicity will be even higher when this therapy is used more broadly under real-world conditions in higher-risk patients, including the elderly with preexisting CV disease and exposure to prior cardiotoxic antineoplastic therapy.

Although it has not been formally studied yet, it is likely that multiple preexisting CV risk factors and diminished CV reserve increases the impact of CRS-related adverse outcomes. There is no standardized protocol for pretherapy CV evaluation, and the work-up may vary from one institution to another, but it is generally geared toward determining whether patients can tolerate a period of hypotension and volume changes, which typically occurs with CAR T-cell therapy and related CRS. **Table 3** lists commonly performed CV evaluations for any patient undergoing CAR T-cell therapy.

Box 1
Risk factors for cytokine release syndrome development

High disease burden

Higher infused CAR T-cell dose

High-intensity lymphodepletion regimen

Preexisting endothelial activation

Severe thrombocytopenia

Fever (within 36 hours of CAR T-cell infusion)

Increased cytokine level (within 36 hours of CAR T-cell infusion)

Table 3
Pre–chimeric antigen receptor T-cell cardiovascular work-up

Cardiac Evaluation	Who Should Undergo?
Detailed review of CV symptoms and examination	All patients
ECG	All patients
Echocardiogram	All patients
Cardio-oncology consult	Patients with any preexisting CVD, multiple CV risk factors, or any active CV symptoms
Imaging stress test	Patients with history of CAD or multiple CV risk factors and poor exercise tolerance
Cardiac biomarkers (cTn, BNP)	Only patients with CV symptoms

Abbreviations: CAD, coronary artery disease; CVD, CV disease.

Table 4
Salient features of chimeric antigen receptor T-cell therapy–associated cytokine release syndrome and cardiotoxicity

What is CAR T-cell therapy?	Patient's own T cells are genetically engineered and infused back to fight against the cancer
What is the most common side effect?	CRS is most prevalent side effect. Severe CRS is reported in 20%–50% of patients receiving CAR T cells
What is CRS?	It is a systemic inflammatory response caused by a large, rapid release of cytokines by activated immune cells and endothelial cells
How does CRS present?	Mild flulike constitutional symptoms to more severe presentation with high-grade fever, hypotension, tachycardia, respiratory failure, distributive shock, DIC, and multiorgan failure
What is the mechanism?	Release of inflammatory cytokines such as IFNγ, IL-6, TNFα, IL-2, GM-CSF, IL-10, IL-8, IL-5 by immune-activated lymphocytes (B cells, T cells, and/or natural killer cells) and/or myeloid cells (macrophages, dendritic cells, and monocytes) as well as endothelial cells
What are associated potential adverse CV effects?	LV systolic dysfunction, hypotension, shock, arrhythmia, myocardial infarction (type II), cardiac arrest. The risk of MACE is likely higher in patients with preexisting CVD. (CAD, systolic or diastolic LV dysfunction, valvular disease, multiple CV risk factors)

What is the mechanism of cardiotoxicity?	Not well understood, but 2 separate mechanisms are thought to play role:
	• On target:
	  ○ Cytokine-induced cardiomyopathy
	  ○ Distributive shock may lead to MI and arrhythmia, especially in patients with preexisting CVD and poor CV reserve
	  ○ TLS-related metabolic derangements may trigger arrhythmia (atrial and ventricular)
	• Off-target cross reactivity against titin, a protein expressed in cardiac tissue

What pretherapy cardiac work-up should be considered?	All patients: Detailed ROS, ECG, Echocardiogram Preexisting CAD or multiple risk factors and poor exercise tolerance: imaging stress test
What is differential diagnosis?	Sepsis, TLS, pulmonary embolism, primary cardiac event
When does it occur?	Median time to development of CRS after CAR T-cell infusion is 2.2 d. Highest risk in first 2 wk after infusion but theoretically it could occur as long as CAR T cells persist in the circulation, which could be years. The delay for CRS development after CAR T-cell infusion is inversely related to the severity of CRS
Who is most likely to develop it?	Any factors that can increase in vivo CAR T-cell numbers, including high disease burden, higher infused CAR T-cell dose, high-intensity lymphodepletion regimen, as well as some patient characteristics, including preexisting endothelial activation and severe thrombocytopenia, may increase the risk of CRS
How to diagnose?	Clinical presentation, particularly fever, which usually presents before CRS, hypoxia, hypotension, tachycardia, increased CRP/ferritin levels
How to treat?	• Supportive care with IV fluid resuscitation and vasopressor for hypotension • Tocilizumab (anti–IL-6 antibody) 8 mg/kg infused over 1 h, maximum 800 mg per dose, repeat every 8 h as needed for patients with severe CRS • ±Corticosteroids for severe CRS refractory to tocilizumab
Are there any late cardiotoxic effects?	This remains unknown at this time. Patients after CAR T-cell therapy should be followed longitudinally to better understand any long-term adverse CV effects

Abbreviations: CRP, C-reactive protein; DIC, disseminated intravascular coagulation; GM-CSF, granulocyte-macrophage colony-stimulating factor, IFNγ, interferon gamma; MI, myocardial infarction; TLS, tumor lysis syndrome; TNFα, tumor necrosis factor alpha.

In addition, for patients with preexisting heart failure, volume status should be optimized before initiation of T-cell therapy, and guidance for close monitoring during the therapy should be provided. As far as antihypertensive medications are concerned, it is reasonable to consider dose reduction or discontinuation given the high risk of hypotension with CRS, sepsis, or tumor lysis syndrome.

Diagnosis

Prompt diagnosis of CRS requires high degree of suspicion and clinical surveillance during CAR T-cell therapy. Close monitoring of heart rate and blood pressure (BP) is required for prompt recognition of CRS. Specific CV testing, such as ECG, echocardiogram, or measurement of cardiac biomarkers (troponin or natriuretic peptide), is performed as required with development of any concerning CV symptoms or high-grade CRS.[67] Although CRS is a frequent cause of hypotension in patients undergoing CAR T-cell therapy, other plausible causes, such as sepsis, tumor lysis syndrome, pulmonary embolism, or primary cardiac events, should be considered.

Treatment

There are no clear guidelines for management of CAR T-cell therapy–related CRS and CV adverse events. **Table 4** lists salient features of CAR T-cell therapy and associated CRS as well as its management.

- Supportive care. Tachycardia, hypotension, and hypoxia are frequently the first manifestations of CRS. If BP is less than the preinfusion baseline, volume resuscitation with IV fluid should be considered. However, the benefit of volume resuscitation must be weighed against the risk of vascular leak and pulmonary congestion. Vasopressors should be considered for persistent hypotension despite volume resuscitation. Patients should be transferred to an intensive care unit if vasopressor or mechanical ventilation is required.
- Tocilizumab is a monoclonal anti–IL-6 receptor antibody and is approved by the FDA as a first-line agent to be used for the management of CRS-related toxicity.[62,63,65,68] There are some concerns that tocilizumab may lessen the efficacy of the CAR T-cell therapy and hence it is usually reserved for patients with hypoxia or hypotension requiring BP support for longer than 24 hours, or those with unstable arrhythmia, evidence of myocardial damage (increased troponin level), or new cardiomyopathy with LVEF less than 40%.[68]

- Corticosteroids are also effective in the treatment of CRS but are generally considered as second-line therapy given similar concern of reduced CAR T-cell efficacy.[69] They are usually reserved for CRS symptoms refractory to tocilizumab. Although exposure to tocilizumab or steroids is thought to potentially decrease CAR T-cell efficacy, results from initial clinical trials did not show an association between the use of either and response rates.[70]

FUTURE DIRECTIONS

The advent of immunotherapy, particularly ICIs and CAR T-cell therapy, has ushered in a promising new era of treatment of patients with a variety of malignancies who historically had a poor prognosis. Although the current indications are limited, they are rapidly expanding. In 2017, 940 immuno-oncology agents were being tested in 3042 clinical trials with a target enrollment of 577,076 patients.[71] However, both ICIs and CAR T-cell therapy are associated with potentially life-threatening CV adverse effects. As immunotherapy evolves to include more patients with a wider variety of malignancies, risk stratification and prompt recognition and treatment of cardiotoxicity will become increasingly important. The best strategies for screening, surveillance, prevention as well as management of cardiotoxicity to minimize major adverse cardiac events are not yet well established but knowledge is evolving. Multidisciplinary collaborations within and across the institutes are pivotal in order to enhance this understanding in a timely fashion and to inform evidence-based practice guidelines allowing improved quality of care and universal benefit. As immunotherapy becomes widely available for patients in community-based practices, to usher patients safely through cancer care, cardio-oncology care needs to expand simultaneously and hence training the next generation of physicians in cardio-oncology is necessary.[72,73]

REFERENCES

1. Coley WB. The treatment of malignant tumors by repeated inoculations of erysipelas. With a report of ten original cases. 1893. Clin Orthop Relat Res 1991;(262):3–11.
2. Decker WK, da Silva RF, Sanabria MH, et al. Cancer immunotherapy: historical perspective of a clinical revolution and emerging preclinical animal models. Front Immunol 2017;8:829.
3. Robert C, Thomas L, Bondarenko I, et al. Ipilimumab plus dacarbazine for previously untreated metastatic melanoma. N Engl J Med 2011;364(26):2517–26.

4. Hodi FS, O'Day SJ, McDermott DF, et al. Improved survival with ipilimumab in patients with metastatic melanoma. N Engl J Med 2010;363(8):711–23.

5. Postow MA, Sidlow R, Hellmann MD. Immune-related adverse events associated with immune checkpoint blockade. N Engl J Med 2018;378(2):158–68.

6. Mahmood SS, Fradley MG, Cohen JV, et al. Myocarditis in patients treated with immune checkpoint inhibitors. J Am Coll Cardiol 2018;71(16):1755–64.

7. Ganatra S, Neilan TG. Immune checkpoint inhibitor-associated myocarditis. Oncologist 2018;23(8):879–86.

8. June CH, Sadelain M. Chimeric antigen receptor therapy. N Engl J Med 2018;379(1):64–73.

9. Brudno JN, Kochenderfer JN. Toxicities of chimeric antigen receptor T cells: recognition and management. Blood 2016;127(26):3321–30.

10. Cameron BJ, Gerry AB, Dukes J, et al. Identification of a Titin-derived HLA-A1-presented peptide as a cross-reactive target for engineered MAGE A3-directed T cells. Sci Transl Med 2013;5(197):197ra103.

11. Linette GP, Stadtmauer EA, Maus MV, et al. Cardiovascular toxicity and titin cross-reactivity of affinity-enhanced T cells in myeloma and melanoma. Blood 2013;122(6):863–71.

12. Spain L, Diem S, Larkin J. Management of toxicities of immune checkpoint inhibitors. Cancer Treat Rev 2016;44:51–60.

13. Johnson DB, Balko JM, Compton ML, et al. Fulminant myocarditis with combination immune checkpoint blockade. N Engl J Med 2016;375(18):1749–55.

14. Berg DD, Vaduganathan M, Nohria A, et al. Immune-related fulminant myocarditis in a patient receiving ipilimumab therapy for relapsed chronic myelomonocytic leukaemia. Eur J Heart Fail 2017;19(5):682–5.

15. Escudier M, Cautela J, Malissen N, et al. Clinical features, management, and outcomes of immune checkpoint inhibitor-related cardiotoxicity. Circulation 2017;136(21):2085–7.

16. Wang DY, Okoye GD, Neilan TG, et al. Cardiovascular toxicities associated with cancer immunotherapies. Curr Cardiol Rep 2017;19(3):21.

17. Reuben A, Petaccia de Macedo M, McQuade J, et al. Comparative immunologic characterization of autoimmune giant cell myocarditis with ipilimumab. Oncoimmunology 2017;6(12):e1361097.

18. Love VA, Grabie N, Duramad P, et al. CTLA-4 ablation and interleukin-12 driven differentiation synergistically augment cardiac pathogenicity of cytotoxic T lymphocytes. Circ Res 2007;101(3):248–57.

19. Nishimura H, Okazaki T, Tanaka Y, et al. Autoimmune dilated cardiomyopathy in PD-1 receptor-deficient mice. Science 2001;291(5502):319–22.

20. Okazaki T, Tanaka Y, Nishio R, et al. Autoantibodies against cardiac troponin I are responsible for dilated cardiomyopathy in PD-1-deficient mice. Nat Med 2003;9(12):1477–83.

21. Grabie N, Gotsman I, DaCosta R, et al. Endothelial programmed death-1 ligand 1 (PD-L1) regulates CD8+ T-cell mediated injury in the heart. Circulation 2007;116(18):2062–71.

22. Sznol M, Ferrucci PF, Hogg D, et al. Pooled analysis safety profile of nivolumab and ipilimumab combination therapy in patients with advanced melanoma. J Clin Oncol 2017;35(34):3815–22.

23. Sarocchi M, Grossi F, Arboscello E, et al. Serial troponin for early detection of nivolumab cardiotoxicity in advanced non-small cell lung cancer patients. Oncologist 2018;23(8):936–42.

24. Johnson DB, Sullivan RJ, Menzies AM. Immune checkpoint inhibitors in challenging populations. Cancer 2017;123(11):1904–11.

25. Moslehi JJ, Salem JE, Sosman JA, et al. Increased reporting of fatal immune checkpoint inhibitor-associated myocarditis. Lancet 2018;391(10124):933.

26. Norwood TG, Westbrook BC, Johnson DB, et al. Smoldering myocarditis following immune checkpoint blockade. J Immunother Cancer 2017;5(1):91.

27. Nakashima H, Honda Y, Katayama T. Serial electrocardiographic findings in acute myocarditis. Intern Med 1994;33(11):659–66.

28. Testani JM, Kolansky DM, Litt H, et al. Focal myocarditis mimicking acute ST-elevation myocardial infarction: diagnosis using cardiac magnetic resonance imaging. Tex Heart Inst J 2006;33(2):256–9.

29. Deluigi CC, Ong P, Hill S, et al. ECG findings in comparison to cardiovascular MR imaging in viral myocarditis. Int J Cardiol 2013;165(1):100–6.

30. Ogawa T, Veinot JP, Kuroski de Bold ML, et al. Angiotensin II receptor antagonism reverts the selective cardiac BNP upregulation and secretion observed in myocarditis. Am J Physiol Heart Circ Physiol 2008;294(6):H2596–603.

31. Abrar S, Ansari MJ, Mittal M, et al. Predictors of mortality in paediatric myocarditis. J Clin Diagn Res 2016;10(6):SC12–6.

32. Awadalla M, Mahmood S, Groarke J, et al. Decreased global longitudinal strain with myocarditis from immune checkpoint inhibitors and occurrence of major adverse cardiac events. J Am Coll Cardiol 2019;73(9 Supplement 1):1532.

33. Friedrich MG, Sechtem U, Schulz-Menger J, et al. Cardiovascular magnetic resonance in myocarditis: a JACC white paper. J Am Coll Cardiol 2009;53(17):1475–87.

34. Farhad H, Staziaki PV, Addison D, et al. Characterization of the changes in cardiac structure and function in mice treated with anthracyclines using serial

cardiac magnetic resonance imaging. Circ Cardiovasc Imaging 2016;9(12) [pii:e003584].

35. Mahrholdt H, Goedecke C, Wagner A, et al. Cardiovascular magnetic resonance assessment of human myocarditis: a comparison to histology and molecular pathology. Circulation 2004;109(10):1250–8.

36. Abdel-Aty H, Boye P, Zagrosek A, et al. Diagnostic performance of cardiovascular magnetic resonance in patients with suspected acute myocarditis: comparison of different approaches. J Am Coll Cardiol 2005;45(11):1815–22.

37. Zhang L, Awadalla M, Mahmood SS, et al. Late gadolinium enhancement in patients with myocarditis from immune checkpoint inhibitors. J Am Coll Cardiol 2019;73(9 Supplement 1):675.

38. Aquaro GD, Perfetti M, Camastra G, et al. Cardiac MR with late gadolinium enhancement in acute myocarditis with preserved systolic function: ITAMY study. J Am Coll Cardiol 2017;70(16):1977–87.

39. Grani C, Eichhorn C, Biere L, et al. Prognostic value of cardiac magnetic resonance tissue characterization in risk stratifying patients with suspected myocarditis. J Am Coll Cardiol 2017; 70(16):1964–76.

40. Hauck AJ, Kearney DL, Edwards WD. Evaluation of postmortem endomyocardial biopsy specimens from 38 patients with lymphocytic myocarditis: implications for role of sampling error. Mayo Clin Proc 1989;64(10):1235–45.

41. Maisch B, Portig I, Ristic A, et al. Definition of inflammatory cardiomyopathy (myocarditis): on the way to consensus. A status report. Herz 2000;25(3):200–9.

42. Suozzi KC, Stahl M, Ko CJ, et al. Immune-related sarcoidosis observed in combination ipilimumab and nivolumab therapy. JAAD Case Rep 2016;2(3): 264–8.

43. Kwon HJ, Cote TR, Cuffe MS, et al. Case reports of heart failure after therapy with a tumor necrosis factor antagonist. Ann Intern Med 2003;138(10): 807–11.

44. Kobashigawa JA, Miller LW, Russell SD, et al. Tacrolimus with mycophenolate mofetil (MMF) or sirolimus vs. cyclosporine with MMF in cardiac transplant patients: 1-year report. Am J Transplant 2006;6(6): 1377–86.

45. Kobashigawa J, Crespo-Leiro MG, Ensminger SM, et al. Report from a consensus conference on antibody-mediated rejection in heart transplantation. J Heart Lung Transplant 2011;30(3):252–69.

46. Rodriguez ER, Skojec DV, Tan CD, et al. Antibody-mediated rejection in human cardiac allografts: evaluation of immunoglobulins and complement activation products C4d and C3d as markers. Am J Transplant 2005;5(11):2778–85.

47. Januzzi JL Jr, Peacock WF, Maisel AS, et al. Measurement of the interleukin family member ST2 in patients with acute dyspnea: results from the PRIDE (Pro-Brain Natriuretic Peptide Investigation of Dyspnea in the Emergency Department) study. J Am Coll Cardiol 2007;50(7):607–13.

48. Sabatine MS, Morrow DA, Higgins LJ, et al. Complementary roles for biomarkers of biomechanical strain ST2 and N-terminal prohormone B-type natriuretic peptide in patients with ST-elevation myocardial infarction. Circulation 2008;117(15):1936–44.

49. Lee GY, Choi JO, Ju ES, et al. Role of soluble ST2 as a marker for rejection after heart transplant. Korean Circ J 2016;46(6):811–20.

50. Nishii M, Inomata T, Takehana H, et al. Serum levels of interleukin-10 on admission as a prognostic predictor of human fulminant myocarditis. J Am Coll Cardiol 2004;44(6):1292–7.

51. Sadelain M, Brentjens R, Riviere I. The basic principles of chimeric antigen receptor design. Cancer Discov 2013;3(4):388–98.

52. Maude SL, Laetsch TW, Buechner J, et al. Tisagenlecleucel in children and young adults with B-cell lymphoblastic leukemia. N Engl J Med 2018; 378(5):439–48.

53. Neelapu SS, Locke FL, Bartlett NL, et al. Axicabtagene ciloleucel CAR T-cell therapy in refractory large B-cell lymphoma. N Engl J Med 2017;377(26): 2531–44.

54. Schuster SJ, Bishop MR, Tam CS, et al. Tisagenlecleucel in adult relapsed or refractory diffuse large B-cell lymphoma. N Engl J Med 2018;380(1):45–56.

55. Ghosh A, Mailankody S, Giralt SA, et al. CAR T cell therapy for multiple myeloma: where are we now and where are we headed? Leuk Lymphoma 2018; 59(9):2056–67.

56. Raje N, Berdeja J, Lin Y, et al. Anti-BCMA CAR T-cell therapy bb2121 in relapsed or refractory multiple myeloma. N Engl J Med 2019;380(18):1726–37.

57. Maldini CR, Ellis GI, Riley JL. CAR T cells for infection, autoimmunity and allotransplantation. Nat Rev Immunol 2018;18(10):605–16.

58. Obstfeld AE, Frey NV, Mansfield K, et al. Cytokine release syndrome associated with chimeric-antigen receptor T-cell therapy: clinicopathological insights. Blood 2017;130(23):2569–72.

59. Teachey DT, Lacey SF, Shaw PA, et al. Identification of predictive biomarkers for cytokine release syndrome after chimeric antigen receptor T-cell therapy for acute lymphoblastic leukemia. Cancer Discov 2016;6(6):664–79.

60. Kochenderfer JN, Dudley ME, Kassim SH, et al. Chemotherapy-refractory diffuse large B-cell lymphoma and indolent B-cell malignancies can be effectively treated with autologous T cells expressing an anti-CD19 chimeric antigen receptor. J Clin Oncol 2015;33(6):540–9.

61. Pathan N, Hemingway CA, Alizadeh AA, et al. Role of interleukin 6 in myocardial dysfunction of meningococcal septic shock. Lancet 2004;363(9404):203–9.

62. Davila ML, Riviere I, Wang X, et al. Efficacy and toxicity management of 19-28z CAR T cell therapy in B cell acute lymphoblastic leukemia. Sci Transl Med 2014;6(224):224ra225.

63. Maude SL, Frey N, Shaw PA, et al. Chimeric antigen receptor T cells for sustained remissions in leukemia. N Engl J Med 2014;371(16):1507–17.

64. Burstein DS, Maude S, Grupp S, et al. Cardiac profile of chimeric antigen receptor T cell therapy in children: a single-institution experience. Biol Blood Marrow Transplant 2018;24(8):1590–5.

65. Lee DW, Kochenderfer JN, Stetler-Stevenson M, et al. T cells expressing CD19 chimeric antigen receptors for acute lymphoblastic leukaemia in children and young adults: a phase 1 dose-escalation trial. Lancet 2015;385(9967):517–28.

66. Hay KA, Hanafi LA, Li D, et al. Kinetics and biomarkers of severe cytokine release syndrome after CD19 chimeric antigen receptor-modified T-cell therapy. Blood 2017;130(21):2295–306.

67. Lee DW, Gardner R, Porter DL, et al. Current concepts in the diagnosis and management of cytokine release syndrome. Blood 2014;124(2):188–95.

68. Le RQ, Li L, Yuan W, et al. FDA approval summary: tocilizumab for treatment of chimeric antigen receptor T cell-induced severe or life-threatening cytokine release syndrome. Oncologist 2018; 23(8):943–7.

69. Brentjens RJ, Davila ML, Riviere I, et al. CD19-targeted T cells rapidly induce molecular remissions in adults with chemotherapy-refractory acute lymphoblastic leukemia. Sci Transl Med 2013; 5(177):177ra138.

70. Locke FL, Neelapu SS, Bartlett NL, et al. Preliminary results of prophylactic tocilizumab after axicabtageneciloleucel (axi-cel; KTE-C19) treatment for patients with refractory, aggressive non-Hodgkin lymphoma (NHL). Blood 2017; 130(Suppl 1):1547.

71. Tang J, Shalabi A, Hubbard-Lucey VM. Comprehensive analysis of the clinical immuno-oncology landscape. Ann Oncol 2018;29(1):84–91.

72. Ganatra S, Hayek SS. Cardio-oncology for GenNext: a missing piece of the training puzzle. J Am Coll Cardiol 2018;71(25):2977–81.

73. Hayek SS, Ganatra S, Lenneman C, et al. Preparing the cardiovascular workforce to care for oncology patients: JACC review topic of the week. J Am Coll Cardiol 2019;73(17):2226–35.

Fluoropyrimidine-Associated Cardiotoxicity

Jaya Kanduri, MD[a], Luis Alberto More, MD[b], Anuradha Godishala, MD[c], Aarti Asnani, MD[d],*

KEYWORDS

• 5-FU • Capecitabine • Fluoropyrimidines • Chemotherapy • Cardiotoxicity • Coronary vasospasm

KEY POINTS

- The fluoropyrimidines, namely 5-fluorouracil (5-FU) and its oral prodrug, capecitabine, are the third most commonly used chemotherapeutic agents for the treatment of solid tumors, such as those involving the head and neck, gastrointestinal tract, and bladder.
- Fluoropyrimidine use is limited by cardiotoxicity in 1% to 19% of exposed patients. A range of clinical presentations has been reported, including chest pain, myocardial infarction, acute cardiomyopathy, arrhythmia, and cardiogenic shock.
- The incidence and precise mechanisms of cardiotoxicity have yet to be elucidated. Proposed mechanisms include coronary vasospasm, coronary endothelial dysfunction, direct myocardial toxicity, myocarditis, and Takotsubo cardiomyopathy.
- Therapeutic and prophylactic interventions primarily target coronary vasospasm.
- Prospective trials are needed to guide risk stratification and cardioprotective strategies in patients receiving fluoropyrimidines.

INTRODUCTION

The fluoropyrimidines, namely 5-fluorouracil (5-FU) and its oral prodrug, capecitabine, are the third most commonly used chemotherapeutic agents for the treatment of solid tumors of glandular and squamous origin, such as those involving the head and neck, gastrointestinal tract, and bladder. Use of fluoropyrimidines is standard of care for treatment of advanced colorectal cancers, and may have synergistic effects with external beam radiation to enhance the radiosensitivity of tumors.[1] However, among conventional cytotoxic chemotherapies, 5-FU is one of the most common agents causing cardiotoxicity, second only to anthracyclines. The classic clinical manifestation of fluoropyrimidine cardiotoxicity is chest pain due to coronary vasospasm, although myocardial infarction, acute cardiomyopathy, arrhythmia, shock, and sudden cardiac death have also been reported.[2]

The mechanisms underlying the antitumor effect of fluoropyrimidines have been well-characterized, but the pathophysiology of fluoropyrimidine cardiotoxicity remains uncertain. 5-FU is a pyrimidine analog that inhibits thymidylate synthase (TS), an enzyme involved in DNA replication. These agents therefore function as S-phase antimetabolites and promote genomic instability by inducing double-strand DNA and single-strand DNA breaks, as well as by interfering with DNA synthesis, repair, and elongation.[3] Capecitabine is metabolized to 5-FU in a series of reactions involving the enzymes cytidine deaminase and thymidine phosphorylase,

Disclosure: The authors have nothing to disclose.
[a] Department of Medicine, Beth Israel Deaconess Medical Center, 330 Brookline Avenue, Boston, MA 02215, USA; [b] CardioVascular Institute, Beth Israel Deaconess Medical Center, 3 Blackfan Circle, Center for Life Sciences 9th Floor, Boston, MA 02215, USA; [c] Division of Cardiovascular Medicine, Beth Israel Deaconess Medical Center, 330 Brookline Avenue, Boston, MA 02215, USA; [d] Cardio-Oncology Program, Division of Cardiovascular Medicine, CardioVascular Institute, Beth Israel Deaconess Medical Center, 3 Blackfan Circle, Center for Life Sciences Room 911, Boston, MA 02215, USA
* Corresponding author.
E-mail address: aasnani@bidmc.harvard.edu

cardiology.theclinics.com

which are overexpressed in tumor cells, thus targeting cancerous rather than normally dividing tissue.[4]

INCIDENCE

Fluoropyrimidine-associated cardiotoxicity was first observed as early as the 1960s. Cardiotoxicity has been estimated to occur in 1% to 19% of exposed patients,[5] although there have been few clinical trials focused specifically on defining the incidence of cardiotoxicity. Reported incidence data are largely based on retrospective studies that lack consistent definitions of cardiotoxicity and have variable reporting of cardiac events. Contemporary studies suggest a similar incidence of 7% to 19%, with most events occurring in patients without a known history of cardiovascular disease.[5,6] Recently, an analysis of 16 clinical trials incorporating 5-FU and capecitabine treatment in the Eastern Cooperative Group Cancer Research Group-American College of Radiology Imaging Network found that most trials excluded patients with known cardiovascular disease.[7] The remaining studies did not account for preexisting cardiovascular disease. Moreover, less than half of the trials reported potential adverse cardiac events related to 5-FU administration, highlighting the need for more robust studies to assess the incidence and mechanisms associated with fluoropyrimidine cardiotoxicity.

CLINICAL MANIFESTATIONS AND RISK FACTORS

Diverse clinical presentations of fluoropyrimidine cardiotoxicity have been described in the literature, including chest pain, myocardial infarction, coronary dissection, heart failure, myopericarditis, arrhythmia, QT prolongation, cardiogenic shock, and cardiac arrest. In a prospective study of patients treated with 5-FU, 19 of 102 patients developed chest pain within 24 hours of 5-FU initiation, defined as severe anginal symptoms.[5] The study population consisted of 69% men with a median age of 62 years. Eighty percent of patients received 5-FU as a continuous infusion, and none had a previous diagnosis of coronary artery disease. Subsequent coronary angiography demonstrated atherosclerotic disease in 11.8% of patients, with no flow-limiting stenoses. Associated electrocardiographic (ECG) changes such as ST depression or ST elevation, which were present in most of the 19 patients, resolved with the chest pain over a 2- to 12-hour period after drug cessation. Two patients demonstrated a reduction in left ventricular ejection fraction on echocardiogram compared with a recent baseline. Similarly, a 2016 study by de Forni and colleagues[6] prospectively enrolled 367 patients treated with high-dose 5-FU. Thirty-two percent of these patients had been previously diagnosed with cardiovascular disease, and there was a 7.6% incidence of 5-FU-associated cardiac events (28 individuals). These events manifested as chest pain (n = 18), arrhythmia (n = 1), and sudden death (n = 1). Of the 28 patients with cardiac events, 75% had persistent symptoms after 5-FU discontinuation.

A diagnosis of fluoropyrimidine cardiotoxicity is typically based on symptoms such as chest pain, palpitations, and shortness of breath, the presence of hemodynamic compromise, dynamic ECG changes, elevated cardiac biomarkers, changes in left ventricular function by echocardiography, and/or abnormal coronary angiography. A study using continuous ambulatory ECG monitoring showed that 68% of patients demonstrated silent ST segment changes ($\geq$1 mm deviation) suggestive of ischemia, therefore highlighting the potential usefulness of this monitoring method to detect cardiotoxicity.[8]

Proposed risk factors for fluoropyrimidine cardiotoxicity include older age, concurrent administration of other cardiotoxic medications, and a history of cardiac disease and/or cardiovascular risk factors including hypertension, hyperlipidemia, and smoking. Continuous infusions of 5-FU have been associated with a higher incidence of cardiotoxicity compared with bolus dosing.[9] Cardiotoxicity most commonly occurs during the first cycle of 5-FU administration, with a mean time to symptoms of 12 hours, although symptoms may develop any time in the course of therapy and have been reported up to 2 days after infusion.[10] Interestingly, oral capecitabine has a similar incidence of cardiotoxicity as intravenous 5-FU.[9]

Finally, some patients may have a genetic predisposition for 5-FU toxicity. A retrospective study of genetic polymorphisms showed that patients with a triple repeat variant of the TS promoter had higher expression levels of TS, the main target of 5-FU.[11] Although the presence of this homozygous variant in patients with colorectal cancer was associated with lower response rates to 5-FU therapy, it was also associated with less 5-FU toxicity. Decreased levels of the primary enzyme that catabolizes 5-FU, dihydropyrimidine dehydrogenase (DYPD), has been associated with predisposition to 5-FU toxicity.[12,13] One case report highlighted a patient who presented with 5-FU-associated coronary vasospasm and was found to have a germline mutation in the DYPD gene on sequencing.[14] Additional studies are needed to elucidate risk factors that can facilitate prediction of 5-FU response, as well as toxicity, on an individualized basis.

PROPOSED MECHANISMS OF CARDIOTOXICITY

Coronary vasospasm is the most well-established mechanism of fluoropyrimidine cardiotoxicity supported by in vivo and in vitro models. In 1991, Luwaert and colleagues[15] demonstrated vasospasm of the left circumflex artery by performing angiography during 5-FU infusion in a patient with stage III squamous cell carcinoma of the palate. This finding resolved with intracoronary injection of isosorbide dinitrate. Similarly, several other case reports have described 5-FU-associated vasospasm in the absence of underlying coronary disease.[16–18]

Fluoropyrimidines have been described to have effects on both vascular smooth muscle cells and endothelial cells (**Fig. 1**). In an in vitro model of vasospasm, rings of aortic tissue isolated from rabbits were treated with 5-FU, resulting in concentration-dependent vasoconstriction of vascular smooth muscle cells.[19] A similar vasoconstrictive response to 5-FU was observed in tissue with and without endothelial cells, suggesting an endothelial cell-independent mechanism. In this model, 5-FU-associated vasoconstriction was attenuated by nitroglycerin, but unchanged by verapamil, diltiazem, propranolol, and phentolamine. Additional studies using chemical inhibitors

and activators of protein kinase C suggested a role for this family of enzymes in the pathogenesis of 5-FU-associated vasoconstriction. Another study using electron microscopy to examine isolated arteries in rabbits treated with 5-FU found evidence of direct toxicity to the coronary endothelial intima, leading to thrombosis.[20] Supporting the endothelial dysfunction hypothesis, increased plasma levels of endothelin-1 and von Willebrand factor have been found in patients receiving 5-FU with or without cardiotoxicity manifestations.[21,22]

In contrast to the aforementioned mechanisms, some patients develop left ventricular systolic dysfunction following 5-FU administration, with global hypokinesis or regional wall motion abnormalities that do not correspond to a typical coronary artery distribution. This suggests that pathways independent of the coronary vasculature may contribute to fluoropyrimidine cardiotoxicity (**Fig. 2**). Direct toxicity to the myocardium has been proposed to be mediated by cardiotoxic metabolites such as fluoroacetate and fluorocitrate. α-Fluoro-β-alanine, a degradation product of 5-FU, is converted to fluoroacetate and, subsequently, fluorocitrate, which competitively inhibits the citric acid cycle. This results in the accumulation of citrate, downstream depletion of high-energy ATP, and subsequent ischemia. In a guinea pig model, 5-FU exposure resulted in ischemic ECG changes, including ST elevation, ST depression, and T wave inversion, as well as depletion of ATP and accumulation of citrate in the

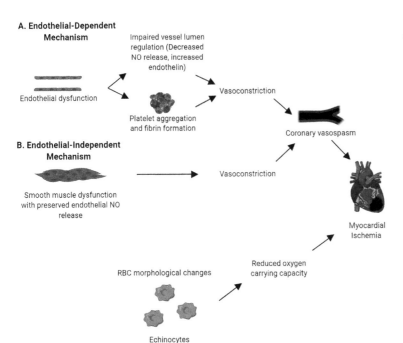

A. Endothelial-Dependent Mechanism

Endothelial dysfunction

Impaired vessel lumen regulation (Decreased NO release, increased endothelin)

Platelet aggregation and fibrin formation

Vasoconstriction

Coronary vasospasm

B. Endothelial-Independent Mechanism

Smooth muscle dysfunction with preserved endothelial NO release

Vasoconstriction

Myocardial Ischemia

RBC morphological changes

Reduced oxygen carrying capacity

Echinocytes

Fig. 1. Proposed mechanisms of cardiotoxicity: myocardial ischemia. NO, nitric oxide; RBC, red blood cells.

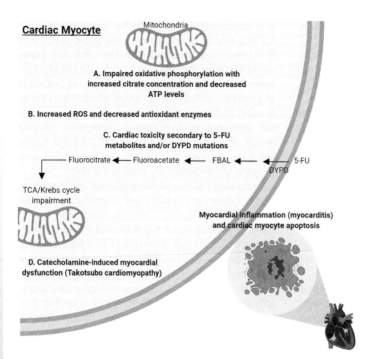

Cardiac Myocyte

Mitochondria

A. Impaired oxidative phosphorylation with increased citrate concentration and decreased ATP levels

B. Increased ROS and decreased antioxidant enzymes

C. Cardiac toxicity secondary to 5-FU metabolites and/or DYPD mutations

Fluorocitrate ← Fluoroacetate ← FBAL ← DYPD ← 5-FU

TCA/Krebs cycle impairment

Myocardial inflammation (myocarditis) and cardiac myocyte apoptosis

D. Catecholamine-induced myocardial dysfunction (Takotsubo cardiomyopathy)

Fig. 2. Proposed mechanisms of cardiotoxicity: cardiomyocyte injury. 5-FU, 5-fluorouracil; ATP, adenosine triphosphate; DYPD, dihydropyrimidine dehydrogenase; FBAL, α-fluoro-β-alanine; TCA, tricarboxylic acid.

ventricular myocardium.[23] An in vivo study in rabbits demonstrated apoptosis of cardiomyocytes, as well as endothelial cells of the distal coronary arteries, as a consequence of low-dose chronic 5-FU treatment. In addition, spasm was observed in the proximal coronary arteries in the setting of high-dose 5-FU treatment.[24]

Oxidative stress has also been implicated in fluoropyrimidine cardiotoxicity. An in vitro study demonstrated increased reactive oxygen species in cardiomyocytes and endothelial cells, leading to 5-FU-induced apoptosis.[25] Electron microscopic evaluation showed destruction of mitochondria, dilation of the endoplasmic reticulum, and autophagic vacuoles. In addition, there was increased activity of senescence-associated β-galactosidase, suggesting cell senescence. Similarly, in guinea pigs treated with 5-FU, levels of superoxide dismutase and glutathione peroxidase were decreased in the heart, further supporting the oxidative stress theory.[26]

Other suggested mechanisms include Takotsubo cardiomyopathy secondary to an exaggerated sympathetic response[27]; transformation of erythrocytes to echinocytes leading to increased blood viscosity, reduced oxygen-carrying capacity, and subsequent ischemia[28]; as well as vasospasm mediated by an allergic reaction to 5-FU, known as Kounis syndrome.[29] More robust studies are necessary to explore the potential mechanisms that contribute to fluoropyrimidine cardiotoxicity.

MANAGEMENT

When acute cardiotoxicity is suspected, prompt discontinuation of fluoropyrimidine therapy is recommended, followed by empiric treatment of coronary vasospasm with aspirin, calcium channel blockers, and nitrates (**Table 1**). Emergent coronary angiography with ad hoc revascularization may be indicated in high-risk patients presenting with 5-FU-related acute coronary syndromes. In lower-risk patients with chest discomfort, exercise stress testing or coronary computed tomography angiography should be considered following symptom resolution.[30]

Generally, fluoropyrimidine rechallenge after a known or suspected cardiotoxic event is not advised because of the risk of recurrence leading to myocardial infarction, cardiogenic shock, or death.[31] However, fluoropyrimidine use may be necessary for some patients in whom alternative chemotherapy regimens of equivalent efficacy are lacking. In a single-center case series, 11 patients with suspected fluoropyrimidine-associated coronary vasospasm were successfully rechallenged with the culprit drug, allowing for completion of planned chemotherapy.[30] Based on their experience, recommendations for rechallenge included the following: (1) switch to a bolus regimen rather than a continuous infusion; (2) pretreatment with extended-release nifedipine and isosorbide mononitrate 3 to 4 hours before 5-FU infusion; (3) treatment during the infusion with short-acting

Table 1
Management of fluoropyrimidine-related cardiotoxicity

Recommendations supported by observational data	

Rechallenge	• Should be avoided whenever possible, given high incidence of recurrence (90%) and risk of death (13%)[6,37]
	• Decision individualized based on risk/benefit ratio
	  ○ Can consider cautious rechallenge in patients with obstructive coronary artery disease who undergo revascularization
	  ○ Bolus regimen preferred[38]
	  ○ Pretreatment with aspirin, CCB, and/or nitrates can be considered[30,38]
	  ○ Requires close clinical and continuous ECG monitoring
	  ○ Prompt discontinuation if any signs/symptoms of cardiotoxicity

Use of alternative nonfluoropyrimidine agents	• Requires discussion with the primary oncologist

Use of alternative fluoropyrimidine agents	• Two agents containing the chemotherapeutic agent tegafur, a prodrug of 5-FU, have been developed but are not currently available in the United States
	  ○ UFT, an oral combination of tegafur/uracil, has a <1% incidence of cardiotoxicity reported to date[34]
	  ○ S-1, combining tegafur/gimeracil/oteracil, has no reported cardiotoxicity to date[35]

Recommendations lacking observational data or with conflicting data	
Dose reduction	• A dose-dependent relationship for fluoropyrimidine cardiotoxicity has not been established • Dose reduction may be considered for capecitabine[39]
Antidote	• Uridine triacetate is approved for severe, life-threatening cardiac or neurologic toxicity[33]
Primary prevention	• Inconclusive data regarding the prophylactic use of CCBs and/or nitrates for cardioprotection ○ No randomized controlled trials to support or refute their role

diltiazem and sublingual nitroglycerin as needed; (4) posttreatment with nifedipine and isosorbide mononitrate 12 hours after the first dose of pretreatment nitrate/CCB; and (5) posttreatment with nifedipine 24 hours after the first dose.[30]

In addition to medications aimed at treating vasospasm, uridine triacetate was approved by the US Food and Drug Administration in 2015 as an antidote for fluoropyrimidine toxicity. Uridine triacetate is an oral prodrug of uridine, a pyrimidine nucleoside that competes with F-UTP incorporation into RNA, thereby attenuating fluoropyrimidine toxicity in normal tissue. Uridine triacetate is efficiently absorbed from the gastrointestinal tract and can be used for early-onset, severe fluoropyrimidine toxicity, including neutropenia, GI toxicity, or cardiac toxicity unresponsive to cessation of the drug and/or initiation of antianginal therapy. In 1 study, 17 patients with 5-FU overdose demonstrated full recovery after administration of uridine triacetate.[32] A subsequent larger cohort included 142 patients treated with 5-FU or capecitabine who experienced overdose or early-onset severe toxicity. These patients were given oral uridine

triacetate within the first 96 hours of fluoropyrimidine administration, at a dose of 10 g every 6 hours for 20 doses. Of these patients, 96% survived and experienced rapid reversal of cardiac and other toxicities, including severe mucositis, hematologic manifestations, acute encephalopathy, and cardiomyopathy.[33]

Interestingly, chemotherapeutic regimens containing tegafur, a prodrug of 5-FU, demonstrate a more favorable side effect profile. UFT, an oral combination of tegafur/uracil, has a documented incidence of cardiotoxicity that is less than 1%.[34] S-1, combining tegafur/gimeracil/oteracil, has no reported cardiotoxicity.[35] These agents are not currently available in the United States.

Although the studies outlined here support the use of medications targeted at preventing coronary vasospasm, as well as uridine triacetate in select patients, larger prospective trials are needed to develop an evidence-based algorithm for the implementation of cardioprotective strategies. Currently, there is no consensus regarding the need for cardioprotective medications before fluoropyrimidine administration in patients with preexisting cardiovascular disease or cardiac risk factors. Based on preclinical evidence, regular exercise could be a potential therapy to counteract the vasoconstrictor effects of 5-FU by enhancing endothelial-dependent vasodilation.[36] Further investigation of polymorphisms in the DYPD and TS genes and other "omics" discoveries may provide ways to stratify use of 5-FU on an individualized basis.

SUMMARY

Fluoropyrimidines are chemotherapeutic agents that confer great benefit to many patients with solid tumors, but their use is limited by cardiotoxicity in a significant portion of patients. The incidence and precise mechanisms of cardiotoxicity have yet to be elucidated. A diverse range of clinical presentations have been reported, including chest pain, myocardial infarction, acute cardiomyopathy, arrhythmias, shock, and cardiac arrest. Proposed mechanisms include coronary vasospasm, coronary endothelial dysfunction, direct myocardial toxicity, myocarditis, and Takotsubo cardiomyopathy. Therapeutic and prophylactic interventions primarily target coronary vasospasm. Prospective trials are needed to guide risk stratification and implementation of cardioprotective strategies in patients receiving fluoropyrimidines.

REFERENCES

1. Bartelink H, Roelofsen F, Eschwege F, et al. Concomitant radiotherapy and chemotherapy is superior to radiotherapy alone in the treatment of locally advanced anal cancer: results of a phase III randomized trial of the European Organization for Research and Treatment of Cancer Radiotherapy and Gastrointestinal Cooperative Groups. J Clin Oncol 1997;15: 2040–9.

2. Sorrentino MF, Kim J, Foderaro AE, et al. 5-Fluorouracil induced cardiotoxicity: review of the literature. Cardiol J 2012;19:453–7.

3. Curtin NJ, Harris AL, Aherne GW. Mechanism of cell death following thymidylate synthase inhibition: 2'-deoxy-5'-triphosphate accumulation, DNA damage, and growth inhibition following exposure to CB3717 and dipyridamole. Cancer Res 1991;51: 2346–52.

4. Layoun ME, Wickramasinghe C, Peralta MV, et al. Fluoropyrimidine-induced cardiotoxicity: manifestations, mechanisms, and management. Curr Oncol Rep 2016;18:35.

5. Wacker A, Lersch C, Scherpinski U, et al. High incidence of angina pectoris in patients treated with 5-fluorouracil. Oncology 2003;65:108–12.

6. de Forni M, Malet-Martino MC, Jaillais P, et al. Cardiotoxicity of high-dose continuous infusion fluorouracil: a prospective clinical study. J Clin Oncol 1992;10:1795–801.

7. Upshaw JN, O'Neill A, Carver JR, et al. Fluoropyrimidine cardiotoxicity: time for contemporaneous appraisal. Clin Colorectal Cancer 2018;18:44–51.

8. Rezkalla S, Kloner RA, Ensley J, et al. Continuous ambulatory ECG monitoring during fluorouracil therapy: a prospective study. J Clin Oncol 1989;7: 509–14.

9. Kosmas C, Kallistratos MS, Kopterides P, et al. Cardiotoxicity of fluoropyrimidines in different schedules of administration: a prospective study. J Cancer Res Clin Oncol 2007;134:75–82.

10. Becker K, Erckenbrecht J, Haussinger D, et al. Cardiotoxicity of the antiproliferative compound fluorouracil. Drugs 1999;57:475–84.

11. Pullarkat ST, Stoehlmacher J, Ghaderi V, et al. Thymidylate synthase gene polymorphism determines response and toxicity of 5-FU chemotherapy. Pharmacogenomics J 2001;1:65–70.

12. Diasio RB, Beavers TL, Carpenter JT. Familial deficiency of dihydropyrimidine dehydrogenase. Biochemical basis for familial pyrimidinemia and severe 5-fluorouracil-induced toxicity. J Clin Invest 1998;81:47–51.

13. Maring JG, van Kuilenburg AB, Haasjes J, et al. Reduced 5-FU clearance in a patient with low DPD activity due to heterozygosity for a mutant allele of the DPYD gene. Br J Cancer 2002;86:1028–33.

14. Shahrokni A, Rajebi MR, Harold L, et al. Cardiotoxicity of 5-fluorouracil and capecitabine in a pancreatic cancer patient with a novel mutation in the dihydropyrimidine dehydrogenase gene. J Pancreas 2009; 10:215–20.

15. Luwaert RJ, Descamps O, Majoist F, et al. Coronary artery spasm induced by fluorouracil. Eur Heart J 1991;12:468–70.

16. Atar A, Korkmaz ME, Ozin B. Two cases of coronary vasospasm induced by 5-fluorouracil. Anadolu Kardiyol Derg 2010;10:461–2.

17. Shoemaker LK, Arora U, Rocha Lima CM. 5-Fluorouracil-induced coronary vasospasm. Cancer Control 2004;11:46–9.

18. Tajik R, Saadat H, Taherkhani M, et al. Angina induced by 5-fluorouracil infusion in a patient with normal coronaries. Am Heart Hosp J 2010;8: E111–2.

19. Mosseri M, Fingert HJ, Varticovski L, et al. In vitro evidence that myocardial ischemia resulting from 5-fluorouracil chemotherapy is due to protein kinase C-mediated vasoconstriction of vascular smooth muscle. Cancer Res 1993;53:3028–33.

20. Cwikiel M, Eskilsson J, Wieslander JB, et al. The appearance of endothelium in small arteries after treatment with 5-fluorouracil. An electron

microscopic study of late effects in rabbits. Scanning Microsc 1996;10:805–18.

21. Jensen SA, Sorensen JB. 5-Fluorouracil-based therapy induces endovascular injury having potential significance to development of clinically overt cardiotoxicity. Cancer Chemother Pharmacol 2012;69: 57–64.

22. Thyss A, Gaspard MH, Marsault R, et al. Very high endothelin plasma levels in patients with 5-FU cardiotoxicity. Ann Oncol 1992;3:88.

23. Matsubara I, Kamiya J, Imai S. Cardiotoxic effects of 5-fluorouracil in the Guinea pig. Jpn J Pharmacol 1980;30:871–9.

24. Tsibiribi P, Bui-Xuan C, Bui-Xuan B, et al. Cardiac lesions induced by 5-fluorouracil in the rabbit. Hum Exp Toxicol 2006;25:305–9.

25. Focaccetti C, Bruno A, Magnani E, et al. Effects of 5-fluorouracil on morphology, cell cycle, proliferation, apoptosis, autophagy, and ROS production in endothelial cells and cardiomyocytes. PLoS One 2015;10:e0115686.

26. Durak I, Karaayvaz M, Kavutcu M, et al. Reduced antioxidant defense capacity in myocardial tissue from Guinea pigs treated with 5-fluorouracil. J Toxicol Environ Health A 2000;59:585–9.

27. Grunwald MR, Howie L, Diaz LA Jr. Takotsubo cardiomyopathy and fluorouracil: case report and review of the literature. J Clin Oncol 2012; 30:e11–4.

28. Spasojevic I, Maksimovic V, Zakrzewska J, et al. Effects of 5-fluorouracil on erythrocytes in relation to its cardiotoxicity: membrane structure and functioning. J Chem Inf Model 2005;45:1680–5.

29. Karabay C, Gecmen C, Aung S, et al. Is 5-fluorouracil-induced vasospasm a Kounis syndrome? A diagnostic challenge. Perfusion 2011;26:543–5.

30. Clasen SC, Ky B, O'Quinn R, et al. Fluoropyrimidine-induced cardiac toxicity: challenging the current paradigm. J Gastrointest Oncol 2017;8:970–9.

31. Clavel M, Simeone P, Grivet B. Cardiac toxicity of 5-fluorouracil: review of the literature, 5 new cases. Presse Med 1988;17:1675–8.

32. Borstel RV, O'Neill J, Bamat M. Vistonuridine: an orally administered, life-saving antidote for 5-fluorouracil (5FU) overdose. J Clin Oncol 2009;155:9616.

33. Ma WW, Saif MW, El-Rayes BF, et al. Emergency use of uridine triacetate for the prevention and treatment of life-threatening 5-fluorouracil and capecitabine toxicity. Cancer 2017;123:345–56.

34. Marsh JC, Catalano P, Huang J, et al. Eastern Cooperative Oncology Group phase II trial (E4296) of oral 5-fluorouracil and eniluracil as a 28-day regimen in metastatic colorectal cancer. Clin Colorectal Cancer 2002;2:43–50.

35. Lee JL, Kang YK, Kang HJ, et al. A randomised multicentre phase II trial of capecitabine vs S-1 as first-line treatment in elderly patients with metastatic or recurrent unresectable gastric cancer. Br J Cancer 2008;99:584–90.

36. Hayward R, Ruangthai R, Schneider CM, et al. Training enhances vascular relaxation after chemotherapy-induced vasoconstriction. Med Sci Sports Exerc 2004;36:428–34.

37. Saif MW, Shah MM, Shah AR. Fluoropyrimidine-associated cardiotoxicity: revisited. Expert Opin Drug Saf 2009;8:191–202.

38. Cianci G, Morelli MF, Cannita K, et al. Prophylactic options in patients with 5-fluorouracil-associated cardiotoxicity. Br J Cancer 2003;88:1507–9.

39. Peng T, Ouyang Y, Tong K. Rechallenge capecitabine after fluoropyrimidine-induced cardiotoxicity in rectal cancer, a case report. Medicine (Baltimore) 2019;98:e14057.

Trastuzumab-Induced Cardiomyopathy

Rachel Barish, MSN, NP[a], Emily Gates, MS[b], Ana Barac, MD, PhD[c],*

KEYWORDS

- Cardiooncology • Cardiotoxicity • Human epidermal growth factor 2 (HER2) • Breast cancer
- Heart failure • Gastric cancer

KEY POINTS

- Human epidermal growth factor receptor 2 (HER2) is a protein that is overexpressed in approximately 20% to 25% of breast cancers in which its presence has been associated with more aggressive disease and significantly worse prognosis before the era of targeted therapies.
- Trastuzumab is a humanized monoclonal antibody that blocks the action of HER2. Addition of trastuzumab to conventional chemotherapy has prolonged survival for patients with HER2-positive (HER2+) breast cancer in both metastatic and early-stage breast cancer.
- In the initial clinical trial in subjects with metastatic breast cancer, use of trastuzumab was associated with cardiac dysfunction in up to 27% of subjects treated with trastuzumab alone, and symptomatic heart failure in 64% of subjects who were treated with concurrent trastuzumab and anthracycline. With changes in administration, avoidance of anthracyclines, and routine cardiac function monitoring in subsequent adjuvant HER2+ breast cancer trials, the incidence of symptomatic heart failure has significantly decreased.
- Current regulatory and clinical practice guidelines recommend routine left ventricular (LV) function assessment before and during treatment with trastuzumab, and holding or stopping treatment in patients with LV dysfunction and/or heart failure.
- Trastuzumab-induced cardiomyopathy adversely affects cardiac and oncology outcomes. Strategies for risk stratification, early diagnosis, and prevention of trastuzumab-induced cardiomyopathy have become an important topic of collaborative trials in cardiooncology.

INTRODUCTION

In recent decades, cancer treatment has been revolutionized by molecular discoveries that have provided new and more specific targets for therapy.[1] Human epidermal growth factor receptor 2 (HER2) was first discovered in the late 1970s and subsequently found to be overexpressed in approximately 25% of breast cancers.[2] More recent investigations identified HER2 overexpression in gastric cancers and other malignancies of primarily epithelial origin.[3] The discovery of HER2 and its role in a particularly aggressive subtype of breast cancer led to the development of a monoclonal antibody that targets the HER2 receptor: trastuzumab. Addition of trastuzumab to standard chemotherapy prolonged survival in patients with metastatic HER2-positive (HER2+) breast cancer and offered new promise to patients with previously very poor prognoses.[2,4] Trastuzumab was, in general, well-tolerated;

Disclosure Statement: A. Barac served as cardiology principal investigator on investigator-initiated study supported by Genentech (no financial support). The other authors have nothing to disclose.
[a] MedStar Georgetown Physicians Group, Division of Cardiology, 3800 Reservoir Road Northwest 5PHC, Washington, DC 20007, USA; [b] MedStar Heart and Vascular Institute, Georgetown University, 3800 Reservoir Road Northwest 5PHC, Washington, DC 20007, USA; [c] CardioOncology Program, MedStar Heart and Vascular Institute, Georgetown University, 110 Irving Street, Northwest, Suite 1218, Washington, DC 20010, USA
* Corresponding author.
E-mail address: Ana.Barac@medstar.net

Cardiol Clin 37 (2019) 407–418
https://doi.org/10.1016/j.ccl.2019.07.005
0733-8651/19/© 2019 Elsevier Inc. All rights reserved.

however, post hoc analysis identified up to 27% higher risk of cardiac dysfunction and symptomatic clinical heart failure in patients who received trastuzumab and chemotherapy compared with chemotherapy alone.[5] Subsequent studies in early breast cancer implemented changes in administration (avoiding concomitant trastuzumab and anthracyclines) and routine cardiac function monitoring, resulting in much improved safety.[6,7] HER2-targeted therapies became the first-line treatment options for essentially all HER2+ breast cancers.[8]

This article summarizes the historical development of trastuzumab, the proposed mechanisms of cardiotoxicity, and approaches to diagnosis and treatment of trastuzumab-induced cardiomyopathy and heart failure. It also explores current controversies regarding trastuzumab-induced cardiotoxicity within the broader field of cardiooncology.

HUMAN EPIDERMAL GROWTH FACTOR RECEPTOR 2–TARGETED THERAPY: DISCOVERY, EARLY TRIALS, AND CURRENT INDICATIONS FOR USE

The development of HER2-targeted therapy was preceded by several steps, most importantly the discovery of HER2 (erbB2/neu) as a receptor tyrosine kinase and a member of the human epidermal growth factor receptor family.[1] HER2 is in humans encoded by the ERBB2 (erythroblastic oncogene B) gene, whereas the name neu reflects its discovery as a protooncogene in rat neuroblastoma cells.[9] HER2 is the most commonly used abbreviation for this receptor. Molecular signaling investigations in the 1980s demonstrated that human neu homologue, HER2/erbB2, was amplified in a significant percentage of human breast cancers. This overexpression and amplification was related to rapid disease progression and increased mortality in patients with breast cancer, with increased levels of the HER2 protein correlated with a greater incidence of metastasis and relapse.[10] These discoveries, along with enhanced understanding of molecular HER2 pathways (**Fig. 1**), led to the hypothesis that blocking the activity of HER2 could improve outcomes in HER2-positive breast cancer.[2,11] Trastuzumab was the first recombinant humanized anti-HER2 antibody that demonstrated powerful antitumor activity in human HER2-overexpressing tumor xenograft models, leading to subsequent translation into breast cancer clinical trials.[12] Many possible mechanisms for antitumor activity of trastuzumab have been proposed including:

- Activation of antibody-dependent cellular cytotoxicity and HER2 degradation

- Antibody-mediated cell death, through attraction of natural killer immune cells to sites that are overexpressing HER2 through CD16-mediated antibody-dependent cellular cytotoxicity[13]
- Inhibition of downstream mitogen-activated phosphor kinase (MAPK) and phosphoinositol 3 kinase (PI3K/Akt) pathways, which halt abnormal proliferation and allow apoptosis
- Tyrosine kinase inhibition via blockade of Src signaling and increased phosphatase and tensin (PTEN) activity.[1]

The role of HER2 amplification and signaling has since been identified in several other malignancies,[3] most notably gastric and gastroesophageal junction cancers, and trastuzumab and other anti-HER2 therapies continue to be investigated in combination with conventional and targeted chemotherapies to improve patient outcomes.[14] As of this writing, trastuzumab has been included as part of the first-line treatment for metastatic gastric cancer and incorporated into existing chemotherapy regimens (**Table 1**),[14] with ongoing interest and investigation into uses in other malignancies.[15]

Following the development of trastuzumab, other targeted anti-HER2 therapies have been developed. Pertuzumab is a humanized monoclonal antibody that binds to domain II of HER2 (in contrast to trastuzumab, which binds to domain IV) and induces antibody-dependent cellular toxicity within cells that express HER2.[16] Pertuzumab has been approved in combination with trastuzumab as therapy for both early-stage and metastatic HER2+ breast cancer[16–18] (see **Table 1**).

Trastuzumab emtansine (T-DM1) is an intravenously delivered antibody-drug conjugate in which trastuzumab is bound to DM1, a toxic chemotherapy agent and derivative of microtubule inhibitor maytansin. The conjugated antibody binds to the extracellular domain of HER2 and allows for targeted delivery of DM1 cytotoxin to HER2+ cells, with decreased toxicity. T-DM1 has been approved for treatment of metastatic and, more recently, adjuvant treatment of HER2+ breast cancer.[19–21] Oral HER2-targeted therapies include lapatinib and neratinib, small tyrosine kinase inhibitors that have activity against HER2[22] and are currently used for metastatic breast cancer.

Proposed Mechanism of Trastuzumab-Induced Cardiotoxicity

Just as the precise mechanism of trastuzumab's action against HER-2 remains unclear and likely involves multiple cellular pathways, its action against cardiomyocytes is not fully understood.[23,24] HER2 and the ErbB family of tyrosine

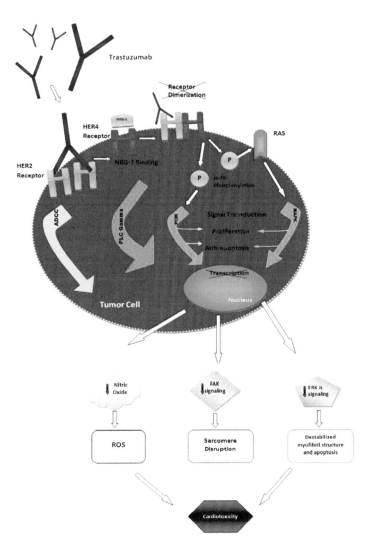

Fig. 1. Molecular mechanisms of HER2 signaling and mechanisms of cardiotoxicity. Trastuzumab acts on breast cancer cells via the HER2 signaling pathway by blocking receptor dimerization to induce apoptosis of the cancer cells. This initiates multiple signaling cascades that can result in damage to cardiomyocytes. ADCC, antibody-dependent cellular cytotoxicity; ERK, extracellular receptor kinase; FAK, focal adhesion kinase; MAPK, mitogen-activated protein kinase; NRG-1, neuregulin-1; P, phosphorylation; PI3K, phosphoinositide 3-kinase; PLC gamma, phospholipase C gamma pathway; RAS, protein family; ROS, reactive oxygen species.

kinase receptors play a significant role in cardiomyocyte development and cellular proliferation,[25] and blocking of downstream intracellular signaling by trastuzumab may affect cellular metabolism, leading to sarcomere disruption, impaired cell proliferation, and survival[26,27] (see **Fig. 1**). It has been recently shown, in a human-induced stem cell cardiomyocyte model, that mitochondrial dysfunction and altered cellular energy metabolism are the primary drivers of trastuzumab-induced cardiomyopathy.[28]

Relevance of HER2 signaling in cardiomyocyte may be of particular importance in the setting of an ongoing injury, such as that induced by anthracyclines. Mice with cardiac myocyte-specific knockout of ERBB2 and ERBB4 genes developed cardiomyopathy with administration of anthracyclines.[29] Similar to mice with heterozygous knockout of neuregulin-1 gene, the upstream

activator of HER2-signaling[30] seems to be activated during times of increased stress. These studies led to the proposed double-hit hypothesis of cardiac injury in which anthracyclines initiate a process of oxidative damage and trastuzumab blocks neuregulin and HER2 downstream signaling required for cellular repair[31] (**Fig. 2**).

Type of Cardiomyopathy: Useful Distinction?

Early recognition of trastuzumab cardiotoxicity occurred in the setting of ongoing anthracycline administration pointing to detrimental effects on cardiac myocytes when 2 agents were administered together. Within cardiooncology, this finding also led to proposed distinction between type I and type II cardiomyopathy.[32] Type I refers to anthracycline-mediated cardiomyopathy, which is dose-dependent, associated with

Table 1
Chemotherapy regimens incorporating trastuzumab

Regimen	Dosing Schedule
Regimens Used for Breast Cancer (Early-Stage or Advanced)	
ACT-H	AC given every 2 wk for 4 cycles, followed by TH every 1 wk for 12 cycles, followed by trastuzumab every 3 wk for a total of 12 mo
ACT-HP	AC given every 2 wk for 4 cycles, followed by paclitaxel every 1 wk with HP every 3 wk for 12 wk, followed by trastuzumab and pertuzumab every 3 wk for a total of 12 mo
TCH	TCH every 3 wk for 6 cycles followed by trastuzumab every 3 wk for total of 1 y
TCHP	TCH every 3 wk for 6 cycles followed by trastuzumab and pertuzumab every 3 wk for total of 1 y
TH	Paclitaxel and trastuzumab every 1 wk for 12 cycles followed by trastuzumab every 3 wk for 40 wk
THP	Paclitaxel, trastuzumab, and pertuzumab every 3 wk
Regimens for Metastatic Breast Cancer	
Trastuzumab monotherapy	Trastuzumab every 1–3 wk, given until disease progression or significant toxicity
Regimens for Gastric Cancer	
HCX	Oral capecitabine for 21 d, with trastuzumab or cisplatin every 3 wk, for a total of 6 cycles
Cisplatin, 5-fluorouracil (5-FU), and trastuzumab	Cisplatin and trastuzumab every 3 wk, with 5-FU daily for 5 d or via continuous pump for 5 d, for a total of 6 cycles

Abbreviations: AC, Adriamycin (doxorubicin), cyclophosphamide; ACT-H, Adriamycin (doxorubicin), cyclophosphamide, Taxol (paclitaxel), Herceptin (trastuzumab); ACT-HP, doxorubicin, cyclophosphamide, paclitaxel, trastuzumab, pertuzumab; HCX, trastuzumab, cisplatin, capecitabine (Xeloda); TCH, Taxotere (docetaxel), cyclophosphamide, trastuzumab; TCHP, docetaxel, cyclophosphamide, trastuzumab, pertuzumab; TH, paclitaxel, trastuzumab; THP, paclitaxel, trastuzumab, pertuzumab; HP, trastuzumab, pertuzumab.

cardiomyocyte necrosis, irreversible, and associated with heart failure symptoms. Type II describes trastuzumab-induced cardiomyopathy, which lacks dose-dependence, is less associated with symptomatic heart failure, and is reversible after drug discontinuation.[32]

Although arguably helpful for clinicians, this concept has been challenged as

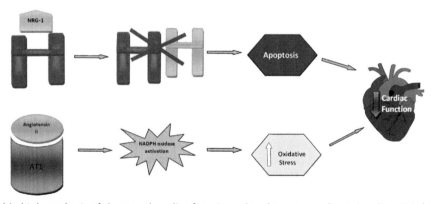

Fig. 2. Double-hit hypothesis of decreased cardiac function related to neuregulin-1 signaling. It is hypothesized that adjuvant use of trastuzumab is able to induce damage to cardiomyocytes via 2 routes: inhibition of the neuregulin-1 signaling pathway by blocking HER2 or HER4 receptor dimerization and/or an increase in oxidative stress as a result of angiotensin II-induced activation of NADPH oxidase. AT1, angiotensin II receptor type 1; NADPH, nicotinamide adenine dinucleotide phosphate.

oversimplified and has recently fallen out of favor for several reasons.[33] Perhaps most importantly, longitudinal studies have identified patients with trastuzumab-induced cardiomyopathy who experience clinical heart failure and/or decrease in left ventricular ejection fraction (LVEF), which does not improve with cessation of trastuzumab treatment.[34,35] Irreversibility of anthracycline-induced cardiomyopathy has also been challenged because early diagnosis and therapy have been shown to improve outcomes.[36] In addition, the number of chemotherapeutic, targeted, and immunologic anticancer agents associated with cardiovascular (CV) cardiotoxicities has increased logarithmically, pointing to the need for more in-depth understanding of mechanisms and creation of clinically relevant subtypes.[33] Newly created

categories would ideally allow individualized clinical assessment and decision-making when determining optimal management in a patient who develops cardiomyopathy during the course of cancer treatment.[13,35]

Monitoring of Cardiac Function During Trastuzumab Treatment

Clinical trials that investigated use of trastuzumab in subjects with early HER2+ breast cancer implemented routine cardiac function monitoring before and during trastuzumab therapy (**Table 2**). They also included prespecified trastuzumab-holding parameters based on changes in LVEF and/or heart failure symptoms, resulting in much improved cardiac safety and a very low number

Table 2
Early trials of trastuzumab for breast cancer

Trial	Treatment Regimen	Oncology Outcomes	Inclusion Criteria and LVEF Assessment	Cardiac Outcomes
HERA[37]	Chemo Or Chemo→H (1 y) Or Chemo→H (2 y)	10-y DFS[37] • 63% for chemo • 69% for 1 y H • 69% for 2 y H 10 y OS[37] • 73% for chemo • 79% for 1 y H • 80% for 2 y H 2 y adjuvant H has no additional benefit	LVEF >55% followed by MUGA or Echo	Class III or IV HF • H (1 y): 0.8% Asx LVEF ↓ • H (1 y): 4.1% H halted (cardiac) • H (1 y): 5.1%
[a]NCCTG 9831 and NSABP B31[38]	AC→T Or AC→TH→H	10-y DFS[39] • 62% for AC→T • 74% for AC→TH→H 10 y OS[39] • 75% for AC→T • 84% for AC→TH→H	LVEF decline ≤15% from baseline followed by MUGA or Echo	Class III/IV HF • AC→T: 0.5% • AC→TH→H: 3.7% Asx LVEF ↓ • AC→T: 4%–5% • AC→TH→H: 6%–10% H halted (cardiac) • AC→T: N/A • AC→TH→H: 18%
BCIRG 006[40]	AC→D Or AC→DH→H Or TCH→H	10 y DFS[41]: • 68% for AC→D • 75% for AC→DH • 73% for TCH→H 10 y OS[41] • 79% for AC→D • 86% for AC→DH • 83% for TCH→H	LVEF ≥50% at baseline followed by MUGA or Echo	Class III/IV HF • AC→D: 0.7% • AC→DH: 2% Asx LVEF ↓ • AC→D: 11.2% • AC→DH: 18.6% H halted (cardiac) • AC→D: N/A • AC→DH: 5.7%

Abbreviations: AC, doxorubicin and cyclophosphamide; Asx, asymptomatic; BCIRG, Breast Cancer International Research Group; D, docetaxel; DFS, disease-free survival; DH, docetaxel and trastuzumab; Echo, echocardiogram; H, Trastuzumab; HERA, Herceptin Adjuvant Trial; HF, heart failure; MUGA, multiple gated acquisition scan; N/A, not applicable; NCCTG, North Central Cancer Treatment Group; NSABP, National Surgical Adjuvant Breast and Bowel Project; OS, overall survival; T, paclitaxel; TCH, docetaxel, carboplatin, trastuzumab.
Arrows indicate continuation of therapy regimen from initial drug to the next.
[a] NCCTG 9831 and NSABP B31 were analyzed jointly.

of heart failure events.[7] In this setting, and with continued evidence of survival benefit with trastuzumab in patients with HER2+ breast cancer, there has been an increased interest in identifying early markers of risk, preventing LVEF decline, and avoiding treatment interruptions (**Fig. 3**).[42]

In patients receiving trastuzumab, echocardiography has become the most widely used tool for cardiac function monitoring because of its availability and lack of radiation exposure. The expert consensus for multimodality imaging evaluation of patients during and after cancer therapy published by the American Society of Echocardiography in 2014 summarized the key components relevant for cardiac imagers, including limitations of reliance on LVEF as a sole measure of cardiac function.[43] In addition to physiologic and technique-related LVEF variability, which reduces the accuracy of detection of pathologic changes, a decrease in LVEF is a late finding that may interrupt trastuzumab treatment and negatively affect cancer outcomes.[13] Global longitudinal strain (GLS) has been identified as an echocardiographic marker of early cardiac dysfunction and predictor of later LVEF decrease in patients with HER2+ breast cancer receiving trastuzumab therapy.[44,45] The key question has been whether intervention based on GLS can guide clinical care. That hypothesis is being prospectively tested in the ongoing Strain sUrveillance of Chemotherapy for improving Cardiovascular Outcomes (SUCCOUR) trial.[46] This international study randomizes subjects receiving trastuzumab and other cardiotoxic therapies to strain-guided

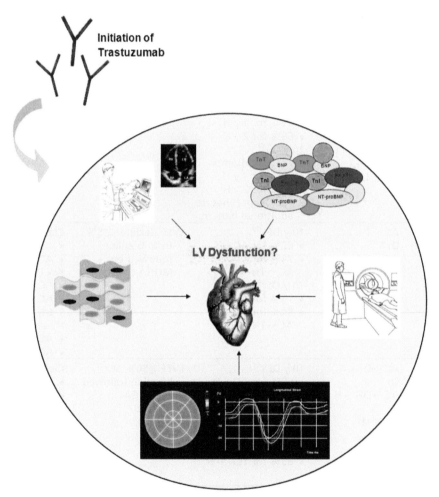

Fig. 3. Monitoring of cardiac function during trastuzumab treatment. Due to the potential cardiotoxic effects of trastuzumab on cardiomyocytes, cardiac function is monitored in all patients receiving this treatment to determine if LV dysfunction is present. Common indications of potential dysfunction are cardiomyocyte damage, increased biomarkers and decreased GLS. This can be determined through echocardiogram and cardiac MRI. BNP, brain natriuretic peptide; GLS, global longitudinal strain; hs-cTn, high-sensitivity cardiac troponin; LV, left ventricle; NT-proBNP, N-terminal pro b-type natriuretic peptide; TnI, troponin I; TnT, troponin T.

versus standard care, and introduces cardiac therapy with beta-blockers and angiotensin inhibitors in patients who experience decline in GLS with the primary outcome of prevention of new LVEF decline.[47]

A different, frequently encountered challenge in serial cardiac function assessment of patients undergoing trastuzumab treatment are limited echocardiographic windows, often related to breast cancer and reconstruction surgeries. Cardiac MRI (cMRI) has been increasingly used as a complementary imaging modality for patients undergoing trastuzumab treatment.[48] cMRI offers superior accuracy in visualization of endocardial border

and is recognized as a gold standard for measurement of left ventricular (LV) and right ventricular volumes and function. In patients with new or previously diagnosed cardiac dysfunction, cMRI can be used to confirm the diagnosis, as well as to provide tissue characterization to exclude other forms of cardiomyopathy.

Serum biomarkers of cardiotoxicity are of significant interest as early predictors of cardiotoxicity because they can be more easily measured in closely timed proximity to delivery of cancer treatment and potentially provide higher accuracy with standardized assays.[49,50] Elevations in cardiac troponin I after trastuzumab therapy have been

Table 3
Summary of trials evaluating cardioprotective strategies for patients treated with trastuzumab

Trial Name (Year)	Study Design	Results
Prevention of Cardiac Dysfunction during Adjuvant Breast Cancer Therapy (PRADA)[53]	N = 130 100% anthracycline 22% trastuzumab Double-blind, randomized Primary endpoint: changes in LVEF by cardiac MRI, 10–64 wk after treatment 2 × 2 design: candesartan or metoprolol vs placebo	LVEF decline was mildly attenuated (2.6%, range 1.5%–3.8%, CI 95%) with candesartan Secondary analysis showed an attenuated troponin elevation with metoprolol for patients who received anthracycline[54]
Multidisciplinary Approach to Novel Therapies in Cardio-Oncology Research (MANTICORE)[55]	N = 94 100% trastuzumab 12%–33% anthracycline 3 arms: bisoprolol, perindopril, placebo Primary endpoint: changes in LVEDVi at 1 y	Negative for primary outcome Secondary data showed mildly attenuated LVEF decline (4%) with bisoprolol
Angiotensin II-Receptor Inhibition With Candesartan to Prevent Trastuzumab-Related Cardiotoxic Effects in Patients With Early Breast Cancer: A Randomized Clinical Trial[56]	N = 206 2 arms: candesartan vs placebo Primary endpoint: LVEF of ≥15%, or below 45% Secondary endpoints: NT-proBNP and hsTnT as surrogate markers; ERBB2 genotype variant as predictive of cardiac dysfunction	Negative for primary outcome Negative for secondary outcome of biomarkers as surrogates Positive for ERBB2 germline Ala1170Pro single nucleotide polymorphism as predictive of cardiac events
Prospective evaluation of the cardiac safety of HER2-targeted therapies in patients with HER2+ breast cancer and compromised heart function (SAFE-HEaRt) (2019)[52]	N = 31 (30) 50% trastuzumab only 46% trastuzumab + pertuzumab 6% TDM1 only LVEF 40%–49% at baseline, without clinical HF Primary endpoint: completion of HER2-targeted therapy without MI, HF, arrhythmia, cardiac death, or significant worsening of LVEF	90% of patients completed anti-HER2 therapy 6% had a cardiac event 3% had an asymptomatic decrease in LVEF to 35%

Abbreviations: HF, heart failure; HsTnT, high-sensitivity troponin T; LVEDVi, left ventricular end diastolic volume index; MI, myocardial infarction; NT-proBNP, N-terminal of the prohormone brain natriuretic peptide.

shown to predict later LVEF decline in a cohort of 251 women treated for HER2+ breast cancer and these subjects were also less likely to have recovered LVEF, even with discontinuation of trastuzumab and initiation of heart failure therapy.[50]

Optimal Strategies for Cardioprotection

The significant benefit of trastuzumab in cancer treatment, balanced against its known potential for inducing cardiomyopathy, has led to increasing research interest in determining how to best prevent trastuzumab-induced cardiomyopathy before initiation of treatment. Several recent prospective randomized trials have used neurohormonal blockade with beta blockers, angiotensin-converting enzyme (ACE)-inhibitors, and angiotensin receptor blockers (ARBs) to prevent decline in LVEF in patients receiving trastuzumab (see **Table 3**). The largest to date is a recently published trial that randomized 468 women with HER2+ breast cancer to receiving placebo, lisinopril, or carvedilol at the time and during administration of trastuzumab treatment.[51] Although the primary endpoint of cardiotoxicity (defined as LVEF decline >10%, or >5% if below 50%) was not significantly different among the groups in the entire cohort. In a stratified analysis

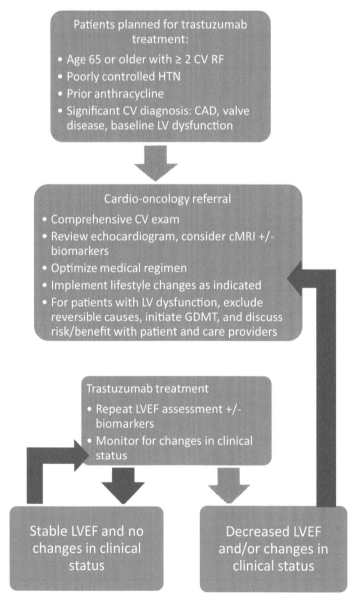

Fig. 4. Algorithm for cardiooncology care during trastuzumab treatment. CAD, coronary artery disease; cMRI, cardiac MRI; CV, cardiovascular; GDMT, guideline-directed medical therapy; RF, risk factors.

of subjects who received anthracycline therapy, there was a significant attenuation of cardiotoxicity in subjects who received lisinopril and carvedilol.[51]

In aggregate, primary prevention trials have shown safety and feasibility of using beta-blockers, ACE-inhibitors, and/or ARBs concomitantly with cancer treatment in early-stage breast cancer; however, the effect size has overall been small and without a clear signal of benefit for a single cardioprotective agent or class. Primary prevention studies excluded subjects at higher cardiac dysfunction risk, such as those with decreased LV function or preexisting cardiomyopathy. The recently completed pilot Study Evaluating the Cardiac Safety of HER2 Targeted Therapy (SAFE-HEaRt)[52] investigated the use of HER2-targeted therapies in subjects with existing LV dysfunction (LVEF 40%–49%) before starting therapy, with optimization of guideline-recommended medical therapy for stage B heart failure and frequent cardiac monitoring during and 6 months after HER2-targeted treatment (**Table 3**). In this trial, 90% (27) of the enrolled subjects met the primary endpoint of successful completion of oncology therapy without development of cardiac event. Two subjects (6%) developed heart failure and 1 subject experienced further decline in LVEF, to 35%, that continued despite treatment holding.[52] This study represents a proof of concept that safe administration of HER2-targeted therapy can be achieved in patients with LV dysfunction in the setting of cardiology and oncology collaborative care. Larger studies in high-risk subjects are needed to investigate implementation of collaborative care in real-world clinical practice and its effect on cardiac and oncology outcomes.

Current Clinical Practice and Shared Decision-Making

The models of shared decision-making and patient-centered care will guide providers to have an informed discussion with patients on the risks and benefits of trastuzumab treatment, balancing the risks of cardiotoxicity with the risks of cancer recurrence. This discussion can be facilitated within a cardiooncology program, in which providers will be aware of the current state of the science regarding risks, benefits, and potential strategies to optimize CV health throughout the cancer treatment process.[52] However, even within cardiooncology, clear guidance regarding when to avoid potentially cardiotoxic therapies remains lacking. Patients with hypertension, diabetes, and/or with a family history of cardiomyopathy

are considered stage A, at risk for developing heart failure, based on current American College of Cardiology guidelines,[57] and should be treated. Models for delivery of comprehensive CV care during ongoing cancer treatment need to be developed together with evidence-based CV interventions in this population. Currently, patients with existing cardiac conditions or multiple cardiac risk factors (**Fig. 4**) should ideally be referred for cardiooncology consultation before starting trastuzumab and a plan for follow-up in survivorship established.

SUMMARY

HER2-targeted therapies have revolutionized cancer treatment and prolonged the survival of many patients with HER2 overexpressing cancers.[2,14] Trastuzumab clinical trials have, for the first time, introduced routine cardiac imaging during active cancer treatment, leading to improved understanding of cardiac function changes and significantly improved safety, and opening several new challenges that are at the core of collaborative cardiooncology care. As the clinical uses of trastuzumab expand, so too will the opportunities for cardiooncology providers and researchers to determine risk-stratification models and optimal cardioprotective strategies to mitigate the risks of trastuzumab-induced cardiomyopathy while ensuring optimal cancer outcomes for patients with HER2+ disease.

REFERENCES

1. Nahta R. Molecular mechanisms of trastuzumab-based treatment in HER2-overexpressing breast cancer. ISRN Oncol 2012;2012:428062.
2. Slamon DJ, Leyland-Jones B, Shak S, et al. Use of chemotherapy plus a monoclonal antibody against HER2 for metastatic breast cancer that overexpresses HER2. N Engl J Med 2001;344(11):783–92.
3. Yan M, Schwaederle M, Arguello D, et al. HER2 expression status in diverse cancers: review of results from 37,992 patients. Cancer Metastasis Rev 2015;34(1):157–64.
4. Giordano SH, Elias AD, Gradishar WJ. NCCN guidelines updates: breast cancer. J Natl Compr Canc Netw 2018;16(5S):605–10.
5. Seidman A, Hudis C, Pierri MK, et al. Cardiac dysfunction in the trastuzumab clinical trials experience. J Clin Oncol 2002;20(5):1215–21.
6. Bowles EJ, Wellman R, Feigelson HS, et al. Risk of heart failure in breast cancer patients after anthracycline and trastuzumab treatment: a retrospective cohort study. J Natl Cancer Inst 2012;104(17):1293–305.

7. Telli ML, Hunt SA, Carlson RW, et al. Trastuzumab-related cardiotoxicity: calling into question the concept of reversibility. J Clin Oncol 2007;25(23):3525–33.

8. Denduluri N, Somerfield MR, Eisen A, et al. Selection of optimal adjuvant chemotherapy regimens for human epidermal growth factor receptor 2 (HER2)-negative and adjuvant targeted therapy for HER2-positive breast cancers: an American Society of Clinical Oncology guideline adaptation of the Cancer Care Ontario clinical practice guideline. J Clin Oncol 2016;34(20):2416–27.

9. Padhy LC, Shih C, Cowing D, et al. Identification of a phosphoprotein specifically induced by the transforming DNA of rat neuroblastomas. Cell 1982;28(4):865–71.

10. Slamon DJ, Clark GM, Wong SG, et al. Human breast cancer: correlation of relapse and survival with amplification of the HER-2/neu oncogene. Science 1987;235(4785):177–82.

11. Zhu YY, Si W, Ji TF, et al. The variation and clinical significance of hormone receptors and Her-2 status from primary to metastatic lesions in breast cancer patients. Tumour Biol 2016;37(6):7675–84.

12. Baselga J, Norton L, Albanell J, et al. Recombinant humanized anti-HER2 antibody (Herceptin) enhances the antitumor activity of paclitaxel and doxorubicin against HER2/neu overexpressing human breast cancer xenografts. Cancer Res 1998;58(13):2825–31.

13. Yu AF, Yadav NU, Lung BY, et al. Trastuzumab interruption and treatment-induced cardiotoxicity in early HER2-positive breast cancer. Breast Cancer Res Treat 2015;149(2):489–95.

14. Bang YJ, Van Cutsem E, Feyereislova A, et al. Trastuzumab in combination with chemotherapy versus chemotherapy alone for treatment of HER2-positive advanced gastric or gastro-oesophageal junction cancer (ToGA): a phase 3, open-label, randomised controlled trial. Lancet 2010;376(9742):687–97.

15. Gunturu KS, Woo Y, Beaubier N, et al. Gastric cancer and trastuzumab: first biologic therapy in gastric cancer. Ther Adv Med Oncol 2013;5(2):143–51.

16. von Minckwitz G, Procter M, de Azambuja E, et al. Adjuvant pertuzumab and trastuzumab in early HER2-positive breast cancer. N Engl J Med 2017;377(2):122–31.

17. Baselga J, Cortes J, Kim SB, et al. Pertuzumab plus trastuzumab plus docetaxel for metastatic breast cancer. N Engl J Med 2012;366(2):109–19.

18. Swain SM, Baselga J, Kim SB, et al. Pertuzumab, trastuzumab, and docetaxel in HER2-positive metastatic breast cancer. N Engl J Med 2015;372(8):724–34.

19. Verma S, Miles D, Gianni L, et al. Trastuzumab emtansine for HER2-positive advanced breast cancer. N Engl J Med 2012;367(19):1783–91.

20. von Minckwitz G, Huang CS, Mano MS, et al. Trastuzumab emtansine for residual invasive HER2-positive breast cancer. N Engl J Med 2019;380(7):617–28.

21. FDA approves Genentech's Kadcyla for adjuvant treatment of people with HER2-positive early breast cancer with residual invasive disease after neoadjuvant treatment [press release]. Available at: https://bit.ly/2UYWOVN. Accessed April 3, 2019.

22. Chia SKL, Martin M, Holmes FA, et al. PIK3CA alterations and benefit with neratinib: analysis from the randomized, double-blind, placebo-controlled, phase III ExteNET trial. Breast Cancer Res 2019;21(1):39.

23. Tripathy D, Seidman A, Keefe D, et al. Effect of cardiac dysfunction on treatment outcomes in women receiving trastuzumab for HER2-overexpressing metastatic breast cancer. Clin Breast Cancer 2004;5(4):293–8.

24. Goldhar HA, Yan AT, Ko DT, et al. The temporal risk of heart failure associated with adjuvant trastuzumab in breast cancer patients: a population study. J Natl Cancer Inst 2016;108(1) [pii:djv301].

25. Lee KF, Simon H, Chen H, et al. Requirement for neuregulin receptor erbB2 in neural and cardiac development. Nature 1995;378(6555):394–8.

26. Du XL, Xia R, Burau K, et al. Cardiac risk associated with the receipt of anthracycline and trastuzumab in a large nationwide cohort of older women with breast cancer, 1998-2005. Med Oncol 2011;28(Suppl 1):S80–90.

27. Milano G, Raucci A, Scopece A, et al. Doxorubicin and trastuzumab regimen induces biventricular failure in mice. J Am Soc Echocardiogr 2014;27(5):568–79.

28. Kitani T, Ong SG, Lam CK, et al. Human induced pluripotent stem cell model of trastuzumab-induced cardiac dysfunction in breast cancer patients. Circulation 2019;139(21):2451–65.

29. Crone SA, Zhao YY, Fan L, et al. ErbB2 is essential in the prevention of dilated cardiomyopathy. Nat Med 2002;8(5):459–65.

30. Liu FF, Stone JR, Schuldt AJ, et al. Heterozygous knockout of neuregulin-1 gene in mice exacerbates doxorubicin-induced heart failure. Am J Physiol Heart Circ Physiol 2005;289(2):H660–6.

31. Cote GM, Sawyer DB, Chabner BA. ERBB2 inhibition and heart failure. N Engl J Med 2012;367(22):2150–3.

32. Ewer MS, Lippman SM. Type II chemotherapy-related cardiac dysfunction: time to recognize a new entity. J Clin Oncol 2005;23(13):2900–2.

33. Witteles RM. Type I and type II cardiomyopathy classifications are complete Nonsense: PRO.

American College of Cardiology. Latest in cardiology Web site 2018. Available at: https://www.acc.org/latest-in-cardiology/articles/2018/05/04/08/41/type-i-and-type-ii-cardiomyopathy-classifications-are-complete-nonsense-pro. Accessed March 19, 2019.

34. Chen J, Long JB, Hurria A, et al. Incidence of heart failure or cardiomyopathy after adjuvant trastuzumab therapy for breast cancer. J Am Coll Cardiol 2012;60(24):2504–12.

35. Dang CT, Yu AF, Jones LW, et al. Cardiac surveillance guidelines for trastuzumab-containing therapy in early-stage breast cancer: getting to the heart of the matter. J Clin Oncol 2016;34(10):1030–3.

36. Cardinale D, Colombo A, Bacchiani G, et al. Early detection of anthracycline cardiotoxicity and improvement with heart failure therapy. Circulation 2015;131(22):1981–8.

37. Cameron D, Piccart-Gebhart MJ, Gelber RD, et al. 11 years' follow-up of trastuzumab after adjuvant chemotherapy in HER2-positive early breast cancer: final analysis of the HERceptin adjuvant (HERA) trial. Lancet 2017;389(10075):1195–205.

38. Perez EA, Romond EH, Suman VJ, et al. Trastuzumab plus adjuvant chemotherapy for human epidermal growth factor receptor 2-positive breast cancer: planned joint analysis of overall survival from NSABP B-31 and NCCTG N9831. J Clin Oncol 2014;32(33):3744–52.

39. Ganz PA, Romond EH, Cecchini RS, et al. Long-term follow-up of cardiac function and quality of life for patients in NSABP protocol B-31/NRG oncology: a randomized trial comparing the safety and efficacy of doxorubicin and cyclophosphamide (AC) followed by paclitaxel with AC followed by paclitaxel and trastuzumab in patients with node-positive breast cancer with tumors overexpressing human epidermal growth factor receptor 2. J Clin Oncol 2017;35(35):3942–8.

40. Subramanian A, Mokbel K. The role of Herceptin in early breast cancer. Int Semin Surg Oncol 2008;5:9.

41. Slamon D, Eirmann W, Robert N, et al. Ten year follow-up of BCIRG-006 comparing doxorubicin plus cyclophosphamide followed by docetaxel (AC→T) with doxorubicin plus cyclophosphamide followed by docetaxel and trastuzumab (AC→TH) with docetaxel, carboplatin and trastuzumab (TCH) in HER2+ early breast cancer. Proceedings of the 38th Annual Meeting of the CTRC-AACR San Antonio Breast Cancer Symposium. San Antonio, TX, December 8-12, 2015. Philadelphia (PA). AACR, 2016.

42. Kenigsberg B, Wellstein A, Barac A. Left ventricular dysfunction in cancer treatment: is it relevant? JACC Heart Fail 2018;6(2):87–95.

43. Plana JC, Galderisi M, Barac A, et al. Expert consensus for multimodality imaging evaluation of adult patients during and after cancer therapy: a report from the American Society of Echocardiography and the European Association of Cardiovascular Imaging. Eur Heart J Cardiovasc Imaging 2014;15(10):1063–93.

44. Sawaya H, Sebag IA, Plana JC, et al. Early detection and prediction of cardiotoxicity in chemotherapy-treated patients. Am J Cardiol 2011;107(9):1375–80.

45. Thavendiranathan P, Poulin F, Lim KD, et al. Use of myocardial strain imaging by echocardiography for the early detection of cardiotoxicity in patients during and after cancer chemotherapy: a systematic review. J Am Coll Cardiol 2014;63(25 Pt A):2751–68.

46. Negishi T, Thavendiranathan P, Negishi K, et al. Rationale and design of the strain surveillance of chemotherapy for improving cardiovascular outcomes: the SUCCOUR trial. JACC Cardiovasc Imaging 2018;11(8):1098–105.

47. Barac A. Optimal treatment of stage B heart failure in cardio-oncology?: the promise of strain. JACC Cardiovasc Imaging 2018;11(8):1106–8.

48. Zamorano J. An ESC position paper on cardio-oncology. Eur Heart J 2016;37(36):2739–40.

49. Yu AF, Ky B. Roadmap for biomarkers of cancer therapy cardiotoxicity. Heart 2016;102(6):425–30.

50. Cardinale D, Colombo A, Torrisi R, et al. Trastuzumab-induced cardiotoxicity: clinical and prognostic implications of troponin I evaluation. J Clin Oncol 2010;28(25):3910–6.

51. Guglin M, Krischer J, Tamura R, et al. Randomized trial of lisinopril versus carvedilol to prevent trastuzumab cardiotoxicity in patients with breast cancer. J Am Coll Cardiol 2019;73(22):2859–68.

52. Lynce F, Barac A, Geng X, et al. Prospective evaluation of the cardiac safety of HER2-targeted therapies in patients with HER2-positive breast cancer and compromised heart function: the SAFE-HEaRt study. Breast Cancer Res Treat 2019;175(3):595–603.

53. Gulati G, Heck SL, Ree AH, et al. Prevention of cardiac dysfunction during adjuvant breast cancer therapy (PRADA): a 2 x 2 factorial, randomized, placebo-controlled, double-blind clinical trial of candesartan and metoprolol. Eur Heart J 2016;37(21):1671–80.

54. Gulati G, Heck SL, Rosjo H, et al. Neurohormonal blockade and circulating cardiovascular biomarkers during anthracycline therapy in breast cancer patients: results from the PRADA (prevention of cardiac dysfunction during adjuvant breast cancer therapy) study. J Am Heart Assoc 2017;6(11) [pii:e006513].

55. Pituskin E, Mackey JR, Koshman S, et al. Multidisciplinary Approach to novel therapies in cardio-oncology research (MANTICORE 101-breast): a randomized trial for the prevention of trastuzumab-associated cardiotoxicity. J Clin Oncol 2017;35(8):870–7.

56. Boekhout AH, Gietema JA, Milojkovic Kerklaan B, et al. Angiotensin II-receptor inhibition with candesartan to prevent trastuzumab-related cardiotoxic effects in patients with early breast cancer: a randomized clinical trial. JAMA Oncol 2016;2(8): 1030–7.

57. Yancy CW, Jessup M, Bozkurt B, et al. 2013 ACCF/AHA guideline for the management of heart failure: a report of the American College of Cardiology Foundation/American Heart Association task Force on practice guidelines. J Am Coll Cardiol 2013;62(16): e147–239.

Echocardiography Imaging of Cardiotoxicity

Yu Kang, MD, PhD, Marielle Scherrer-Crosbie, MD, PhD*

KEYWORDS

- Echocardiography • Cardiotoxicity • Cancer • Imaging • Strain • Speckle tracking imaging

KEY POINTS

- Echocardiography plays a big role in cancer treatment-induced cardiotoxicity.
- Additional research is critical to clarify a uniformly accepted definition of cancer therapy-induced cardiotoxicity, and define the value of conventional and novel indices in guiding clinical management of cancer treatment-induced cardiotoxicity.

INTRODUCTION

The US National Cancer Institute estimates that more than 15.5 million Americans with a history of cancer were alive in 2016 and this number is projected to reach 20.3 million by 2026.[1] With longer survival, attention to the chronic and long-term comorbidities has become increasingly important. Based on the National Cancer Institute's Surveillance, Epidemiology, and End Results (SEER) program, the risk of noncancer death has now surpassed the risk of cancer death in patients with cancer; heart disease is the most important cause of noncancer death (40%) for patients with cancer.[2] Addressing the cardiotoxic effects of anticancer therapies to prevent increased cardiovascular risk in this population is therefore crucial.

One of the most common manifestations of cardiotoxicity associated with exposure to anticancer therapies is the development of left ventricular (LV) dysfunction and overt heart failure. The major role of echocardiography in patients treated with cardiotoxic therapies is the identification of cardiac dysfunction; hence, we focus our study of cardiotoxicity on this complication. The risk of LV dysfunction varies according to the type and intensity of cancer treatment. Among antineoplastic

agents, anthracyclines have been studied most extensively, with dose-dependent LV dysfunction rates ranging from 4.7% to 48%.[3] LV dysfunction may also be caused by other classes of chemotherapeutic agents, such as alkylating agents (risk ranging from 7% to 28%),[4,5] monoclonal antibodies (risk with trastuzumab monotherapy from 3% to 12%),[3,6,7] tyrosine kinase inhibitors (risk ranging from 8% to 12.5%),[8,9] and the novel checkpoint inhibitors (2.0%).[10]

Transthoracic echocardiography, a noninvasive and cost-effective strategy, is currently the cornerstone for monitoring cardiac function, before, during, and after the potentially cardiotoxic cancer treatment. Whereas LV ejection fraction (LVEF) is currently the most widely used index to quantify cardiac function, other emerging indices such as Doppler-derived indices, speckle-tracking imaging (STI), and 3-dimensional (3D)-derived parameters may offer additional values to detect subtle cardiac injury.

DEFINITION OF CANCER THERAPY-RELATED LEFT VENTRICULAR DYSFUNCTION

Current strategies to identify antineoplastic therapy-related LV dysfunction primarily consist of LVEF assessment by echocardiography or

Disclosure: The authors have nothing to disclose.
Division of Cardiovascular Diseases, Department of Medicine, Hospital of the University of Pennsylvania, 3400 Spruce Street, Philadelphia, PA 19104, USA
* Corresponding author.
E-mail address: marielle.scherrer-crosbie@pennmedicine.upenn.edu

Cardiol Clin 37 (2019) 419–427
https://doi.org/10.1016/j.ccl.2019.07.006

multigated acquisition scan (MUGA scan). Cardiac MRI (CMRI) shows promise but is currently used if LVEF cannot be determined using more easily available techniques. At present, a consensus definition for cardiotoxicity is still lacking. The diagnostic criteria for cardiac dysfunction, as defined by the Cardiac Review and Evaluation Committee, are any one of the following: (1) cardiomyopathy characterized by a global decrease in LVEF; (2) signs or symptoms of heart failure; or (3) decline in LVEF of at least 5% to less than 55% with signs or symptoms of heart failure or decline in LVEF of at least 10% to less than 55% without signs or symptoms.[6] In a joint position paper, the American Society of Echocardiography and the European Association of Cardiovascular Imaging suggest a homogeneous definition as a decrease in the LVEF of greater than 10% points, to a value less than 53%, confirmed by a repeated study 2 to 3 weeks after the first diagnostic imaging study.[11] However, the HERA study uses a decrease in the LVEF of greater than 10% points, to a value less than 50%, to indicate cardiotoxicity.[12]

Although LVEF is a robust predictor of symptomatic heart failure in patients treated with chemotherapy,[13,14] the accuracy of LVEF calculated by conventional 2-dimensional echocardiography (2DE) is limited by the image quality, inadequate visualization of the true LV apex, LV geometric assumptions, the presence of regional wall motion abnormalities, and the inherent variability of the measurement.[15] Otterstad and colleagues[16] reported that 2DE was able to recognize differences in sequential measurements of LVEF of 8.9%, close to the 10% threshold of LVEF change used to define cardiotoxicity in several studies and consensus,[11,12] explaining why 2DE LVEF may fail to detect small variations in LV function attributable to cardiotoxicity.

The American Society of Echocardiography recommends the use of contrast echocardiography if 2 or more segments of the LV are not well visualized.[17] Microbubble administration has been shown to result in significant improvement in endocardial border definition and reader confidence in regional and global LV function assessment, reducing intraobserver and interobserver variability of LVEF measurement, in patients with normal or reduced LV function.[18–22] In a study of 110 patients, the accuracy of contrast 2DE was significantly better than unenhanced tissue harmonic imaging in comparison with CMRI, even in patients with good image quality.[23]

Three-dimensional echocardiography (3DE) is of great interest in cardio-oncology for the serial monitoring of LVEF changes over time. 3DE provides more accurate LV volumes and LVEF than 2D echocardiography, with higher agreement with CMRI.[15,18,19,24,25] In a recent meta-analysis of 174 studies comparing 3DE, 2DE, MUGA scan, cardiac computed tomography (CT), gated single-photon emission CT, and invasive cardiac cine ventriculography, with CMRI as the gold standard, CT and 3DE had the best agreement with CMRI for LVEF measurement.[26] In an ideal 3DE, the potential errors inherent to 2DE LVEF measurement, including geometric assumption, foreshortened apical views, or suboptimal orthogonal apical 4- and 2-chamber views should not be present. However, despite the apparent benefits, 3DE is frequently hampered by suboptimal image quality. Several studies have examined the role of contrast-enhanced real-time 3DE in different patient populations.[18,19] In a multicenter study in patients with various degrees of LV dysfunction, contrast 3DE improved the accuracy of LV volumes assessment and reduced interobserver variation for volumes and LVEF, over unenhanced 3DE.[18]

DOPPLER-DERIVED PARAMETERS

Tissue Doppler imaging (TDI) uses Doppler echocardiography in the analysis of real-time myocardial velocity in systolic and diastolic periods. Several studies have demonstrated an early decrease in peak mitral annular systolic velocity (S′) in patients receiving anthracyclines, which remained reduced several years thereafter.[27,28]

Tei myocardial performance index, which is defined as the sum of isovolumetric contraction and relaxation time divided by the ejection time,[29] combines systolic and diastolic echocardiographic parameters. The Tei index has been shown to correlate well with other invasive and noninvasive measures of LV function,[30] and to be a powerful predictor of outcome in several diseases.[31,32] A rise of Tei index has been observed in 75% to 100% patients treated with anthracyclines.[33,34] In 100 patients who received anthracycline-based chemotherapy, Dodos and colleagues[35] illustrated that the Tei index significantly increased 1 month after anthracycline chemotherapy in most patients, that is, in 78.8%, whereas 17.7% had a significant decline of LVEF. The changes of Tei index detected earlier than alterations of the E/A ratio, however, did not correlate with the deterioration of LVEF. From a technical point of view, all Doppler-derived parameters are angle dependent. TDI is also influenced by the passive translational and tethering motion of the myocardium, which could hinder the identification of regional function and contractility. It remains unclear whether the Tei index could provide long-term clinical relevance in individuals.

SPECKLE-TRACKING IMAGING

Unlike TDI, STI, which tracks the speckles in gray scale of B mode images, is angle independent, has better spatial resolution, and is less sensitive to signal noise than TDI: it is, however, of limited temporal resolution.[36] Strain is a dimensionless parameter of myocardial tissue deformation, reflecting the fractional change in the length of a myocardial segment (reported as percentage). Strain rate is the rate of deformation or stretch (reported as s^{-1}).[37] Both strain and strain rate have the ability to differentiate active versus passive movement, allowing for the analysis of myocardial deformation independent of the translational motion of the heart. A growing body of literature supports the use of STI to detect early myocardial injury after exposure to cancer therapy, both in animal models and patients.[38–40] An early study showed that in 67 patients with lymphoma, global longitudinal strain (GLS), global circumferential strain (GCS), and global radial strain were reduced shortly after anthracycline exposure (mean cumulative doses of anthracycline as low as 170 mg/m^2), whereas LVEF and diastolic function remained normal.[41] The real value of deformation indices, however, depends on their ability to predict subsequent LV systolic dysfunction or development of heart failure.

The value of pretreatment GLS in patients treated with anthracyclines has been studied in patients with hematological malignancies[42,43] and in patients with low normal LVEF.[42,43] In both populations, pretreatment GLS was associated with symptomatic heart failure after anthracycline exposure. In patients with hematological malignancies, GLS brought additional value to the measurement of LVEF.[42,43] In patients with low normal LVEF, GLS was associated with symptomatic heart failure, whereas LVEF was not.

A growing body of studies, several of them prospective in nature, have demonstrated the prognostic value of measurement of speckle tracking-derived indices during and shortly after anthracycline treatment, and are summarized in **Table 1**. The outcome in these studies was the subsequent decrease in LVEF.

STI cannot only measure myocardial deformation in longitudinal, circumferential and radial dimensions, but also track the wringing movement (rotation) of the left ventricle. LV twist is defined as the difference in rotation between base and apex. Two case-control studies have assessed the rotational deformation in childhood cancer survivors treated with anthracycline. At a segmental level, the apical rather than basal rotational deformation seems to be more sensitive to the exposure of cardiotoxic agents.[44,45] In a study of 25 adult patients receiving anthracyclines, torsion, twisting, and untwisting rates decreased significantly 1 month after chemotherapy, whereas the LVEF and Tei index remained unchanged.[46] Mornos and Petrescu[47] reported that, in 74 patients with anthracyclines, both changes of GLS (ΔGLS) and twist (Δtwist) 6 weeks after anthracycline treatment predicted a subsequent decrease in LVEF. However, ΔGLSxtwist, which could indicate rotational and longitudinal deformation, was superior to each component (ΔGLS or Δtwist), and was identified as the best early independent predictor of future development of cardiotoxicity, with a sensitivity of 90% and specificity of 82%.

Some limitations have to be recognized when using STI. An important limitation is intervendor variability. Different echocardiography software packages and machines can produce different results, making serial comparisons over time unreliable unless done using the same machine.[48] The American Society of Echocardiography and the European Association of Cardiovascular Imaging[11] recommend using the same vendor's machine and software version to compare individual patients with cancer when using 2D STI for the serial evaluation of systolic function. Strain values also decrease with age,[48] and are lower in men compared with women. Based on these concerns, it is not yet possible to recommend universal cut-off values to detect cardiotoxicity. Tables may be used for software, ages, and gender. Alternatively, an absolute value of ≤−16% is most often abnormal, and has been used in clinical practice.[49] The expert consensus of the American Society of Echocardiography has agreed that a decrease of 15% in the absolute strain value measured on the same vendor's machine is most likely a sign of cardiotoxicity.[11]

The optimal surveillance timing and strategy, which will most likely depend on the population, type of cancer, and cardiotoxic treatment, is also unknown. The task force for cancer treatments and cardiovascular toxicity of the European Society of Cardiology recommends that cancer treatment should not be stopped, interrupted, or reduced in dose based on a new GLS reduction alone.[50]

One important practical concern is whether speckle tracking could not only identify higher-risk individuals but directly inform a specific intervention to prevent further compromise in cardiac function. The SUCCOUR study is a multicenter, randomized controlled trial, which was initiated in April 2014 and continued until January 2018, which followed a total of 185 patients.[51] It assessed whether a strain-guided cardioprotective strategy could prevent subsequent cardiac dysfunction compared with

Table 1
Summary of studies using STI to predict cardiotoxicity

First Author	Cancer Type	n	Age (y)	Treatment	Mean Anthracycline Dose	Echo Timing	Cardiotoxicity Definition	Cardiotoxicity Rate (%)	Deformation Indices Predict Toxicity	Vendor Reproducibility
Mornos & Petrescu,[47] 2013	Breast, lymphoma, acute leukemia, osteosarcoma	74	51 ± 11	Anthracycline	259 mg/m²	Pre-, 6 wk, 12 wk, 24 wk, 52 wk after	LVEF decrease ≥5% to <55% with symptoms or asymptomatic reduction of LVEF ≥10% to <55%	13	ΔGLS × twist >71%: sensitivity (sen), 90%; specificity (spe), 82% (Δ between baseline and 6 wk after)	EchoPAC (GE)
Negishi et al,[28] 2013	Breast	81	50 ± 11	Trastuzumab, doxorubicin, radiotherapy	Not known	Pre-, 6 and 12 mo after	LVEF reduction ≥10%	30	Percentage of GLS change >11% at 6 mo: sen, 65%; spe. 94%	EchoPAC (GE) Intra-/interobserver variation for GLS: 0.85/0.71
Baratta et al,[57] 2013	Breast, lymphoma, leukemia, and other disease	36	47 ± 16	Doxorubicin, trastuzumab	Adriamycin 294 mg/m² for cardiotoxicity/ 102 mg/m² for noncardiotoxicity	Pre-, 2, 3, 4 and 6 mo after	LVEF decrease ≥5% to <55% with symptoms or asymptomatic reduction of LVEF ≥10% to <55%	19.4	Percentage of longitudinal strain (LS) reduction ≥15% at 2 mo: sen, 86%; spe, 86%	EchoPAC (GE) Intra-/interobserver variability for LS: -0.20% ± 1.1%/-0.6% ± 1.4%
Sawaya et al,[56] 2012	Breast	81	50 ± 10	Anthracycline, trastuzumab, paclitaxel, radiotherapy	88% with doxorubicin 240 mg/m², 12% with epirubicin 300 mg/m²	Pre-, 3, 6, 9, 12 and 15 mo after	LVEF decrease ≥5% to <55% with symptoms or asymptomatic reduction of LVEF ≥10% to <55%	32	GLS <19% after anthracycline: sen, 74%; spe, 73%	EchoPAC (GE)
Fallah-Rad et al,[58] 2011	Breast	42	47 ± 9	Anthracycline, trastuzumab, radiotherapy	Not known	Pre-anthracycline, pre-trastuzumab, 3, 6, 9, and 12 mo after	LVEF decrease ≥10% to <55% with symptoms or signs and discontinuation of chemotherapy	10	Absolute LS decrease >2% at 3 mo: sen, 0.79; spe, 0.82	EchoPAC (GE) Intra-/interobserver variability for LS: 0.94/0.90

Study	Cancer	N	Age	Chemotherapy	Dose	Timing	LVEF criteria	%	GLS/LS findings	Software / ICC
Kang et al,[55] 2014	Lymphoma	75	53 ± 13	Epirubicin	Epirubicin: 300 mg/m²	Pre-, 3 cycles, completion of chemotherapy, 4–6 mo after	LVEF decrease ≥5% to <55% with symptoms or asymptomatic reduction of LVEF ≥10% to <55%	18.7	Percentage of GLS decrease >15.9% after 3 cycles: sen, 86%; spe, 75%	QLAB (Philips) Inter-/intraobserver interclass correlation coefficient (ICC) for LS: 0.93/0.88
Florescu et al,[59] 2014	Breast	40	51 ± 8	Epirubicin	Epirubicin: 268 mg/m²	Pre-, 3 cycles, 6 cycles	Decrease in LVEF of ≥10% to <55%	35	Percentage of LS reduced >9% at 3 cycles sen, 84%; spe, 80%	EchoPAC (GE) Inter-/intraobserver/test-retest variability for LS: ±4.2%/±3.3%/±7.2%
Arciniegas Calle et al,[60] 2018	Breast	66	52 ± 9	Anthracycline, trastuzumab	Anthracycline: 252 mg/m²	Pre- (T0), T1, T2 (T1, T2, not specified)	LVEF decrease ≥10%	20	LV GLS ≤ −14.06% + RV GLS ≤ −14.83% at T1: sen, 100%; spe, 73%	EchoPAC (GE) Inter-/intraobserver ICC for LS: 0.969/0.956
Hatazawa et al,[61] 2018	Lymphoma	73	64 ± 15	Anthracycline	Doxorubicin: 265 mg/m²	Pre-, after termination of treatment	LVEF decrease ≥5% to <53% with symptoms or asymptomatic decrease LVEF ≥10% to <53%	14	Baseline GLS ≤ −19%: sen, 60%; spe, 87%	QLAB (Philips) Inter-/intraobserver ICC for LS: 0.979/0.926

current LVEF-guided management in patients receiving cardiotoxic cancer therapy.

FUTURE DIRECTIONS

Many uncertainties remain about the role of echocardiography in the identification and management of cancer treatment-related cardiotoxicity. Recently, several additional techniques have been investigated in an attempt to overcome the limitations of existing methods. The use of 3D STI has been developed. It has potential benefits over 2D strain, such as lack of apical foreshortening, the ability to track speckles in all 3 directions without concern for out-of-plane motion, and the opportunity to measure multiple directions of strain using the same acquisition.[52] Zhang and colleagues[53] investigated the use of 3D echocardiography to assess the cardiac consequence of anthracycline therapy in 142 women with breast cancer. In this, the largest study to date, describing temporal changes in 3D LVEF and 3D myocardial strain, the investigators found that changes in 3D parameters, including 3D LVEF, GCS, and longitudinal and principal strain, were more pronounced than 2D changes, and the abnormalities persisted at 2 years of follow-up. Post-anthracycline 3D LVEF and GCS predicted subsequent 2D LVEF decrease, even after adjustment for the respective 2D parameters. However, the absence of complete and consistent data in approximately two-thirds of the study population is an important limitation. Clearly, more studies are needed to validate the findings.

The role of cardiac biomarkers, such as troponin, NT-proBNP, and myeloperoxidase has been investigated in providing diagnostic and prognostic information in patients undergoing cancer treatment.[54] The combination of cardiac biomarkers may increase the positive predictive value and negative predictive value. In a study of 75 patients with non-Hodgkin lymphoma,[55] the combination of longitudinal strain (LS) decrease greater than 15.9% and high-sensitive troponin T increase greater than 4 pg/mL increased the positive predictive value to 61%, from 44% (considering LS alone) and 38% (considering high-sensitive troponin T alone). The absence of either abnormality had a 95% negative predictive value. A similar increase in sensitivity and specificity has been reported using ultrasensitive troponin I with LS in patients with breast cancer treated with anthracycline and trastuzumab.[56] However, the optimal timing of obtaining biomarker measurements is not clear, and the clinical significance of the combined assessment strategy has not yet been established.

SUMMARY

In this review, we highlight the role of echocardiography in the cancer treatment-induced cardiotoxicity. Additional research is critical to clarify a uniformly accepted definition of cancer therapy-induced cardiotoxicity, and to define the value of both conventional and novel indices in guiding clinical management of cancer treatment-induced cardiotoxicity.

REFERENCES

1. Miller KD, Siegel RL, Lin CC, et al. Cancer treatment and survivorship statistics, 2016. CA Cancer J Clin 2016;66:271–89.
2. Zaorsky NG, Churilla TM, Egleston BL, et al. Causes of death among cancer patients. Ann Oncol 2017; 28:400–7.
3. Doyle JJ, Neugut AI, Jacobson JS, et al. Chemotherapy and cardiotoxicity in older breast cancer patients: a population-based study. J Clin Oncol 2005; 23:8597–605.
4. Curigliano G, Cardinale D, Suter T, et al. Cardiovascular toxicity induced by chemotherapy, targeted agents and radiotherapy: ESMO Clinical Practice Guidelines. Ann Oncol 2012;23(Suppl 7):vii155–66.
5. Senkus E, Jassem J. Cardiovascular effects of systemic cancer treatment. Cancer Treat Rev 2011;37: 300–11.
6. Seidman A, Hudis C, Pierri MK, et al. Cardiac dysfunction in the trastuzumab clinical trials experience. J Clin Oncol 2002;20:1215–21.
7. Cameron D, Piccart-Gebhart MJ, Gelber RD, et al. 11 years' follow-up of trastuzumab after adjuvant chemotherapy in HER2-positive early breast cancer: final analysis of the HERceptin Adjuvant (HERA) trial. Lancet 2017;389:1195–205.
8. Chu TF, Rupnick MA, Kerkela R, et al. Cardiotoxicity associated with tyrosine kinase inhibitor sunitinib. Lancet 2007;370:2011–9.
9. Hutson TE, Figlin RA, Kuhn JG, et al. Targeted therapies for metastatic renal cell carcinoma: an overview of toxicity and dosing strategies. Oncologist 2008;13:1084–96.
10. Hu YB, Zhang Q, Li HJ, et al. Evaluation of rare but severe immune related adverse effects in PD-1 and PD-L1 inhibitors in non-small cell lung cancer: a meta-analysis. Transl Lung Cancer Res 2017;6: S8–20.
11. Plana JC, Galderisi M, Barac A, et al. Expert consensus for multimodality imaging evaluation of adult patients during and after cancer therapy: a report from the American Society of Echocardiography and the European Association of Cardiovascular Imaging. J Am Soc Echocardiogr 2014;27: 911–39.

12. Procter M, Suter TM, de Azambuja E, et al. Longer-term assessment of trastuzumab-related cardiac adverse events in the Herceptin Adjuvant (HERA) trial. J Clin Oncol 2010;28:3422–8.

13. Romond EH, Jeong JH, Rastogi P, et al. Seven-year follow-up assessment of cardiac function in NSABP B-31, a randomized trial comparing doxorubicin and cyclophosphamide followed by paclitaxel (ACP) with ACP plus trastuzumab as adjuvant therapy for patients with node-positive, human epidermal growth factor receptor 2-positive breast cancer. J Clin Oncol 2012;30:3792–9.

14. Cardinale D, Colombo A, Bacchiani G, et al. Early detection of anthracycline cardiotoxicity and improvement with heart failure therapy. Circulation 2015;131:1981–8.

15. Jacobs LD, Salgo IS, Goonewardena S, et al. Rapid online quantification of left ventricular volume from real-time three-dimensional echocardiographic data. Eur Heart J 2006;27:460–8.

16. Otterstad JE, Froeland G, St John Sutton M, et al. Accuracy and reproducibility of biplane two-dimensional echocardiographic measurements of left ventricular dimensions and function. Eur Heart J 1997;18:507–13.

17. Porter TR, Abdelmoneim S, Belcik JT, et al. Guidelines for the cardiac sonographer in the performance of contrast echocardiography: a focused update from the American Society of Echocardiography. J Am Soc Echocardiogr 2014;27:797–810.

18. Hoffmann R, Barletta G, von Bardeleben S, et al. Analysis of left ventricular volumes and function: a multicenter comparison of cardiac magnetic resonance imaging, cine ventriculography, and unenhanced and contrast-enhanced two-dimensional and three-dimensional echocardiography. J Am Soc Echocardiogr 2014;27:292–301.

19. Hoffmann R, von Bardeleben S, Barletta G, et al. Comparison of two- and three-dimensional unenhanced and contrast-enhanced echocardiographies versus cineventriculography versus cardiac magnetic resonance for determination of left ventricular function. Am J Cardiol 2014;113:395–401.

20. Alherbish A, Becher H, Alemayehu W, et al. Impact of contrast echocardiography on accurate discrimination of specific degree of left ventricular systolic dysfunction and comparison with cardiac magnetic resonance imaging. Echocardiography 2018;35:1746–54.

21. Gurunathan S, Karogiannis N, Senior R. Imaging the heart failure patient-need for accurate measurements of left ventricular volumes and ejection fraction: the role of three-dimensional and contrast echocardiography. Curr Opin Cardiol 2016;31:459–68.

22. Kurt M, Shaikh KA, Peterson L, et al. Impact of contrast echocardiography on evaluation of ventricular function and clinical management in a large prospective cohort. J Am Coll Cardiol 2009;53:802–10.

23. Malm S, Frigstad S, Sagberg E, et al. Accurate and reproducible measurement of left ventricular volume and ejection fraction by contrast echocardiography: a comparison with magnetic resonance imaging. J Am Coll Cardiol 2004;44:1030–5.

24. Walker J, Bhullar N, Fallah-Rad N, et al. Role of three-dimensional echocardiography in breast cancer: comparison with two-dimensional echocardiography, multiple-gated acquisition scans, and cardiac magnetic resonance imaging. J Clin Oncol 2010;28:3429–36.

25. Sugeng L, Mor-Avi V, Weinert L, et al. Quantitative assessment of left ventricular size and function: side-by-side comparison of real-time three-dimensional echocardiography and computed tomography with magnetic resonance reference. Circulation 2006;114:654–61.

26. Pickett CA, Cheezum MK, Kassop D, et al. Accuracy of cardiac CT, radionucleotide and invasive ventriculography, two- and three-dimensional echocardiography, and SPECT for left and right ventricular ejection fraction compared with cardiac MRI: a meta-analysis. Eur Heart J Cardiovasc Imaging 2015;16:848–52.

27. Ho E, Brown A, Barrett P, et al. Subclinical anthracycline- and trastuzumab-induced cardiotoxicity in the long-term follow-up of asymptomatic breast cancer survivors: a speckle tracking echocardiographic study. Heart 2010;96:701–7.

28. Negishi K, Negishi T, Hare JL, et al. Independent and incremental value of deformation indices for prediction of trastuzumab-induced cardiotoxicity—ClinicalKey. J Am Soc Echocardiogr 2013;20:493–8.

29. Tei C. New non-invasive index for combined systolic and diastolic ventricular function. J Cardiol 1995;26:135–6.

30. Tei C, Nishimura RA, Seward JB, et al. Noninvasive Doppler-derived myocardial performance index: correlation with simultaneous measurements of cardiac catheterization measurements. J Am Soc Echocardiogr 1997;10:169–78.

31. Dujardin KS, Tei C, Yeo TC, et al. Prognostic value of a Doppler index combining systolic and diastolic performance in idiopathic-dilated cardiomyopathy. Am J Cardiol 1998;82:1071–6.

32. Yeo TC, Dujardin KS, Tei C, et al. Value of a Doppler-derived index combining systolic and diastolic time intervals in predicting outcome in primary pulmonary hypertension. Am J Cardiol 1998;81:1157–61.

33. Eidem BW, Sapp BG, Suarez CR, et al. Usefulness of the myocardial performance index for early detection of anthracycline-induced cardiotoxicity in children. Am J Cardiol 2001;87:1120–2. a9.

34. Ishii M, Tsutsumi T, Himeno W, et al. Sequential evaluation of left ventricular myocardial performance in children after anthracycline therapy. Am J Cardiol 2000;86:1279–81. a9.

35. Dodos F, Halbsguth T, Erdmann E, et al. Usefulness of myocardial performance index and biochemical markers for early detection of anthracycline-induced cardiotoxicity in adults. Clin Res Cardiol 2008;97:318–26.

36. Pokharel PFK, Bella JN. Clinical applications and prognostic implications of strain and strain rate imaging. PubMed-NCBI. Expert Rev Cardiovasc Ther 2015;13:853–66.

37. Mor-Avi V, Chicago I, Padua N, et al. Current and evolving echocardiographic techniques for the quantitative evaluation of cardiac mechanics: ASE/EAE consensus statement on methodology and indications endorsed by the Japanese Society of Echocardiography. Eur J Echocardiogr 2019;12:167–205.

38. Wang W, Kang Y, Shu XH, et al. Early detection of the cardiotoxicity induced by chemotherapy drug through two-dimensional speckle tracking echocardiography combined with high-sensitive cardiac troponin T. Zhonghua Zhong Liu Za Zhi 2017;39:835–40.

39. Coppola CRG, Barbieri A, Monti MG, et al. Antineoplastic-related cardiotoxicity, morphofunctional aspects in a murine model: contribution of the new tool 2D-speckle tracking. Onco Targets Ther 2016;9:6785–94.

40. Kang Y, Wang W, Zhao H, et al. Assessment of subclinical doxorubicin-induced cardiotoxicity in a rat model by speckle-tracking imaging. Arq Bras Cardiol 2017;0.

41. Kang Y, Cheng L, Li L, et al. Early detection of anthracycline-induced cardiotoxicity using two-dimensional speckle tracking echocardiography. Cardiol J 2013;20:592–9.

42. Ali MT, Yucel E, Bouras S, et al. Myocardial strain is associated with adverse clinical cardiac events in patients treated with anthracyclines. J Am Soc Echocardiogr 2016;29:522–7.e3.

43. Mousavi N, Tan TC, Ali M, et al. Echocardiographic parameters of left ventricular size and function as predictors of symptomatic heart failure in patients with a left ventricular ejection fraction of 50–59% treated with anthracyclines. Eur Heart J Cardiovasc Imaging 2015;16:977–84.

44. Cheung YF, Li SN, Chan GC, et al. Left ventricular twisting and untwisting motion in childhood cancer survivors. Echocardiography 2011;28:738–45.

45. Yu W, Li SN, Chan GC, et al. Transmural strain and rotation gradient in survivors of childhood cancers. Eur Heart J Cardiovasc Imaging 2013;14:175–82.

46. Motoki H, Koyama J, Nakazawa H, et al. Torsion analysis in the early detection of anthracycline-mediated cardiomyopathy. Eur Heart J Cardiovasc Imaging 2012;13:95–103.

47. Mornos C, Petrescu L. Early detection of anthracycline-mediated cardiotoxicity: the value of considering both global longitudinal left ventricular strain and twist. Can J Physiol Pharmacol 2013;91:601–7.

48. Takigiku K, Takeuchi M, Izumi C, et al, JUSTICE Investigators. Normal range of left ventricular 2-dimensional strain: Japanese Ultrasound Speckle Tracking of the Left Ventricle (JUSTICE) study. Circ J 2012;76:2623–32.

49. Liu J, Banchs J, Mousavi N, et al. Contemporary role of echocardiography for clinical decision making in patients during and after cancer therapy. JACC Cardiovasc Imaging 2018;11:1122–31.

50. Zamorano JL, Lancellotti P, Rodriguez Munoz D, et al. 2016 ESC Position Paper on cancer treatments and cardiovascular toxicity developed under the auspices of the ESC Committee for Practice Guidelines: the Task Force for cancer treatments and cardiovascular toxicity of the European Society of Cardiology (ESC). Eur Heart J 2016;37:2768–801.

51. Negishi T, Thavendiranathan P, Negishi K, et al. Rationale and design of the strain surveillance of chemotherapy for improving cardiovascular outcomes: the SUCCOUR trial. JACC Cardiovasc Imaging 2018;11:1098–105.

52. Thavendiranathan P. Is there added value of the third imaging dimension in cardio-oncology? JACC Cardiovasc Imaging 2018;11:1069–71.

53. Zhang KW, Finkelman BS, Gulati G, et al. Abnormalities in 3-dimensional left ventricular mechanics with anthracycline chemotherapy are associated with systolic and diastolic dysfunction. JACC Cardiovasc Imaging 2018;11:1059–68.

54. Cardinale D, Colombo A, Torrisi R, et al. Trastuzumab-induced cardiotoxicity: clinical and prognostic implications of troponin I evaluation. J Clin Oncol 2010;28:3910–6.

55. Kang Y, Xu X, Cheng L, et al. Two-dimensional speckle tracking echocardiography combined with high-sensitive cardiac troponin T in early detection and prediction of cardiotoxicity during epirubicine-based chemotherapy. Eur J Heart Fail 2014;16:300–8.

56. Sawaya H, Sebag IA, Plana JC, et al. Assessment of echocardiography and biomarkers for the extended prediction of cardiotoxicity in patients treated with anthracyclines, taxanes, and trastuzumab. Circ Cardiovasc Imaging 2012;5:596–603.

57. Baratta S, Damiano MA, Marchese ML. Serum markers, conventional Doppler echocardiography and two-dimensional systolic strain in the diagnosis of chemotherapy-induced myocardial toxicity. Rev Argent Cardiol 2013;81:151–8.

58. Fallah-Rad N, Walker JR, Wassef A, et al. The utility of cardiac biomarkers, tissue velocity and strain imaging, and cardiac magnetic resonance imaging in predicting early left ventricular dysfunction in patients with human epidermal growth factor receptor II-positive breast cancer treated with adjuvant trastuzumab therapy. J Am Coll Cardiol 2011;57: 2263–70.

59. Florescu M, Magda LS, Enescu OA, et al. Early detection of epirubicin-induced cardiotoxicity in patients with breast cancer. J Am Soc Echocardiogr 2014;27:83–92.

60. Arciniegas Calle MC, Sandhu NP, Xia H, et al. Two-dimensional speckle tracking echocardiography predicts early subclinical cardiotoxicity associated with anthracycline-trastuzumab chemotherapy in patients with breast cancer. BMC Cancer 2018;18: 1037.

61. Hatazawa K, Tanaka H, Nonaka A, et al. Baseline global longitudinal strain as a predictor of left ventricular dysfunction and hospitalization for heart failure of patients with malignant lymphoma after anthracycline therapy. Circ J 2018;82: 2566–74.

MRI of Cardiotoxicity

Jennifer Hawthorne Jordan, PhD, MS[a],*, William Gregory Hundley, MD[b]

KEYWORDS

- Cardiovascular magnetic resonance • Cardiotoxicity • Imaging • Tissue characterization
- Left ventricular ejection fraction • Myocardial strain

KEY POINTS

- Cardiovascular magnetic resonance imaging is a safe, nonionizing imaging modality to noninvasively and comprehensively assess myocardial structure, function, and tissue changes in cardio-oncology patients.
- Accurate quantification of LVEF and LV strain may be performed with CMR and should be considered in cases in whom values from other modalities (echo, multigated acquisition scan) are borderline or of poor imaging quality.
- Acute cardiotoxic changes in the myocardium involving edema and inflammation may be identified using T2-based tissue characterization; in the absence of T2-based changes, late cardiotoxic changes may be identified using T1-based methods such as LGE and ECV.
- Noncontrasted and contrasted tissue characterization can identify underlying myopathic processes such as inflammation, edema, and fibrosis in cardio-oncology patients and may precede LV systolic dysfunction.

INTRODUCTION

This article discusses the current clinical and research landscape with respect to cardiovascular magnetic resonance (CMR) imaging in several types of cardiotoxicity related to cancer therapy, because cardio-oncology is a heterogeneous indication for CMR (**Boxes 1–4**). CMR imaging can provide valuable, noninvasive diagnostic assessments of myocardial function and composition as well as vascular assessments (**Fig. 1**). Because CMR does not use ionizing radiation, its use in oncology patients who receive external radiation therapy is advantageous compared with other imaging modalities that may repetitively expose patients to additional radiation for serial cardio-oncology evaluations. This, combined with the high spatial and temporal resolutions associated with CMR imaging, make it an increasingly valued tool in cardio-oncology assessments.

Although several recent position papers and guidelines have been published in cardio-oncology,[1–4] there remains a lack of consensus on the appropriate clinical and research use of CMR in cardio-oncology screening and surveillance. A point of agreement, however, is that CMR examinations should be considered secondary to poor echocardiographic measures where acoustic windows may be poor or that the LVEF may be borderline.[2] The use of CMR for screening and surveillance of cardiotoxicity extends beyond looking at systolic function measures, such as LVEF, for identifying the underlying cause of changes in tissue characterization properties, assessments of vasculature and perfusion, and characterization of masses within the left ventricle (LV)

Disclosure: The authors have nothing to disclose.
[a] Department of Biomedical Engineering, Virginia Commonwealth University, Pauley Heart Center, Virginia Commonwealth University Health Sciences, 8-119B, 1200 East Broad Street, Richmond, VA 23298, USA;
[b] Pauley Heart Center, Virginia Commonwealth University Health Sciences, 8-124, 1200 East Broad Street, Richmond, VA 23298, USA
* Corresponding author.
E-mail address: jennifer.jordan@vcuhealth.org
twitter: @jenjordanphd (J.H.J.)

Box 1
When CMR is useful after echocardiography

- Poor acoustic windows and difficult imaging by echocardiography
- Borderline LVEF assessment by echocardiography

(see **Fig. 1**).[5] We refer to other sections in this issue with regard to mechanisms of action for these examples of cardiotoxicity. This article summarizes current knowledge surrounding the use of CMR in cardiotoxicity to evaluate functional capacity, anatomic and structural abnormalities, and both noncontrasted and contrasted tissue characterization techniques. Although imaging of cardiotoxicity related to anthracyclines is presented in most of the literature and in this review, we also discuss CMR imaging of cardiotoxicity related to radiation therapy, trastuzumab, and immune checkpoint inhibitors (ICIs) used in immunotherapy.

FUNCTIONAL MEASURES

The LVEF is the primary imaging marker of cardiotoxicity and may be measured noninvasively using modalities such as 2D or 3D echocardiography, radionuclide ventriculography or multigated acquisition scans, or CMR imaging. CMR imaging is advantageous for measuring LVEF because of its high temporal and spatial resolutions and the use of Simpson's rule to quantify LV volumes that does not require geometric assumptions. Furthermore, CMR does not use ionizing radiation and, thus, may be beneficial for monitoring LVEF in serial settings that may be necessitated by the long-term care of patients with cancer in survivorship. The LVEF is quantified from a short-axis cine stack of steady-state free-precession (SSFP) images in which the left ventricular end-diastolic (LVEDV) and left ventricular end-systolic (LVESV) volumes are identified, and the endocardial surface is contoured in postprocessing software. The discs of volumes are summed by Simpson's rule and the LVEF is then calculated as the difference in LVEDV

Box 2
Functional assessment pearls

- Assess for large changes in LVEF (>10% decline) and/or to a value <50%
- Assess for relative strain changes >15%
- Evaluate both LVEDV and LVESV in the context of LVEF and strain changes

---

Box 3
Noncontrast tissue characterization

- Increased native T1 indicates many pathologic changes, whereas increased T2 indicates an acute process with myocardial edema
- Establish local normative native T1 and T2 values
- Normative values are effected by field strength, version of acquisition sequence, and local field inhomogeneities

---

and LVESV and divided by the LVEDV. Baseline and serial screening of cardiotoxicity with risk-based algorithms have been proposed by Panjrath and Jain[6] for monitoring trastuzumab cardiotoxicity, and by Hall and colleagues[7] for monitoring cardiotoxicity from targeted therapies; in general, echocardiographic or radionuclide measures of LVEF are proposed. Although the American Society of Echocardiography and the European Association of Cardiovascular Imaging consensus statement recommends screening of the LVEF with echocardiography, CMR is recommended in circumstances where poor acoustic windows or body habitus may limit the quality of the study, or if a borderline LVEF is measured and CMR may provide additional clarity.[2]

When the LVEF drops to a value below normal (50%–53%) or changes by more than 10 absolute points without other intervening factors (such as sepsis or myocardial infarction), cancer therapy-related cardiotoxicity should be considered when chemotherapy that has been associated with myocellular injury has been administered. Before confirming this diagnosis, however, the cause for a change in LVEF should be investigated. In a cohort of 112 patients with cancer receiving potentially cardiotoxic chemotherapy regimens (72% anthracycline-based), Melendez and colleagues[8] demonstrated that nearly 20% of patients experienced a cardiotoxic LVEF drop (>10 absolute points or to a value <50%) owing to a large decline in LVEDV. These findings may suggest potential

---

Box 4
Contrasted tissue characterization

- Diffuse and focal LGE have been reported in studies related to inflammation, edema, and fibrosis
- Extracellular volume (ECV) calculated from native and contrasted T1 mapping may aid in identifying myocardial fibrosis late after cancer-related treatment

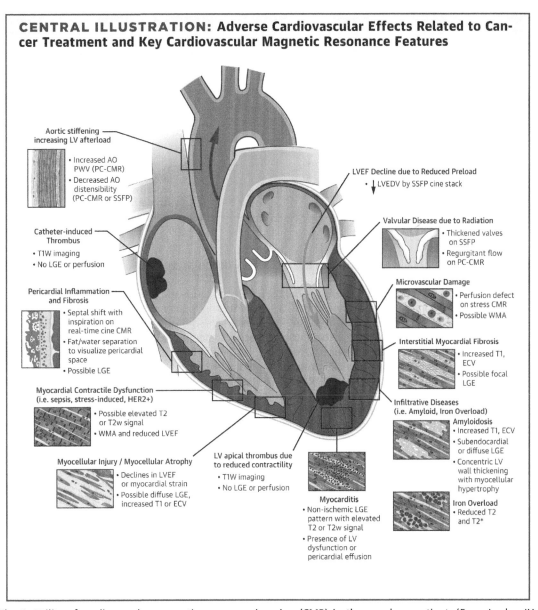

CENTRAL ILLUSTRATION: Adverse Cardiovascular Effects Related to Cancer Treatment and Key Cardiovascular Magnetic Resonance Features

Aortic stiffening increasing LV afterload
- Increased AO PWV (PC-CMR)
- Decreased AO distensibility (PC-CMR or SSFP)

LVEF Decline due to Reduced Preload
- ↓ LVEDV by SSFP cine stack

Valvular Disease due to Radiation
- Thickened valves on SSFP
- Regurgitant flow on PC-CMR

Catheter-induced Thrombus
- T1W imaging
- No LGE or perfusion

Microvascular Damage
- Perfusion defect on stress CMR
- Possible WMA

Pericardial Inflammation and Fibrosis
- Septal shift with inspiration on real-time cine CMR
- Fat/water separation to visualize pericardial space
- Possible LGE

Interstitial Myocardial Fibrosis
- Increased T1, ECV
- Possible focal LGE

Myocardial Contractile Dysfunction (i.e. sepsis, stress-induced, HER2+)
- Possible elevated T2 or T2w signal
- WMA and reduced LVEF

Infiltrative Diseases (i.e. Amyloid, Iron Overload)
Amyloidosis
- Increased T1, ECV
- Subendocardial or diffuse LGE
- Concentric LV wall thickening with myocellular hypertrophy

Myocellular Injury / Myocellular Atrophy
- Declines in LVEF or myocardial strain
- Possible diffuse LGE, increased T1 or ECV

LV apical thrombus due to reduced contractility
- T1W imaging
- No LGE or perfusion

Myocarditis
- Non-ischemic LGE pattern with elevated T2 or T2w signal
- Presence of LV dysfunction or pericardial effusion

Iron Overload
- Reduced T2 and T2*

Fig. 1. Utility of cardiovascular magnetic resonance imaging (CMR) in the oncology patient. (*From* Jordan JH, Todd RM, Vasu S, Hundley WG. Cardiovascular magnetic resonance in the oncology patient. *JACC Cardiovasc Imaging.* 2018;11(8):1150-1172; with permission.)

intravascular volume depletion 3 months after initiating treatment.[8] Additional unanswered questions regarding imaging LVEF with CMR after anthracyclines include whether acute changes recover after cessation of treatment and if early subclinical changes (changes of <10 points or to a value >50%) portend worse outcomes later in survivorship.

Deteriorations in LV myocardial strain after anthracyclines have been observed with CMR imaging in several studies.[9–14] Several myocardial strain techniques exist for CMR, including spatially modulated magnetization with line or grid tags, feature tracking from SSFP cine images, displacement encoding with stimulated echoes, and strain-encoded imaging. Values of CMR strain are oriented to planes of the LV and include global radial strain (GRS), global circumferential strain (GCS), and global longitudinal strain (GLS) (**Fig. 2**).[15] The GCS and GLS are most widely used and reported in CMR because of the technical limitations in measuring GRS.[15] In a prospective assessment of GCS in 53 patients receiving low to moderate doses of anthracyclines (50–375 mg/m² of doxorubicin equivalent), early subclinical deteriorations in

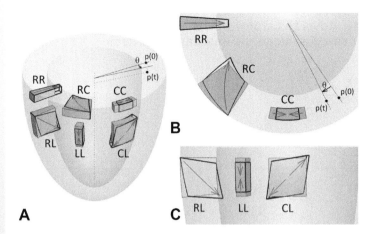

Fig. 2. Cardiovascular magnetic strain directions shown (*A*) in 3D, (*B*) short axis, and (*C*) long axis. Global circumferential strain (GCS) is calculated from circumferential changes (CC) and deformation in the long-axis planes (LL), and is used to calculate global longitudinal strain (GLS). (*From* Zhong X, Gibberman LB, Spottiswoode BS, et al. Comprehensive cardiovascular magnetic resonance of myocardial mechanics in mice using three-dimensional cine DENSE. *J Cardiovasc Magn Reson.* 2011;13:83; with permission.)

GCS tracked concurrently with subclinical declines in LVEF (**Fig. 3**).[9]

Similar to LVEF, the LVEDV and LVESV should be considered when interpreting changes in GCS with the administration of anthracyclines. In a cohort of 101 patients receiving cardiotoxic chemotherapies (71% anthracycline-based regimens), Jordan and colleagues[16] found that up to 16% of individuals experienced a deterioration in circumferential myocardial strain mediated by a decline in LVEDV rather than an increase in LVESV. Recent data from Haslbauer and colleagues[10] demonstrated that, although GCS changes only trended toward being higher than in controls, GLS did significantly increase (or worsen) early (<3 months) and late (>12 months) after treatment (21% ± 8% and 17% ± 11%, respectively) when compared with controls (24% ± 5%, *P*<.001) using feature tracking strain analysis.

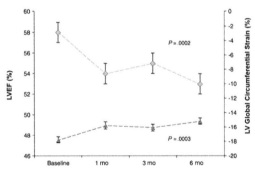

Fig. 3. Reduced LV global circumferential strain occurred concurrent with subclinical left ventricular ejection fraction changes early after initiation of chemotherapy. (*From* Drafts BC, Twomley KM, D'Agostino R, Jr., et al. Low to moderate dose anthracycline-based chemotherapy is associated with early noninvasive imaging evidence of subclinical cardiovascular disease. *JACC Cardiovasc Imaging.* 2013;6(8):877-885; with permission.)

Although studies have demonstrated the usefulness of CMR to identify subclinical cardiac dysfunction with LVEF and strain,[8–11,14,16,17] the usefulness of imaging to intervene and guide therapy remains uncertain. The ongoing SUCCOUR Trial, although echocardiography based, may answer this gap in knowledge because it is evaluating the hypothesis that cardioprotective therapy guided by GLS rather than LVEF would benefit patients at risk of developing future declines in LVEF.[18]

ANATOMY AND STRUCTURE

CMR imaging is also useful for investigating anatomic and structural features in the heart and surrounding structures that may occur in oncology patients. For instance, CMR images may be useful for identifying the causes of masses in the cardiac field of view or to identify thickening of the pericardial space (see **Fig. 1**).

An LV mass can be quantified from the SSFP cine stack images (acquired for the assessment of LV volumes) by adding an additional endocardial border to contour the myocardial tissue. Anthracyclines such as doxorubicin may be associated to atrophic remodeling due to the mechanisms of action which include topoisomerase IIβ-mediated myocellular death, downregulation of myocellular GATA4 expression, and DNA oxidant damage.[19–24] Several recent studies have demonstrated early and late decreases in LV mass in response to anthracyclines.[1,25–30] However, these findings are not uniform and may be related to the timing of measurement in the cycle of remodeling.

Using a novel method of noninvasively measuring cardiomyocyte size with CMR, called intracellular water lifetime (τ_{ic}), de Souza and colleagues[31] demonstrated that women with breast cancer treated with anthracyclines had a decrease in LV mass resulting from cardiomyocyte atrophy.

Importantly, other studies have demonstrated that declines in the LV mass of anthracycline-treated patients with cancer portended increased risk of future cardiac events[27] and were more associated with heart failure symptoms than with changes in LVEF early after treatment.[30] Willis and colleagues[32] recently suggested that this atrophic mechanism following doxorubicin exposure may be dependent on the striated muscle-specific ubiquitin ligase MuRF1. The compensatory mechanism following atrophic responses remains to be determined and is likely due to multifactorial processes.

TISSUE CHARACTERIZATION: NONCONTRAST TECHNIQUES

One of the major advantages of CMR imaging in cardio-oncology patients is the ability to assess both functional capacity and changes in tissue characteristics in a single, noninvasive examination. Increases in noncontrasted T1, or native T1, are associated with pathology in the myocardium including edema, inflammation, and fibrosis.[33] T2 relaxation is a water-sensitive process, and increases above normal myocardial T2 values are therefore strongly associated with acute processes and myocardial edema.[33,34]

Historical work in nuclear magnetic resonance spectroscopy of rodents exposed to cardiotoxic drugs demonstrated that histologic changes in myocardial tissue were associated with an increase in myocardial T1 and T2 relaxation.[35,36] Because T2 relaxation is tightly linked to myocardial water content and edema, the ability to identify changes in myocardial T2 is thus dependent on timing of the CMR examination with respect to the cardiotoxic remodeling process.[34]

Quantitative parametric mapping of myocardial T1 and T2 relaxation may be accomplished in a single breath hold that characterizes the myocardial relaxation constants in a voxel-by-voxel basis. As MRI scanner vendors provide motion-corrected registration of these maps and sites, and establish normative/abnormal values for their specific scanner, parametric mapping may be used to identify myocardial tissue characteristics associated with cardiotoxicity.[10,33,34] For example, using a cut point of T2 greater than 59 ms, Thavendiranathan and colleagues[37] demonstrated that quantitative T2 mapping was elevated in HER2-positive patients with breast cancer treated with sequential anthracycline and trastuzumab treatment who were diagnosed with subclinical cardiotoxicity. A recent communication from Lustberg and colleagues[38] followed 29 patients with breast cancer with a preserved LVEF and normal baseline T2 (51.8 ± 3.5 ms); after the first anthracycline treatment there was no change in functional measures; however, T2 increased by 3.3 ± 0.8 ms ($P<.001$) and continued to increase by 5.4 ± 0.8 ms after the fourth anthracycline treatment (**Fig. 4**). Although LVEF declined in the overall group, early changes in T2 were not associated with LVEF decline, thus the prognostic significance of identifying acute cardiotoxicity with T2 mapping remains unclear.[38]

Haslbauer and colleagues[10] sought to answer these gaps in knowledge regarding early and late noncontrasted tissue characterization features in 115 patients receiving cancer-related therapy. Early cardiotoxic changes were demonstrated as increased native T1 and T2 in the first 3 months of therapy, whereas late after treatment, the acute processes resolved and increased T1 in absentia of T2 changes indicated myocardial fibrosis (**Fig. 5**).

The results of that work produced an algorithm of phenotypical signatures for cardiac involvement after cancer treatment in which early involvement, defined as native T1 $\geq$ 2 SD and native T2 $\geq$ 2 SD, and late involvement, defined as native T1 $\geq$ 2 SD, and normal T2 and/or GLS $\leq$ 17%, led to a detection rate of 84% in their cohort. Importantly, both native T1 and T2 outperformed functional

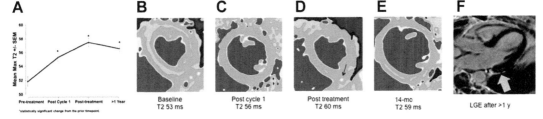

Fig. 4. (A) Serial increases in a population of patients with breast cancer during and after treatment (*B–E*), and representative T2 images from a woman in whom T2 increased significantly (denoted by *arrow* in *D*) and who developed subepicardial scarring on late gadolinium enhancement (LGE) images 1 year after treatment (denoted by *arrow* in *F*). (*From* Lustberg MB, Reinbolt R, Addison D, et al. Early detection of anthracycline-induced cardiotoxicity in breast cancer survivors with T2 cardiac magnetic resonance. Circ Cardiovasc Imaging 2019;12(5):e008777; with permission.)

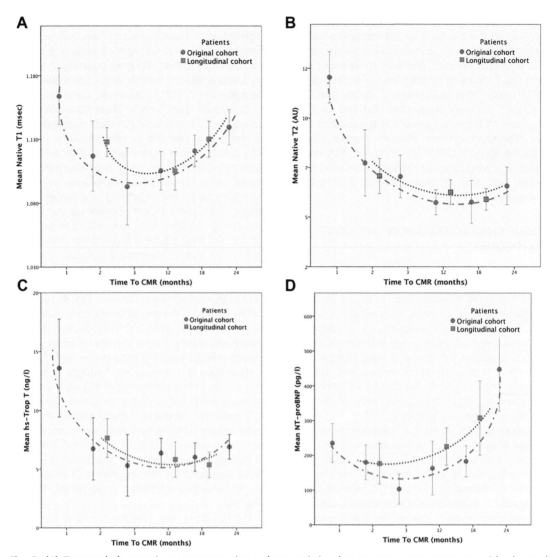

Fig. 5. (*A*) Temporal changes in noncontrast tissue characteristics demonstrate acute processes with elevated native T1 (*B*) and T2 are then followed by a resolution in T2 values, when late increased native T1 is associated with myocardial fibrosis. Biomarker data (shown in *C* and *D*) follow the CMR imaging findings. (*From* Haslbauer JD, Lindner S, Valbuena-Lopez S, et al. CMR imaging biosignature of cardiac involvement due to cancer-related treatment by T1 and T2 mapping. *Int J Cardiol.* 2019;275:179-186; with permission.)

measures such as LVEF and GLS in identifying patients with cardiotoxicity (**Fig. 6**).

TISSUE CHARACTERIZATION: CONTRASTED TECHNIQUES

Myocardial tissue characterization with CMR imaging may also involve one of several contrasted techniques with an extracellular gadolinium contrast agent. Of note, contrasted tissue characterization has limited use in patients with contraindications to gadolinium contrast or with renal insufficiency, and noncontrasted techniques must be used. Qualitative contrasted imaging

using T1-weighted sequences assesses the infiltration of contrast to identify areas with early and late signal enhancement, generally highlighting areas in which underlying pathologic conditions such as inflammation, edema, and fibrosis may exist.[39,40] Wassmuth and colleagues[39] were able to show that an increase of more than 5 times in the relative early enhancement on T1-weighted images identified future LVEF declines after the first month of an anthracycline-based regimen. Anthracyclines have also been associated with acute, diffuse late gadolinium enhancement (LGE) in several studies. In an animal model of anthracycline cardiotoxicity, increased diffuse myocardial

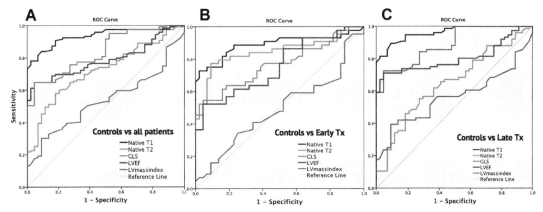

Fig. 6. ROC curve from all patients (*A*) demonstrating noncontrasted CMR tissue characterization (native T1 and T2) outperform functional measures such as left ventricular ejection fraction (LVEF) and global longitudinal strain (GLS) in identifying cardiotoxicity following cancer-related therapy. Native T1 outperformed other CMR measures whether early after treatment (*B*) or late after treatment (*C*). (*From* Haslbauer JD, Lindner S, Valbuena-Lopez S, et al. CMR imaging biosignature of cardiac involvement due to cancer-related treatment by T1 and T2 mapping. *Int J Cardiol.* 2019;275:179-186; with permission.)

signal intensity in LGE images was associated with future LV systolic dysfunction and evidence of vacuolization and extracellular volume (ECV) on histopathologic examination (**Fig. 7**).[40] Similar imaging results were confirmed in a clinical study of patients receiving anthracyclines and other cardiotoxic chemotherapy regimens.[41]

Limited reports of focal LGE have been observed following anthracyclines (see **Fig. 4**)[38,42] and trastuzumab therapy, predominantly in a subepicardial linear pattern.[43,44] Of interest to many may be the that the increasing use of ICIs in the treatment of cancer[45–47] has resulted in an increase in case reports of

fulminant ICI-associated myocarditis.[27,48,49] Zhang and colleagues[50] recently reported initial findings from the International ICI Myocarditis Study involving a registry from 19 sites and a total of 102 ICI-associated cases of myocarditis. Only half of the myocarditis patients in the registry had LGE noted on CMR imaging, and LGE was not associated with outcomes, emphasizing that an LGE-only approach would not be sufficient in ICI-associated myocarditis patients with preserved LVEF (**Fig. 8**).[50]

The quantitative contrasted characterization equivalent to qualitative LGE imaging is considered to be ECV mapping, in which a native T1

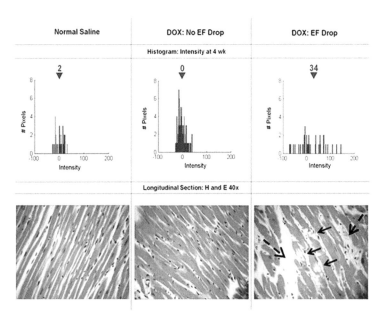

Fig. 7. Serial histograms of myocardial LGE signal intensity (*top*, mean intensity shown above the *inverted black triangles*) and corresponding histopathology (*bottom*) of individual animals 4 weeks after receipt of normal saline (*left*), doxorubicin without an LVEF drop (*middle*), and doxorubicin with an LVEF drop (*right*). Vacuolization (*arrows*) and increased extracellular space (*dashed arrows*) were observed in animals with doxorubicin cardiotoxicity. (*From* Lightfoot JC, D'Agostino RB, Jr., Hamilton CA, et al. Novel approach to early detection of doxorubicin cardiotoxicity by gadolinium-enhanced cardiovascular magnetic resonance imaging in an experimental model. *Circ Cardiovasc Imaging.* 2010;3(5):550-558; with permission.)

International ICI Myocarditis Cohort Study

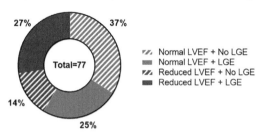

Fig. 8. Data recently presented at the 2019 American College of Cardiology on behalf of the International ICI Myocarditis Cohort Study demonstrating that roughly only half of ICI-associated myocarditis patients have LGE and more than half have a preserved LVEF. (*Data from* Zhang L, Awadalla M, Mahmood SS, et al. Late gadolinium enhancement in patients with myocarditis from immune checkpoint inhibitors. *J Am Coll Cardiol.* 2019;73(9 Supplement 1):675.)

map and a postcontrast T1 map are acquired and the relaxivities of the tissue and LV blood pool are compared and adjusted to the hematocrit.[33,51,52] Each voxel in an ECV map corresponds to the percentage of extracellular space in the imaged tissue. Extracellular space may increase acutely because of interstitial edema and inflammation; however, increases in ECV late after injury (or cancer treatment) are considered to be due to myocardial fibrosis.[33,34,52] A major advantage of ECV is the ability to readily identify diffuse myocardial fibrosis that is not easily identified visually with LGE imaging, a claim that has been histologically validated by several groups.[53–56]

Interestingly, an increased myocardial ECV has been observed both in survivors diagnosed with anthracycline cardiomyopathy[57] and in asymptomatic cancer survivors years after treatment with anthracycline-based chemotherapies compared with healthy individuals and untreated patients with cancer.[58] Although those late changes are attributable to myocardial fibrosis, prospective measurements of acute increases in ECV have been observed after initiation of anthracyclines, which are likely more associated with edema and acute injury processes.[59]

SUMMARY AND FUTURE DIRECTIONS

CMR imaging is useful for identifying systolic dysfunction, particularly in patients in whom echocardiographic imaging is not acceptable because of poor acoustic windows or that the LVEF is inconclusive by other modalities and an accurate LVEF or strain measurement is needed. Of particular advantage is capability of CMR to perform tissue characterization (noncontrasted or contrasted

techniques) to noninvasively identify changes in pathologic conditions related to cancer therapy or to discriminate causes of disease that may confound presentation in cardio-oncology patients (ie, regional wall abnormalities from ischemia or downregulation of contractility secondary to trastuzumab administration).

CMR imaging does not use ionizing radiation and is the gold standard for many cardiovascular measurements, making it a great serial imaging option if equipment and expertise are available. As cardio-oncology grows, more research with regard to screening and surveillance guidelines specific to CMR is needed, because most data are produced by other imaging modalities. The scope of cardio-oncology is wide and includes many types of diseases and therapies, and an ever-changing landscape of emerging therapies that need to be considered when developing these guidelines. Given the advantages of CMR imaging in screening and surveillance, CMR certainly has a role to play in the future of cardio-oncology.

ACKNOWLEDGMENTS

The authors wish to acknowledge the following National Institutes of Health grants for their efforts: R01CA199167, R21CA226960, and R01HL118740.

REFERENCES

1. Armstrong GT, Plana JC, Zhang N, et al. Screening adult survivors of childhood cancer for cardiomyopathy: comparison of echocardiography and cardiac magnetic resonance imaging. J Clin Oncol 2012; 30(23):2876–84.
2. Plana JC, Galderisi M, Barac A, et al. Expert consensus for multimodality imaging evaluation of adult patients during and after cancer therapy: a report from the American Society of Echocardiography and the European Association of Cardiovascular Imaging. Eur Heart J Cardiovasc Imaging 2014; 15(10):1063–93.
3. Armenian SH, Lacchetti C, Barac A, et al. Prevention and monitoring of cardiac dysfunction in survivors of adult cancers: American Society of Clinical Oncology clinical practice guideline. J Clin Oncol 2017;35(8):893–911.
4. Eschenhagen T, Force T, Ewer MS, et al. Cardiovascular side effects of cancer therapies: a position statement from the heart failure association of the European Society of Cardiology. Eur J Heart Fail 2011;13(1):1–10.
5. Jordan JH, Todd RM, Vasu S, et al. Cardiovascular magnetic resonance in the oncology patient. JACC Cardiovasc Imaging 2018;11(8):1150–72.

6. Panjrath GS, Jain D. Trastuzumab-induced cardiac dysfunction. Nucl Med Commun 2007;28(2): 69–73.

7. Hall PS, Harshman LC, Srinivas S, et al. The frequency and severity of cardiovascular toxicity from targeted therapy in advanced renal cell carcinoma patients. JACC Heart Fail 2013;1(1):72–8.

8. Melendez GC, Sukpraphrute B, D'Agostino RB Jr, et al. Frequency of left ventricular end-diastolic volume-mediated declines in ejection fraction in patients receiving potentially cardiotoxic cancer treatment. Am J Cardiol 2017;119(10):1637–42.

9. Drafts BC, Twomley KM, D'Agostino R Jr, et al. Low to moderate dose anthracycline-based chemotherapy is associated with early noninvasive imaging evidence of subclinical cardiovascular disease. JACC Cardiovasc Imaging 2013;6(8):877–85.

10. Haslbauer JD, Lindner S, Valbuena-Lopez S, et al. CMR imaging biosignature of cardiac involvement due to cancer-related treatment by T1 and T2 mapping. Int J Cardiol 2019;275:179–86.

11. Thavendiranathan P, Wintersperger BJ, Flamm SD, et al. Cardiac MRI in the assessment of cardiac injury and toxicity from cancer chemotherapy: a systematic review. Circ Cardiovasc Imaging 2013;6(6): 1080–91.

12. Jolly MP, Jordan JH, Melendez GC, et al. Automated assessments of circumferential strain from cine CMR correlate with LVEF declines in cancer patients early after receipt of cardio-toxic chemotherapy. J Cardiovasc Magn Reson 2017;19(1):59.

13. Nakano S, Takahashi M, Kimura F, et al. Cardiac magnetic resonance imaging-based myocardial strain study for evaluation of cardiotoxicity in breast cancer patients treated with trastuzumab: a pilot study to evaluate the feasibility of the method. Cardiol J 2016;23(3):270–80.

14. Ong G, Brezden-Masley C, Dhir V, et al. Myocardial strain imaging by cardiac magnetic resonance for detection of subclinical myocardial dysfunction in breast cancer patients receiving trastuzumab and chemotherapy. Int J Cardiol 2018;261:228–33.

15. Zhong X, Gibberman LB, Spottiswoode BS, et al. Comprehensive cardiovascular magnetic resonance of myocardial mechanics in mice using three-dimensional cine DENSE. J Cardiovasc Magn Reson 2011;13:83.

16. Jordan JH, Sukpraphrute B, Melendez GC, et al. Early myocardial strain changes during potentially cardiotoxic chemotherapy may occur as a result of reductions in left ventricular end-diastolic volume: the need to interpret left ventricular strain with volumes. Circulation 2017;135(25):2575–7.

17. Fallah-Rad N, Walker JR, Wassef A, et al. The utility of cardiac biomarkers, tissue velocity and strain imaging, and cardiac magnetic resonance imaging in predicting early left ventricular dysfunction in patients with human epidermal growth factor receptor II–positive breast cancer treated with adjuvant trastuzumab therapy. J Am Coll Cardiol 2011; 57(22):2263–70.

18. Negishi T, Thavendiranathan P, Negishi K, et al. Rationale and design of the strain surveillance of chemotherapy for improving cardiovascular outcomes: the SUCCOUR trial. JACC Cardiovasc Imaging 2018; 11(8):1098–105.

19. Childs AC, Phaneuf SL, Dirks AJ, et al. Doxorubicin treatment in vivo causes cytochrome C release and cardiomyocyte apoptosis, as well as increased mitochondrial efficiency, superoxide dismutase activity, and Bcl-2:Bax ratio. Cancer Res 2002;62(16): 4592–8.

20. An J, Li P, Li J, et al. ARC is a critical cardiomyocyte survival switch in doxorubicin cardiotoxicity. J Mol Med (Berl) 2009;87(4):401–10.

21. Sorensen BS, Sinding J, Andersen AH, et al. Mode of action of topoisomerase II-targeting agents at a specific DNA sequence: uncoupling the DNA binding, cleavage and religation events. J Mol Biol 1992;228(3):778–86.

22. Zhu S-G, Kukreja RC, Das A, et al. Dietary nitrate supplementation protects against doxorubicin-induced cardiomyopathy by improving mitochondrial function. J Am Coll Cardiol 2011;57(21): 2181–9.

23. Kim Y, Ma AG, Kitta K, et al. Anthracycline-induced suppression of GATA-4 transcription factor: implication in the regulation of cardiac myocyte apoptosis. Mol Pharmacol 2003;63(2):368–77.

24. Menna P, Salvatorelli E, Minotti G. Anthracycline degradation in cardiomyocytes: a journey to oxidative survival. Chem Res Toxicol 2010;23(1): 6–10.

25. Ganame J, Claus P, Eyskens B, et al. Acute cardiac functional and morphological changes after anthracycline infusions in children. Am J Cardiol 2007; 99(7):974–7.

26. Tham EB, Haykowsky MJ, Chow K, et al. Diffuse myocardial fibrosis by T1-mapping in children with subclinical anthracycline cardiotoxicity: relationship to exercise capacity, cumulative dose and remodeling. J Cardiovasc Magn Reson 2013;15:48.

27. Neilan TG, Coelho-Filho OR, Pena-Herrera D, et al. Left ventricular mass in patients with a cardiomyopathy after treatment with anthracyclines. Am J Cardiol 2012;110(11):1679–86.

28. De Wolf D, Suys B, Maurus R, et al. Dobutamine stress echocardiography in the evaluation of late anthracycline cardiotoxicity in childhood cancer survivors. Pediatr Res 1996;39(3):504–12.

29. Iarussi D, Galderisi M, Ratti G, et al. Left ventricular systolic and diastolic function after anthracycline chemotherapy in childhood. Clin Cardiol 2001; 24(10):663–9.

30. Jordan JH, Castellino SM, Melendez GC, et al. Left ventricular mass change after anthracycline chemotherapy. Circ Heart Fail 2018;11(7):e004560.

31. de Souza TF, Silva TQA, Costa FO, et al. Anthracycline therapy is associated with cardiomyocyte atrophy and preclinical manifestations of heart disease. JACC Cardiovasc Imaging 2018;11(8):1045–55.

32. Willis MS, Parry TL, Brown DI, et al. Doxorubicin exposure causes subacute cardiac atrophy dependent on the striated muscle-specific ubiquitin ligase MuRF1. Circ Heart Fail 2019;12(3):e005234.

33. Messroghli DR, Moon JC, Ferreira VM, et al. Clinical recommendations for cardiovascular magnetic resonance mapping of T1, T2, T2* and extracellular volume: a consensus statement by the Society for Cardiovascular Magnetic Resonance (SCMR) endorsed by the European Association for Cardiovascular Imaging (EACVI). J Cardiovasc Magn Reson 2017;19(1):75.

34. Ferreira VM, Schulz-Menger J, Holmvang G, et al. Cardiovascular magnetic resonance in nonischemic myocardial inflammation: expert recommendations. J Am Coll Cardiol 2018;72(24):3158–76.

35. Thompson RC, Canby RC, Lojeski EW, et al. Adriamycin cardiotoxicity and proton nuclear-magnetic-resonance relaxation properties. Am Heart J 1987;113(6):1444–9.

36. Cottin Y, Ribuot C, Maupoil V, et al. Early incidence of adriamycin treatment on cardiac parameters in the rat. Can J Physiol Pharmacol 1994;72(2):140–5.

37. Thavendiranathan P, Amir E, Bedard P, et al. Regional myocardial edema detected by T2 mapping is a feature of cardiotoxicity in breast cancer patients receiving sequential therapy with anthracyclines and trastuzumab. J Cardiovasc Magn Reson 2014;16(Suppl 1):P273.

38. Lustberg MB, Reinbolt R, Addison D, et al. Early detection of anthracycline-induced cardiotoxicity in breast cancer survivors with T2 cardiac magnetic resonance. Circ Cardiovasc Imaging 2019;12(5):e008777.

39. Wassmuth R, Lentzsch S, Erdbruegger U, et al. Subclinical cardiotoxic effects of anthracyclines as assessed by magnetic resonance imaging - a pilot study. Am Heart J 2001;141(6):1007–13.

40. Lightfoot JC, D'Agostino RB Jr, Hamilton CA, et al. Novel approach to early detection of doxorubicin cardiotoxicity by gadolinium-enhanced cardiovascular magnetic resonance imaging in an experimental model. Circ Cardiovasc Imaging 2010;3(5):550–8.

41. Jordan JH, D'Agostino RB Jr, Hamilton CA, et al. Longitudinal assessment of concurrent changes in left ventricular ejection fraction and left ventricular myocardial tissue characteristics after administration of cardiotoxic chemotherapies using T1-weighted and T2-weighted cardiovascular magnetic resonance. Circ Cardiovasc Imaging 2014;7(6):872–9.

42. Lunning MA, Kutty S, Rome ET, et al. Cardiac magnetic resonance imaging for the assessment of the myocardium after doxorubicin-based chemotherapy. Am J Clin Oncol 2013;21(12):1283–9.

43. Fallah-Rad N, Lytwyn M, Fang T, et al. Delayed contrast enhancement cardiac magnetic resonance imaging in trastuzumab induced cardiomyopathy. J Cardiovasc Magn Reson 2008;10(1):1–4.

44. Lawley C, Wainwright C, Segelov E, et al. Pilot study evaluating the role of cardiac magnetic resonance imaging in monitoring adjuvant trastuzumab therapy for breast cancer. Asia Pac J Clin Oncol 2012;8(1):95–100.

45. Pardoll DM. The blockade of immune checkpoints in cancer immunotherapy. Nat Rev Cancer 2012;12(4):252.

46. Topalian SL, Drake CG, Pardoll DM. Immune checkpoint blockade: a common denominator approach to cancer therapy. Cancer Cell 2015;27(4):450–61.

47. Sharma P, Allison JP. Immune checkpoint targeting in cancer therapy: toward combination strategies with curative potential. Cell 2015;161(2):205–14.

48. Moslehi JJ, Salem J-E, Sosman JA, et al. Increased reporting of fatal immune checkpoint inhibitor-associated myocarditis. Lancet 2018;391(10124):933.

49. Mahmood SS, Fradley MG, Cohen JV, et al. Myocarditis in patients treated with immune checkpoint inhibitors. J Am Coll Cardiol 2018;71(16):1755–64.

50. Zhang L, Awadalla M, Mahmood SS, et al. Late gadolinium enhancement in patients with myocarditis from immune checkpoint inhibitors. J Am Coll Cardiol 2019;73(9 Supplement 1):675.

51. Ugander M, Oki AJ, Kellman P, et al. Myocardial extracellular volume imaging allows quantitative assessment of atypical late gadolinium enhancement. J Cardiovasc Magn Reson 2010;12(1):100.

52. Ugander M, Oki AJ, L H, et al. Myocardial extracellular volume imaging by CMR quantitatively characterizes myocardial infarction and subclinical myocardial fibrosis. J Cardiovasc Magn Reson 2011;13(1):148.

53. Flett AS, Hayward MP, Ashworth MT, et al. Equilibrium contrast cardiovascular magnetic resonance for the measurement of diffuse myocardial fibrosis: preliminary validation in humans. Circulation 2010;122(2):138–44.

54. Bandula S, White SK, Flett AS, et al. Measurement of myocardial extracellular volume fraction by using equilibrium contrast-enhanced CT: validation against histologic findings. Radiology 2013;269(2):396–403.

55. Fontana M, White SK, Banypersad SM, et al. Comparison of T1 mapping techniques for ECV quantification. Histological validation and reproducibility of ShMOLLI versus multibreath-hold T1 quantification equilibrium contrast CMR. J Cardiovasc Magn Reson 2012;14(1):88.

56. Broberg CS, Chugh SS, Conklin C, et al. Quantification of diffuse myocardial fibrosis and its association with myocardial dysfunction in congenital heart disease. Circ Cardiovasc Imaging 2010; 3(6):727–34.

57. Neilan TG, Coelho-Filho OR, Shah RV, et al. Myocardial extracellular volume by cardiac magnetic resonance imaging in patients treated with anthracycline-based chemotherapy. Am J Cardiol 2013;111(5):717–22.

58. Jordan JH, Vasu S, Morgan TM, et al. Anthracycline-associated T1 mapping characteristics are elevated independent of the presence of cardiovascular comorbidities in cancer survivors. Circ Cardiovasc Imaging 2016;9(8) [pii:e004325].

59. Melendez GC, Jordan JH, D'Agostino RB Jr, et al. Progressive 3-month increase in LV myocardial ECV after anthracycline-based chemotherapy. JACC Cardiovasc Imaging 2017;10(6): 708–9.

Cardiomyopathy Prevention in Cancer Patients

Tarek Barbar, MD[a], Syed S. Mahmood, MD, MPH[b], Jennifer E. Liu, MD[c,d],*

KEYWORDS

- Cardiomyopathy • Heart failure • Anthracyclines • Trastuzumab • Prevention strategies
- Neurohormonal blockades • Cardiovascular risk factors

KEY POINTS

- Cancer therapy–induced cardiomyopathy is a serious complication of cancer treatment, threatening to limit the tremendous gains in cancer survival achieved with modern cancer care.
- Several interventions have been identified to prevent cancer-induced cardiomyopathy.
- Anthracyclines is a major culprit, and prevention strategies with limiting cumulative dose, continuous infusion, dexrazoxane, and liposomal formulation have been shown to decrease the risk of cardiotoxicity.

BACKGROUND

Advances in cancer therapies have resulted in significant improvement in cancer-specific survival, transforming many once-fatal cancers into chronic diseases. Currently, there are more than 16 million cancer survivors in the United States,[1,2] and this number is expected to increase as early cancer screening improves, treatments advance, and the population ages. The accomplishment in cancer survival, however, is often offset by the cardiotoxicity associated with cancer treatment. Left ventricular systolic dysfunction (LVSD) and overt heart failure are well known manifestations of chemotherapy-induced cardiotoxicity. The development of LVSD is clinically significant because it can impact the delivery of lifesaving chemotherapy and increase the risk of developing heart failure, compromising quality of life and survival years after cure of the cancer. Understanding how to improve the prevention, recognition, and treatment of cancer therapy–related cardiac dysfunction has become an important priority. This article reviews the current strategies and best practices on primary prevention of cancer therapy–related cardiomyopathy before, during, and after cancer therapy.

CANCER AGENTS ASSOCIATED WITH CARDIOMYOPATHY

Cancer treatment–related cardiomyopathy is most commonly associated with anthracyclines and trastuzumab. Discovered in the 1960s, anthracyclines remain the cornerstone of contemporary cancer regimen for a variety of cancers. It is estimated that more than half of childhood cancer survivors have received prior anthracycline treatment.

Disclosures: S.S. Mahmood: Funding support New York Academy of Medicine's Glorney-Raisbeck Fellowship Award in Cardiovascular Diseases; consulting fees from Medicure, OMR Globus, Alpha Detail, and Opinion Research Team. The rest of the authors have nothing to disclose.

[a] Department of Medicine, New York Presbyterian Hospital, Weill Cornell Medical Center, 525 East 68th Street, New York, NY 10065, USA; [b] Cardiology Division, New York Presbyterian Hospital, Weill Cornell Medical Center, Starr Pavilion, 520 East 70th Street, 4th Fl, New York, NY 10021, USA; [c] Cardiology Service, Department of Medicine, Memorial Sloan Kettering Cancer Center, 1275 York Avenue, New York, NY 10065, USA; [d] Department of Medicine, Weill Cornell Medical College, New York, NY, USA
* Corresponding author. Cardiology Service, Department of Medicine, Memorial Sloan Kettering Cancer Center, 1275 York Avenue, New York, NY 10065.
E-mail address: liuj1234@mskcc.org

Cardiol Clin 37 (2019) 441–447
https://doi.org/10.1016/j.ccl.2019.07.009
0733-8651/19/© 2019 Elsevier Inc. All rights reserved.

The key mediator of anthracycline-induced cardiotoxicity is thought to be inhibition of topoisomerase 2b with mitochondrial dysfunction and oxidative stress, causing myocyte necrosis.[3] The spectrum of anthracycline cardiomyopathy ranges from asymptomatic decline in left ventricular ejection fraction (LVEF) to development of signs and symptoms of overt heart failure. It is typically a dilated cardiomyopathy with thinned left ventricular (LV) walls and abnormal systolic and diastolic indices, which, in pediatric survivors, can progress over time to a restrictive cardiomyopathy.[4] The most consistent risk factor for developing anthracycline-induced cardiomyopathy is cumulative dose with cardiac event rates of 7%, 18%, and 65% at 150 mg/m^2, 350 mg/m^2, and 550 mg/m^2, respectively.[5] Other risk factors include female gender, extreme age at treatment (<5 and >65 years old), baseline LV dysfunction, concomitant exposure to chest radiation and/or trastuzumab therapy, preexisting cardiovascular conditions, and possible genetic factors. Hypertension in particular has been shown to increase the risk by 7- to 12-fold in childhood and adult cancer survivors.[6] Most LV systolic dysfunction or heart failure occur within the first year after anthracycline therapy, but the elevated risk can persist over decades after cure of the cancer among the long-term cancer survivorship population.[7]

Human epidermal growth factor 2 (HER2) is a cell surface tyrosine kinase receptor overexpressed in 15% to 20% of primary invasive breast cancer and is associated with an aggressive cancer phenotype and poor clinical outcome. Trastuzumab, a humanized monoclonal antibody against the extracellular domain of HER2, has significantly improved the outcome of patients with HER2-positive breast cancer with 50% reduction in the 3-year recurrence of breast cancer and 33% reduction in the risk of death from breast cancer.[8,9] However, significant cardiotoxicity was noted in the pivotal trial of concurrent anthracycline and trastuzumab–based therapy for metastatic breast cancer. LV dysfunction was observed in 27% of patients and severe heart failure (New York Heart Association class III or IV) was observed in 16% of patients.[9] When trastuzumab was administered sequentially after completion of anthracyclines with implementation of surveillance cardiac monitoring during trastuzumab treatment, the incidence of LV dysfunction and severe heart failure decreased to 7% to 18% and 0.4% to 4.1%, respectively.[8,10] The risk of cardiotoxicity was further decreased when trastuzumab is administered without anthracyclines (3.2% asymptomatic LV dysfunction and 0.5% symptomatic heart failure).[11] The cardiotoxic mechanism of HER2-targeted therapies is not well understood. It has been shown in animal models that HER2 is involved in the signaling of cardiac development in embryos as well as providing protection against cardiotoxins.[12,13] When HER2 genes were knocked out in animal models, dilated cardiomyopathy was observed.[13] It is hypothesized that trastuzumab blocks HER2 signaling pathway in the heart, disabling myocardial cellular protective and repair mechanism, thereby compromising the stress response of the heart. In contrast to anthracycline-associated cardiotoxicity, LV dysfunction is largely reversible in most cases with interruption or discontinuation of trastuzumab therapy.[10]

PREVENTATIVE STRATEGIES

Successful prevention of cancer therapy–related cardiotoxicity requires a multidisciplinary approach that involves the collaboration between the treating oncologist/hematologist, internist, and cardiologist. Limited data from small studies are available to guide prevention strategies. The following approach is based on available evidence, good clinical judgment, and expert opinion.[14]

BEFORE TREATMENT

Consideration should be given to avoidance or modification of anthracycline chemotherapy if alternatives exist that would not compromise cancer-specific outcome, particularly in a patient at moderate or high risk. All patients planning to receive potentially cardiotoxic therapies should undergo comprehensive cardiovascular evaluation that includes a history and physical examination, assessment of cardiovascular risk factors, and an echocardiogram (echo) to assure adequate cardiac function before starting treatment. Cardiac MRI or multigated acquisition (MUGA) scan can also be used to assess LV systolic function if echo is inadequate or not available. Cardiovascular disease, hypertension, in particular, should be optimally managed. These recommendations are based on evidence from epidemiologic studies that pretreatment cardiovascular disease status and impaired or even low normal LVEF are important prognosticators of cardiac events in patients treated with anthracyclines.[15,16]

DURING TREATMENT

Several cardioprotective strategies have been used in preventing LV dysfunction during anthracycline-based therapy with varying levels of success.

Dexrazoxane

Dexrazoxane is the only Food and Drug Administration (FDA) -approved agent specifically to prevent anthracycline-induced cardiotoxicity. It is thought to chelate intracellular iron and disrupt doxorubicin-iron complex formation, thereby preventing oxygen free radical formation and inhibiting topoisomerase II beta isoenzyme.[17–19] In a meta-analysis of 10 randomized controlled trials, dexrazoxane showed a 5-fold decrease in risk of developing clinical heart failure when compared with placebo in the setting of anthracycline therapy.[20] Although much evidence supports the safety of dexrazoxane as a cardioprotectant, its effect on cancer-related cancer outcomes remains controversial with concerns that dexrazoxane might reduce antitumor response rates and increase the risk of secondary hematologic malignancies.[19] As a result, the FDA restricts its use to patients with metastatic or advanced breast cancer who have reached a cumulative anthracycline dose of greater than300 mg/m^2 and who are continuing to receiving doxorubicin.

Statins

Statins decrease inflammation and oxidative stress. It has been postulated that it might prevent anthracycline cardiotoxicity mediated in part by increased reactive oxygen species via its "pleotropic effects." A small trial of 20 patients randomized to prophylactic atorvastatin before anthracycline therapy showed no change in LVEF (61.3% $\pm$ 7.9% vs 62.6% $\pm$ 9.3%, P = .144), whereas patients in the control arm had a significant drop in LVEF (62.9% $\pm$ 7.0% vs 55.0% $\pm$ 9.5%, P<.0001) at 6 months of therapy.[21] In addition, a retrospective study of patients with breast cancer showed that incidental statin treatment was associated with significantly decreased risk of heart failure hospitalizations.[22] These initial results are promising, and 2 larger prospective randomized clinical trials, PREVENT and STOP-CA, are currently underway to investigate the efficacy of prophylactic statin therapy for the prevention of anthracycline-induced cardiomyopathy in patients with breast cancer and nonHodgkin's lymphoma.[23,24]

Dosing and Administration

Given that the risk of anthracycline-induced cardiomyopathy increases with increasing cumulative dose, the lifetime cumulative dose should be limited to 450 to 550 mg/m^2 or less to minimize cardiotoxicity, particularly among high-risk patients. Higher doses may be considered on an individualized basis for patients with limited options who have not developed signs of cardiotoxicity. Such cases would constitute high risk and should be monitored closely for signs of cardiotoxicity during and after treatment. Infusional rather than bolus dosing of anthracycline has been used as a cardioprotective strategy. Peak anthracycline plasma level correlates with the risk of developing cardiotoxicity. Longer infusion durations lead to lower anthracycline plasma level and have been associated with reduced risk of heart failure and subclinical cardiotoxicity compared with bolus regimens. Studies have shown prolonging infusion times over 48 to 96 hours resulted in less myocardial injury on endomyocardial biopsy than administering the medication as boluses.[25] The efficacy of the treatment was similar whether by continuous infusion or bolus administration.[26] However, despite having less cardiotoxicity, longer duration infusions remain controversial given the increased risk of extravasation and tissue necrosis.

Liposomal formulation of doxorubicin is available to reduce cardiotoxicity. Compared with conventional doxorubicin, liposomal doxorubicin is associated with lower incidence of both asymptomatic and symptomatic cardiomyopathy (odds ratio = 0.46; 95% confidence interval, 0.23–0.92; P = .03) without compromise of the antitumor efficacy.[27] These drugs preferentially accumulate in the cancer tissue because of the frail microvasculature of the tumor, while the vessel permeability with tight capillary junctions of the myocardium prevents the extravasation of the encapsulated liposome into the cardiomyocytes. Most studies with liposomal doxorubicin have included patients with advanced cancer, predominantly breast cancer. As such, no conclusion on the effect of treatment between liposomal doxorubicin and conventional doxorubicin can be drawn for patients receiving treatment in the setting of curative intent. Routine use of liposomal doxorubicin is limited by the increased risk of hand-foot syndrome and higher cost.

Neurohormonal Antagonist

There has been much interest in assessing the efficacy of neurohormonal blockade in preventing cancer therapy–induced cardiomyopathy given the established benefit of such treatment in patients with systolic heart failure. Beta-blockade, angiotensin-converting enzyme inhibitor, and angiotensin receptor blockers have been evaluated in randomized control trials for the prevention of anthracycline and trastuzumab–induced cardiomyopathy (**Table 1**). Several of these studies

Table 1
Summary of randomized controlled trials using angiotensin-converting enzyme inhibitor, angiotensin receptor blocker, and beta-blockade to prevent anthracycline and/or trastuzumab induced cardiotoxicity

Trial Name Study Population	Cancer Treatment	Intervention Study Design	Results
OVERCOME Study[28] N = 90	High-dose chemotherapy (anthracyclines) (80%)	1:1 enalapril and carvedilol combined vs placebo	LVEF unchanged with enalapril + carvedilol vs ↓3.1% (echo) and ↓3.4% (CMR) with control
Cardinale et al,[29] 2006 N = 473	High-dose chemotherapy (anthracyclines mean dose 332–338 mg/m^2)	1:1 enalapril vs no enalapril	LVEF unchanged with enalapril vs ↓ 9.7% control (echo)
PRADA[30] N = 130	All epirubicin; 22% trastuzumab	2 × 2 metoprolol and candesartan	LVEF ↓ 0.8% with candesartan vs 2.6% with placebo (CMR)
MANTICORE[31] N = 94	All trastuzumab; 33% anthracycline	1:1:1 bisoprolol, perindopril, placebo	LVEF ↓1% with bisoprolol vs 3% w/perindopril vs 5% with placebo (CMR)
CECCY[32] N = 200	All doxorubicin	1:1 carvedilol and placebo	No difference in LVEF decline >10% (13.5% vs 14.5%) (echo)
USF study[33] N = 486	All trastuzumab; 40% anthracycline	1:1:1 carvedilol, lisinopril, placebo	No difference in LVEF decline >10% (30% lisinopril vs 29% carvedilol vs 32% placebo) (echo) Subgroup analysis of patients treated with anthracycline and trastuzumab: LVEF decline >10% (37% lisinopril vs 31% carvedilol vs 47% placebo)

Abbreviation: CMR, cardiac magnetic resonance imaging.

suggest that prophylactic treatment with neurohormonal blockade attenuated LVEF decline but were not adequately powered to detect a difference in clinical heart failure events and have used surrogate endpoints, such as a change in LVEF. Furthermore, the clinical significance of the modest attenuation in LVEF decline is uncertain. These trials involve administration of cardioprotective medication to all patients receiving cancer therapy. This nonselective treatment approach necessitates overtreatment because only a minority of patients will develop cardiotoxicity, which can dilute the cardioprotective effect and may be missed in small trials. There are 2 ongoing trials with study design targeting treatment among selected high-risk patients with

imaging or biomarker-based evidence of subclinical LV dysfunction. The SUCCOUR study is an ongoing international prospective randomized clinical trial assessing if echo strain imaging-guided use of ACE inhibitors and beta-blockers will limit the development of reduced LVEF in patients receiving potentially cardiotoxic therapy.[34] The ICOS ONE study is another ongoing multicenter study randomizing patients to 1 of 2 treatment arms: enalapril started concomitantly with anthracycline versus selective administration of enalapril in patients with elevated troponin.[35] The objective of the study is to investigate whether the strategy of administering enalapril to all patients is more effective in preventing cardiotoxicity than enalapril administered only to patients with an increase in troponin during or after anthracycline therapy. The primary endpoint is the incidence of the troponin elevation above the laboratory threshold at any time during the study up to 1 year. The results of these prospective randomized studies will contribute to informing therapeutic strategies, although more multicenter randomized trials are needed to conclusively assess the efficacy of prophylactic neurohormonal blockade for prevention of cancer therapy–induced cardiomyopathy. At the present time, there are insufficient data to support routine administration of neurohormonal antagonist for all patients, but it may be appropriate for selected high-risk patients receiving potentially cardiotoxic therapy.

Exercise Strategy

It is well established that cardiorespiratory fitness (CRF) is a strong prognostic factor for cardiovascular and all-cause mortality. Among more than 4000 participants in the Women's Health Study followed for a median of nearly 13 years, participants who were able to complete ≥9 metabolic equivalent of task (METS) of activity per week had a 27% reduction in cardiovascular events compared with those who were only able to perform less than 9 METS of exercise.[36] Low CRF in patients with cancer is associated with treatment-related toxicities and increased risk of all-cause and cancer-specific mortality, and exercise training after the completion of adjuvant therapy has been shown to significantly increase CRF compared with standard care.[37] In addition, observational data have indicated that both physical activity and structured exercise may be associated with enhanced response to standard anticancer therapy.[38] As such, recommendations are now being made on the use of cardiac rehabilitation to provide structured exercise to patients with cancer and survivors.[39] However, the role of exercise therapy for prevention of cancer therapy–induced cardiomyopathy during and after cancer therapy remains uncertain.

AFTER TREATMENT

Cancer survivors who were treated with prior anthracycline chemotherapy or chest-directed radiotherapy are at increased risk of developing cardiomyopathy years after treatment. Among adult survivors of childhood cancer, the development of traditional cardiovascular risk factors, such as hypertension, dyslipidemia, obesity, and diabetes, increase risk for heart failure in a multiplicative fashion, at a risk higher than the simple addition of another risk factor.[6] This occurrence suggests that survivors who were treated with cardiotoxic agents at a young age have decreased cardiac reserve and are particularly vulnerable to further myocardial injury. Thus, a heart-healthy lifestyle is incredibly important for survivors to prevent or mitigate the risk of developing cardiomyopathy. Prevention, diagnosis, and aggressive management of modifiable risk factors need to be a high priority in the survivorship care plan. Routine imaging surveillance has not been incorporated into standard practice. The American Society of Clinical Oncology guideline recommends consideration of a single echo between 6 and 12 months after completion of treatment in adult cancer survivors considered to be at high risk for cardiac dysfunction, diligent clinical assessment, and follow-up testing dictated by patient risk profile and clinical suspicion,[14] whereas the Children Oncology Group long-term follow-up guideline recommends lifetime echo or MUGA surveillance of late effects for survivors of childhood cancer based on age of exposure, cumulative anthracycline dose, and radiation therapy with cardiac involvement.

SUMMARY

Cancer therapy–induced cardiomyopathy is a serious complication of cancer treatment, threatening to limit the tremendous gains in cancer survival achieved with modern cancer care. Several interventions have been identified to prevent cancer-induced cardiomyopathy. Anthracyclines is a major culprit, and prevention strategies with limiting cumulative dose, continuous infusion, dexrazoxane, and liposomal formulation have been shown to decrease the risk of cardiotoxicity. Concurrent administration of neurohormonal blockade with anthracycline treatment has demonstrated a significant but modest attenuation of LVEF decline, although the clinical significance of such observation remains uncertain. Currently, there are insufficient data to recommend prophylactic neurohormonal antagonists in all patients receiving potentially cardiotoxic therapy, but selected high-risk patients may benefit from prophylactic treatment. Identifying effective preventive/therapeutic strategies is an ongoing area of active investigation with multiple randomized trials underway that it is hoped will inform best practice approach and improve patient outcome.

REFERENCES

1. Bluethmann SM, Mariotto AB, Rowland JH. Anticipating the "silver tsunami": prevalence trajectories and comorbidity burden among older cancer survivors in the United States. Cancer Epidemiol Biomarkers Prev 2016;25:1029–36.

2. National Cancer Institute at the National Institutes of Health: Surveillance, Epidemiology and End Results Program, U.S. Department of Health and Human Services. Reports on cancer: cancer stat facts. Available at: https://seer.cancer.gov/statfacts/html/all.html. Accessed April 16, 2019.

3. Zhang S, Liu X, Bawa-Khalfe T, et al. Identification of the molecular basis of doxorubicin-induced cardiotoxicity. Nat Med 2012;18(11):1639.

4. Lipshultz SE, Lipsitz SR, Sallan SE, et al. Chronic progressive cardiac dysfunction years after doxorubicin therapy for childhood acute lymphoblastic leukemia. J Clin Oncol 2005;23(12):2629–36.

5. Swain SM, Whaley FS, Ewer MS. Congestive heart failure in patients treated with doxorubicin: a retrospective analysis of three trials. Cancer 2003; 97(11):2869–79.

6. Armstrong GT, Oeffinger KC, Chen Y, et al. Modifiable risk factors and major cardiac events among adult survivors of childhood cancer. J Clin Oncol 2013;31(29):3673.

7. Cardinale D, Colombo A, Bacchiani G, et al. Early detection of anthracycline cardiotoxicity and improvement with heart failure therapy. Circulation 2015;131(22):1981–8.

8. Romond EH, Perez EA, Bryant J, et al. Trastuzumab plus adjuvant chemotherapy for operable HER2-positive breast cancer. N Engl J Med 2005; 353(16):1673–84.

9. Slamon DJ, Leyland-Jones B, Shak S, et al. Use of chemotherapy plus a monoclonal antibody against HER2 for metastatic breast cancer that overexpresses HER2. N Engl J Med 2001;344(11):783–92.

10. Slamon D, Eiermann W, Robert N, et al. Adjuvant trastuzumab in HER2-positive breast cancer. N Engl J Med 2011;365(14):1273–83.

11. Tolaney SM, Barry WT, Dang CT, et al. Adjuvant paclitaxel and trastuzumab for node-negative, HER2-positive breast cancer. N Engl J Med 2015; 372(2):134–41.

12. Erickson SL, O'Shea KS, Ghaboosi N, et al. ErbB3 is required for normal cerebellar and cardiac development: a comparison with ErbB2-and heregulin-deficient mice. Development 1997;124:4999.

13. Crone SA, Zhao YY, Fan L, et al. ErbB2 is essential in the prevention of dilated cardiomyopathy. Nat Med 2002;8:459.

14. Armenian SH, Lacchetti C, Barac A, et al. Prevention and monitoring of cardiac dysfunction in survivors of adult cancers: American Society of Clinical Oncology clinical practice guideline. J Clin Oncol 2016;35(8):893–911.

15. Romond EH, Jeong JH, Rastogi P, et al. Seven-year follow-up assessment of cardiac function in NSABP B-31, a randomized trial comparing doxorubicin and cyclophosphamide followed by paclitaxel (ACP) with ACP plus trastuzumab as adjuvant therapy for patients with node-positive, human epidermal growth factor receptor 2–positive breast cancer. J Clin Oncol 2012;30(31):3792.

16. Hershman DL, Till C, Shen S, et al. Association of cardiovascular risk factors with cardiac events and survival outcomes among patients with breast cancer enrolled in SWOG clinical trials. J Clin Oncol 2018;36(26):2710–7.

17. Ichikawa Y, Ghanefar M, Bayeva M, et al. Cardiotoxicity of doxorubicin is mediated through mitochondrial iron accumulation. J Clin Invest 2014;124(2): 617–30.

18. Lyu YL, Kerrigan JE, Lin CP, et al. Topoisomerase IIβ–mediated DNA double-strand breaks: implications in doxorubicin cardiotoxicity and prevention by dexrazoxane. Cancer Res 2007;67(18):8839–46.

19. Ganatra S, Nohria A, Shah S, et al. Upfront dexrazoxane for the reduction of anthracycline-induced cardiotoxicity in adults with preexisting cardiomyopathy and cancer: a consecutive case series. Cardio Oncol 2019;5(1):1.

20. Van Dalen EC, Caron HN, Dickinson HO, et al. Cardioprotective interventions for cancer patients receiving anthracyclines. Cochrane Database Syst Rev 2011;(6):CD003917.

21. Acar Z, Kale A, Turgut M, et al. Efficiency of atorvastatin in the protection of anthracycline-induced cardiomyopathy. J Am Coll Cardiol 2011;58(9):988–9.

22. Seicean S, Seicean A, Plana JC, et al. Effect of statin therapy on the risk for incident heart failure in patients with breast cancer receiving anthracycline chemotherapy: an observational clinical cohort study. J Am Coll Cardiol 2012;60(23):2384–90.

23. Preventing anthracycline cardiovascular toxicity with statins (PREVENT). 2013 (ClinicalTrials.gov Identifier: NCT01988571). Available at: https://clinicaltrials.gov/ct2/show/NCT01988571. Accessed April 22, 2019.

24. Statins to prevent the cardiotoxicity from anthracyclines (STOP-CA). 2016. ClinicalTrials.gov Identifier: NCT02943590). Available at: https://clinicaltrials.gov/ct2/show/NCT02943590. Accessed May 11, 2019.

25. Valdivieso M, Burgess MA, Ewer MS, et al. Increased therapeutic index of weekly doxorubicin in the therapy of non-small cell lung cancer: a prospective, randomized study. J Clin Oncol 1984;2: 207–14.

26. Pacciarini MA, Barbieri B, Colombo T, et al. Distribution and antitumor activity of adriamycin given in a high-dose and a repeated low-dose schedule to mice. Cancer Treat Rep 1978;62:791–800.

27. Gabizon AA. Stealth liposomes and tumor targeting: one step further in the quest for the magic bullet. Clin Cancer Res 2001;7:223–5.

28. Bosch X, Rovira M, Sitges M, et al. Enalapril and carvedilol for preventing chemotherapy-induced left

ventricular systolic dysfunction in patients with malignant hemopathies: the OVERCOME trial (prevenтiOn of left Ventricular dysfunction with Enalapril and caRvedilol in patients submitted to intensive ChemOtherapy for the treatment of Malignant hEmopathies). J Am Coll Cardiol 2013;61(23):2355–62.

29. Cardinale D, Colombo A, Sandri MT, et al. Prevention of high-dose chemotherapy–induced cardiotoxicity in high-risk patients by angiotensin-converting enzyme inhibition. Circulation 2006;114:2474–81.

30. Gulati G, Heck SL, Ree AH, et al. Prevention of cardiac dysfunction during adjuvant breast cancer therapy (PRADA): a 2 × 2 factorial, randomized, placebo-controlled, double-blind clinical trial of candesartan and metoprolol. Eur Heart J 2016;37:1671.

31. Pituskin E, Mackey JR, Koshman S, et al. Multidisciplinary approach to novel therapies in cardiooncology research (MANTICORE 101–Breast): a randomized trial for the prevention of trastuzumab-associated cardiotoxicity. J Clin Oncol 2016;35(8): 870–7.

32. Avila MS, Ayub-Ferreira SM, de Barros Wanderley MR, et al. Carvedilol for prevention of chemotherapy-related cardiotoxicity: the CECCY trial. J Am Coll Cardiol 2018;71(20):2281–90.

33. Guglin M, Munster P, Fink A, et al. Lisinopril or Coreg CR in reducing cardiotoxicity in women with breast cancer receiving trastuzumab: a rationale and design of a randomized clinical trial. Am Heart J 2017;188:87–92.

34. Negishi T, Thavendiranathan P, Negishi K, et al. Rationale and design of the strain surveillance of chemotherapy for improving cardiovascular outcomes: the SUCCOUR trial. JACC Cardiovasc Imaging 2018;11(8):1098–105.

35. Cardinale D, Ciceri F, Latini R, et al. Anthracycline-induced cardiotoxicity: a multicenter randomised trial comparing two strategies for guiding prevention with enalapril: the International CardioOncology Society-one trial. Eur J Cancer 2018;94: 126–37.

36. Palomo A, Ray RM, Johnson L, et al. Associations between exercise prior to and around the time of cancer diagnosis and subsequent cardiovascular events in women with breast cancer: a Women's Health Initiative (WHI) analysis. J Am Coll Cardiol 2017;69(11 Supplement):1774.

37. Scott JM, Zabor EC, Schwitzer E, et al. Efficacy of exercise therapy on cardiorespiratory fitness in patients with cancer: a systematic review and meta-analysis. J Clin Oncol 2018;36(22):2297–305.

38. Ashcraft KA, Warner AB, Jones LW, et al. Exercise as adjunct therapy in cancer. Semin Radiat Oncol 2019;29(1):16–24. WB Saunders.

39. Gilchrist SC, Barac A, Ades PA, et al. Cardio-oncology rehabilitation to manage cardiovascular outcomes in cancer patients and survivors: a scientific statement from the American Heart Association. Circulation 2019;139(21):e997–1012.

Cardiotoxicity Related to Radiation Therapy

Sana Shoukat, MD[a], Danyi Zheng, MD[a], Syed Wamique Yusuf, MD[b],*

KEYWORDS

- Cardiotoxicity • Radiation • Therapy

KEY POINTS

- With increasing survival from cancer, the incidence of cardiovascular diseases is increasing as a chronic side effect of radiation therapy.
- Prevention, early recognition, and prompt intervention should be the major focus in the care of these patients.

INTRODUCTION

In recent decades, cancer treatment modalities have advanced significantly, with radiation therapy (RT) becoming an essential aspect of treatment of many malignancies, including lung, breast, and head and neck.[1,2] One-half of the patients who are diagnosed with cancer would undergo RT as neoadjuvant or adjuvant treatment.[1,2] With improvement in cancer treatment, patients are living longer. In 2016, there were an estimated 15.5 million cancer survivors in the United States. This number of cancer survivors is expected to increase to 20.3 million by 2026.[3] Among patients suffering from malignancy and survivors of Hodgkin lymphoma, who have received RT, cardiovascular disease is one the most common causes of non–cancer-related death[4,5]

RT is thought to cause microvascular changes and promote inflammation leading to endothelial dysfunction and acceleration of the atherosclerotic process in the coronary vessels.[5–9] The long-term side effects manifest as coronary artery disease (CAD), valvular disease, conduction system defects, and diseases involving the pericardium and myocardium.[10,11] The extent of cardiac effects and risk of developing cardiovascular disease seem to be directly related to the amount of radiation received and proximity of the heart to the field of exposure.[12–15]

This review outlines the pathophysiologic processes related to RT and its possible clinical effects on the cardiovascular system. With improved survival rate among patients with cancer, it is important to understand the chronic complications of RT on the cardiovascular system because early detection and prompt treatment are crucial for the care of cancer survivors.

EPIDEMIOLOGY AND DISEASE BURDEN

Risk Factors for Radiation-Induced Cardiovascular Disease

Studies suggest that the cumulative dose of radiation, number of treatments, high daily fraction dose, cardiac volume exposed to radiation, and location of radiation/tumor (anterior or left sided) play key roles in the development of radiation-induced cardiovascular diseases (RICVD).[14–19] Significant clinical damage to the heart was seen with radiation doses of greater than 30 Gy.[17] A decrease in the incidence of pericarditis from 20.0% to 2.5% was observed in patients with a radiation dose of less than 30 Gy and cardiac shielding.[17] In patients with breast cancer, younger age (<35 years old) at the time of RT seems to be associated with increased risk of developing RICAD.[18]

Disclosure: None.
[a] University of Texas Health Science Center at Houston, 6410 Fannin Street, Houston, TX 77030, USA;
[b] University of Texas MD Anderson Cancer Center, 1515 Holcombe Boulevard, Houston, TX 77030, USA
* Corresponding author.
E-mail address: syusuf@mdanderson.org

In addition, the presence of traditional risk factors, including smoking, diabetes, hyperlipidemia, hypertension, and obesity, may influence the overall risk of developing RICVD (**Table 1**).

PATHOPHYSIOLOGY

There are several proposed mechanisms as to how RT can lead to the development of cardiovascular diseases in its recipients. The endothelium damage is the key initial component, with atherosclerosis as the end result of chronic inflammation of endothelial vessels. The inflammatory process leads to the release of a large array of cytokines that, in turn, activate and attract circulating monocytes to enter endothelial walls. The activated macrophages ingest lipoproteins and subsequently lead to the formation of atherosclerotic plaques.[22,23] Radiation is thought to stimulate and accelerate this atherogenic process.[22,24,25] This phenomenon is likely the basis of increased incidence of cardiovascular disease in survivors of the Hiroshima and Nagasaki atomic bombings.[26] Radiation promotes atherosclerosis in animal models who were fed with a high-fat, diet suggesting that cardiovascular risk factors are contributing constituents for RICVD.[27] Cytokine-mediated inflammatory processes are also seen in patients receiving RT. Altogether, the release of cytokines such as tumor necrosis factor, IL-1, IL-6, IL-8, platelet-derived growth factor, and transforming growth factor-β1 lead to a chronic process of collagen deposition and fibrosis. In addition, radiation creates a state of oxidative stress, which leads to activation of nuclear factor-κB. Persistent elevation of nuclear factor-κB in postirradiated tissues promote fibrotic changes by upregulating proinflammatory cytokines and adhesive modules, which in turn activates an inflammatory process.[6,28] **Fig. 1** shows the proposed mechanisms of RICVD.

TYPE OF CARDIOVASCULAR DISEASE
Coronary Artery Disease

Clinical symptoms and signs of RICVD include chest pain, dyspnea, heart failure, syncope, and rarely sudden death.[29,30] Radiation accelerates the atherosclerotic process by inducing endothelial dysfunction in the coronary vessels, eventually leading to plaque formation.[31]

In a study of patients with esophageal cancer, Gayed and colleagues[14] reported that the myocardial perfusion imaging (MPI) defects in the inferior segments were more prevalent in the RT group (14 patients [54%]) than the NRT group (4 patients [16%]; $P = .001$). In the RT group, the majority of myocardial perfusion defects (70%) were encompassed by RT isodose lines of greater than 45 Gy. This finding likely reflects the proximity of the heart to the location of irradiated cancer and suggests that toxicity is directly associated with the radiation dose as well as the extent of myocardium involved during treatment.[14]

Another study by Gayed and colleagues[15] looked at the development of perfusion defects

Table 1
Summary of studies demonstrating ischemic heart disease related to RT

Study	Patient Population/Cancer Type	Outcome
Gayed et al,[14] 2006	Esophagus	Higher prevalence of inferior segment ischemia after RT.
Gayed et al,[15] 2009	Lung	Perfusion abnormality mostly involving Anterior/anteroseptal wall after RT. Higher incidence of perfusion abnormalities after RT in centrally located lung cancer.
Van Nimwegen et al,[20] 2015	Hodgkin lymphoma	Survivors treated with mediastinal RT had increased risk for any cardiovascular events compared with general population. Higher risk of coronary artery disease was associated with treatment at younger age.
Marks et al,[21] 2005	Left-sided breast cancer	New myocardial perfusions and wall motion abnormality seen in 40% of patients after RT, mostly involving anterior segments of the LV.
Hancock et al,[17] 1993	Hodgkin lymphoma	Mediastinal radiation of 40–45 Gy increased the risk of death from coronary artery disease.

Abbreviations: CAD, coronary artery disease; LV, left ventricle.

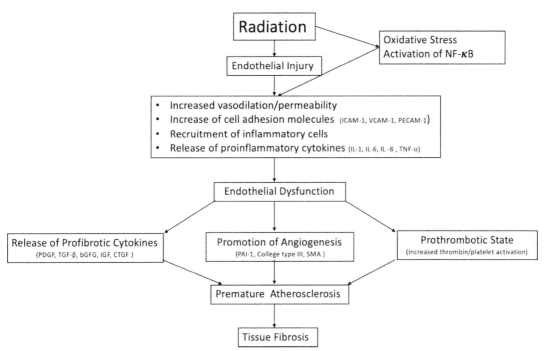

Fig. 1. Proposed pathogenetic mechanisms of RICVD. bFGF, basic fibroblast growth factor; CTGF, connective tissue growth factor; ICAM-1, intercellular adhesion molecule 1; IGF, insulin-like growth factor; PAI, plasminogen activator inhibitor; PECAM-1, platelet endothelial cell adhesion molecule; PGDF, platelet-derived growth factor; SMA, smooth muscle actin; TGF-β, transforming growth factor β; VCAM-1, vascular cell adhesion molecule 1.

after chemoradiation (CRT)/RT in patients with lung cancer. CRT/RT and control groups had similar baseline risk factors. In patients with centrally located tumors, MPI defects were found in 7 of 18 patients (39%) in CRT/RT group versus 1 of 15 patients (7%) in the control group (*P* = .04). Most of the perfusion abnormalities in the CRT/RT group involved the anterior/anteroseptal and septal wall of the left ventricle (LV). Segments with perfusion defect in CRT/RT received a mean radiation dose of 39 Gy. The average time between end of therapy and MPI defects was about 1 year.

A prospective study was conducted by Marks and colleagues[21] to evaluate potential RT-induced cardiotoxicity in 114 patients with left-sided breast cancer. Patients were treated with a total dose of 45 to 50 Gy to the breast or chest wall. LV regional myocardial perfusion, regional wall motion abnormalities, and LV ejection fraction were assessed via single photon emission computed tomography (SPECT) MPI scans at 6, 12, 18, and 24 months after radiation exposure. Forty percent of patients had new MPI defects within 2 years after RT and it directly correlated with volume of LV exposed to RT field.

Van Nimwegen and colleagues[32] examined the relative and absolute risks for cardiovascular diseases in survivors of Hodgkin lymphoma treated with mediastinal RT (MRT) and/or chemotherapy up to 40 years. The incidence was compared with that of the general population. The retrospective study consisted of 2524 patients treated from 1965 to 1995 who survived for 5 years after initial diagnosis. Among these patients, 2052 (81.3%) received MRT and 773 (30.6%) received chemotherapy. There were 1713 cardiovascular events occurred in 797 patients. CAD, valvular heart disease, and heart failure were the 3 most common diseases. In these cancer survivors, the risk of CAD was 3 times higher than the general population. The risk was higher in patients who were treated at a younger age (<25 years of age). The 40-year cumulative risk of any cardiovascular disease for patients treated with mediastinal radiotherapy was 54.6% (95% confidence interval [CI], 51.2%-57.9%) compared with 24.7% (95% CI, 17.2%-32.9%) in patients without any treatments. The risk for the first CAD postmediastinal radiotherapy was significantly higher after 20 to 47 years of follow-up than in the 5- to 20-year follow-up period.

Hancock and colleagues[17] also showed that mediastinal irradiation for Hodgkin disease increased the risk of subsequent death from heart disease. In a retrospective study with 9.5 years of follow-up, including 2232 patients, 88 (3.9%) died of heart disease, 55 from acute myocardial infarction, and 33 from other cardiac diseases, including congestive heart failure, radiation pericarditis or pancarditis, cardiomyopathy, or valvular heart disease. The risk for acute myocardial infarction was highest after irradiation before 20 years of age (**Box 1**).

Valvular Diseases

Radiation-induced valvular disease is a common latent side effect of MRT. The disease typically manifests years after exposure and the risk progressively increases over time. A study by Hull and colleagues[33] demonstrated that the incidence of valvular disease was 1% at 10 years, 4% at 15 years, and 6% at 20 years after the completion of treatment. Compared with patients who were 10 years post MRT, the incidences of valvular dysfunctions were found to be higher in those who received MRT more than 20 years ago: aortic regurgitation (60 vs 4%; $P<.0001$), tricuspid regurgitation (4 vs 0%; $P = .06$), and aortic stenosis (16 vs 0%; $P = .0008$).[34] Among asymptomatic patients, aortic regurgitation is the commonest valvular dysfunction.[35] According to a review analysis of several clinical studies, the prevalence of valvular disease was found in between 2% and 37% of patients with Hodgkin lymphoma who received MRT.[35] The risk of developing valvular dysfunction increased proportionately with the radiation dose. A study with 1852 Hodgkin lymphoma survivors showed a positive correlation between the rate of developing valvular disease and doses to the affected valve ($P<.001$).[36] An autopsy study of valves from patients who received MRT showed that about 71% of patients (12/17) had valvular diseases with diffuse fibrosis with and without calcifications.[37] The working hypothesis was that radiation led to the activation and upregulation transforming growth factor-ß, fibroblasts, and myofibroblasts resulting in increased collagen synthesis and

deposition in the extracellular matrix. In addition, radiation induced an osteogenic phenotype with increased production of osteogenic factors, alkaline phosphatase, Runx2, and osteopontin resulting in calcification of valves in the field of radiation.[38,39] Echocardiography remains the most common modality to evaluate valvular dysfunction.[40] Early findings can include diffuse thickening of leaflets with normal or unchanged functions. Calcification of valves tends to happen in the later stage with left-sided valves, such as the aortic and mitral valves, as well as the mitral–aortic curtain, being affected predominantly.[34,41,42] The left side of the heart is more commonly affected after MRT, with the aortic valve being the most commonly involved.[43]

Pericardial Disease

RT-induced pericardial disease is a common complication of MRT, and includes acute pericarditis, chronic pericardial effusion, and constrictive pericarditis. An autopsy report examining pericardial specimens found that 70% of patients had pericardial disease.[37] Post-MRT pericardial disease is thought to be caused by the inflammatory process and fibrin deposition.[44–47] Initially driven by microvascular damages to the pericardium, neovascularization further causes ischemia and fibrosis. These changes also impair venous and lymphatic system function, leading to the accumulation of exudative fluid in the pericardial sac. Several studies have suggested that the incidence of RT-induced pericardial disease was related to the dose and volume of pericardium involved. In a study including 635 patients with Hodgkin lymphoma from 1961 to 1991, most patients with severe pericardial disease after RT received treatment before the introduction of subcarinal blocking.[48] Using subcarinal blocking led to a decrease in the incidence of acute pericarditis or pericardial effusion from 20% to 7.5% during the post-treatment follow-up period.[49]

Acute pericarditis usually happens during or soon after RT, with clinical symptoms and signs of chest pain and fever; however, electrocardiography may not show the classic findings of pericarditis.[45] Regardless, treatment remains the same as non–MRT-induced acute pericarditis with nonsteroidal anti-inflammatory drugs and colchicine. Acute pericarditis may progress to the development of pericardial effusion, which typically occur months or even years after MRT. One study report that the median time frame for developing pericardial effusion in patients with esophageal cancer treated with MRT was 5.3 months with time range between 1 to 17 months.[50] The risk of developing pericardial effusion increases with greater than

---

Box 1
Risk factors for developing heart disease after RT

- Cumulative radiation dose (>30 Gy)
- Cardiac volume exposed to radiation and tumor location
- Younger age at the time of RT
- Preexisting cardiovascular disease or risk factors
- No shielding or blocking during RT

30 Gy of radiation and a radiation field width of the mediastinum exceeding 8 cm.[50,51] Patients may be completely asymptomatic or may present with shortness of breath, chest discomfort, elevated jugular venous pulsations, and hypotension.[45,52] Echocardiogram is used to diagnose pericardial effusion, evaluate its extent, and rule out emergencies such as cardiac tamponade. Pericardial effusions can be self-limiting and may not warrant any additional intervention. However, if the effusion is large enough to cause symptoms or cardiac tamponade, then pericardiocentesis or pericardial window will be required to drain the fluid.

Constrictive pericarditis is the result of chronic inflammatory changes and fibrosis of pericardium.[53] It typically manifests months to years after the completion of RT. Hemodynamic and echocardiographic features of constrictive pericarditis are listed in **Table 2**. In a study of 86 patients treated with MRT for Hodgkin lymphoma, 7% developed constrictive pericarditis with medium time frame being 15 months, ranging from 3 months to 3 years.[5] The incidence of developing constrictive pericardium was associated with delivery technique (ortho-voltage) and total dose of radiation to the pericardium. Clinical features include symptoms and signs of congestive heart failure. Aside from medical management of symptoms, pericardiotomy is the definitive treatment.[54] After pericardiectomy, the long-term survival depends on the etiology and preexisting comorbidities. Patients with postradiation constrictive pericarditis were found to have worse survival rate after pericardiotomy with a 7-year survival rate of 27%.[54] Overall, the development of constrictive pericarditis after MRT is associated with a poor prognosis and a high mortality rate.[54,55]

Dysfunction of the Conducting System

Radiation-induced conduction abnormalities are less common. The underlying mechanism is likely related to myocardial fibrosis and ischemia or direct damage to the sinoatrial or atrioventricular nodes by radiation. Right bundle branch block is a common clinical finding seen in patients after MRT owing to the close proximity of the right bundle to the myocardium and fibrotic lesions as result of radiation.[56,57] Complete atrioventricular block requiring a permanent pacemaker has been reported in patients treated with MRT.[57,58] These patients also have other RT-related cardiac injuries, such as CAD, valvular dysfunction, and pericardial disease.[57] In general, patients with complete atrioventricular block related to RT received a total dose of radiation of more than 40 Gy, presented with late onset of disease (>10 years after RT), bundle branch block as part of electrocardiogram findings, and had other cardiac injuries, especially pericardial disease.[59] Among childhood cancer survivors who receive RT, persistent sinus tachycardia is present, suggesting possible autonomic dysfunction after MRT.[56,60] In patients with breast cancer receiving trastuzumab, left side RT was associated with significantly higher incidence of arrhythmia compared with the right side: 14.2% versus 1% (P<.001).[61]

Table 2
Features of RT induced constrictive pericarditis when compared with restrictive cardiomyopathy

	RT-Induced Constrictive Pericarditis	Restrictive Cardiomyopathy
Clinical examination	Pericardial knock present Signs of heart failure	Pericardial knock absent Signs of heart failure
Echocardiographic features	Increased pericardial thickness Pericardial calcification Pericardial effusion Ventricular interdependence Respiratory variation >25% in mitral inflow Diastolic flow reversal in hepatic vein on expiration Normal/increased mitral annulus medial e' velocity	Increased wall thickness Biatrial enlargement Systolic and diastolic dysfunction Elevated pulmonary artery systolic pressure Decreased mitral annulus medial e' velocity
Invasive hemodynamics	Discordant respirophasic ventricular pressure changes LVEDP – RVEDP <5 mm Hg	Concordant respirophasic ventricular pressure changes LVEDP – RVEDP >5 mm Hg

Abbreviations: LVEDP, left ventricular end-diastolic pressure; RVEDP, right ventricular end-diastolic pressure.

Cardiomyopathy

RT to the mediastinum can cause myocardial fibrosis, which may eventually lead to cardiomyopathy and heart failure years after treatment. In an autopsy report of 27 patients, about 63% of the patients with available samples were found to have myocardial fibrosis.[37] Perivascular and pericellular fibrosis were the predominant patterns. The findings were likely the end results of microischemia caused by damages and loss of capillaries and myocytes subsequently.[37] RT also increases the concentration of collagen deposition, particularly type I, which is associated with impaired diastolic distensibility.[62] Collagen content plays an important role in the integrity and elasticity of the myocardium, suggesting that this change in its composition may lead to myocardium dysfunction.[62] In a cohort study of 1362 survivors of childhood cancer diagnosed between 1966 and 1996 who had received anthracyclines only, cardiac RT only, or combination therapy, congestive heart failure was the most common complication, with a 30-year overall risk of 2.7% (95% CI, 1.6–3.8).[63] Survivors treated with anthracyclines and RT were at the highest risk for developing cardiac events.[63] In a study of 229 patients after RT and anthracycline treatments, the risk for heart failure at 20 years was 18% (95% CI, 10%–34%) in those who received an average radiation dose of greater than 3.7 Gy.[64] In a case-control study including 2617 5-year survivors of Hodgkin lymphoma diagnosed before age 51 years from 1965 to 1995, it was found that the risk of heart failure increases significantly with the radiation dose.[65] In particular, the risk increases steeply as the mean heart dose increases to greater than 25 Gy.[65] Treatment for congestive heart failure caused by RT is the same as heart failure owing to other causes. Medications like ß-blockers and angiotensin-converting enzyme inhibitors or angiotensin receptor blockers are generally used for treatment. However, good evidence-based data for the use of these medications for radiation-induced cardiomyopathy is still lacking.

SCREENING, DIAGNOSIS, AND FOLLOW-UP

There is lack of evidence-based guidelines with respect to screening and surveillance for cardiovascular disease in asymptomatic patients after MRT. Most recommendations are based on expert consensus and opinions; thus, large-scale studies are warranted to determine potential strategies for screening modalities, frequencies, and most appropriate interventions.[19] Cancer survivors should have a comprehensive screening and long-term routine follow-up for cardiovascular disease after RT, especially given the long latency period between exposure and onset of diseases. It is important to be aware of patients who are at an increased

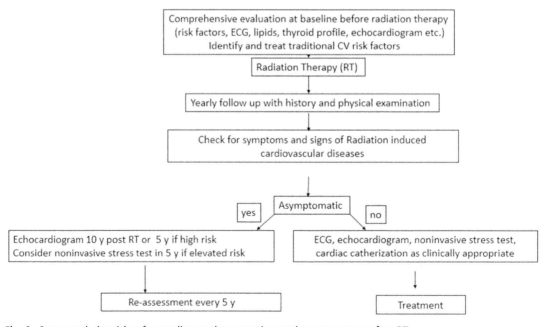

Fig. 2. Suggested algorithm for cardiovascular screening and management after RT.

risk for developing RICVD and would likely benefit from early and routine screening or follow-up: for example, younger age at time of RT, exposure to a higher radiation dose, radiation to anterior or left chest, and lack of shielding or blocking.[16–19] In addition, aggressive treatments of preexisting and modifiable traditional cardiovascular risk factors, such as hypertension, obesity, diabetes, hyperlipidemia, and smoking may improve long-term outcomes and decrease cardiac events in these patients.

An expert consensus from the European Association of Cardiovascular Imaging and the American Society of Echocardiography recommends comprehensive clinic assessment for cardiovascular risk factors and electrographic evaluation at baseline in all patients before RT.[19] Electrocardiographic findings are typically nonspecific.[66] Yearly history and physical examinations should be obtained with focus on symptoms and signs suggestive of new onset cardiovascular disease. Surveillance echocardiogram should be obtained for screening 5 years after RT in asymptomatic high-risk patients or 10 years in others, then every 5 years thereafter. In these high-risk patients it may be reasonable to consider noninvasive stress test to assess for CAD (**Fig. 2**).

The noninvasive cardiac imaging such as echocardiogram, cardiac MRI, cardiac CT, and SPECT are available modalities to screen for structural and functional abnormalities. Echocardiography has a central role in the evaluation of heart disease as the imaging of choice in evaluating pericardial diseases (constrictive and effusive diseases), LV function, and valvular structures.[33,34,67,68] Serial imaging is useful for disease surveillance. Cardiac MRI or CT are more sensitive at detecting anatomic changes and preferred over echocardiography in the evaluation of pericardial thickening and calcifications. Patchy myocardial fibrosis on cardiac MRI, perfusion abnormalities via SPECT, and decreased global longitudinal strain on echocardiogram can be used as markers for subclinical myocardial disease with preserved ventricular systolic function.[21,37,69,70] Stress echocardiography can be used to detect changes in LvV contractility and monitor LV dysfunction. If wall motion abnormalities are detected or there is new onset of symptoms, a stress echocardiogram, perfusion SPECT, cardiac MRI, and coronary angiography are available to assess for inducible ischemia[71] (**Table 3**).

Table 3 Imaging modalities for evaluation of RICVD	
Echocardiogram	Evaluation of pericardial disease LV systolic and diastolic dysfunctions (first line) CAD: wall motion abnormalities Valvular disease
Cardiac MRI	Pericardial constriction Myocardial fibrosis LV systolic dysfunction Valvular disease
Cardiac coronary CT angiography	CAD
Stress echocardiogram	LV dysfunction CAD
SPECT perfusion	LV dysfunction CAD

SUMMARY

With increasing survival from cancer, the incidence of cardiovascular diseases is increasing as a chronic side effect of RT. Prevention, early recognition and prompt intervention should be the major focus in the care of these patients.

REFERENCES

1. Baskar R, Lee KA, Yeo R, et al. Cancer and radiation therapy: current advances and future directions. Int J Med Sci 2012;9(3):193–9.
2. Delaney G, Jacob S, Featherstone C, et al. The role of radiotherapy in cancer treatment: estimating optimal utilization from a review of evidence-based clinical guidelines. Cancer 2005;104(6):1129–37.
3. Cancer Statistics [online article]. 2018. Available at: https://www.cancer.gov/about-cancer/understanding/statistics. Accessed August 28, 2019.
4. Ng AK, Bernardo MP, Weller E, et al. Long-term survival and competing causes of death in patients with early-stage Hodgkin's disease treated at age 50 or younger. J Clin Oncol 2002;20(8):2101–8.
5. Greenwood RD, Rosenthal A, Cassady R, et al. Constrictive pericarditis in childhood due to mediastinal irradiation. Circulation 1974;50(5):1033–9.
6. Halle M, Gabrielsen A, Paulsson-Berne G, et al. Sustained inflammation due to nuclear factor-kappa B activation in irradiated human arteries. J Am Coll Cardiol 2010;55(12):1227–36.
7. Hayashi T, Kusunoki Y, Hakoda M, et al. Radiation dose-dependent increases in inflammatory response

markers in A-bomb survivors. Int J Radiat Biol 2003; 79(2):129–36.

8. Kruse JJ, Bart CI, Visser A, et al. Changes in transforming growth factor-beta (TGF-beta 1), procollagen types I and II mRNA in the rat heart after irradiation. Int J Radiat Biol 1999;75(11):1429–36.

9. Schultz-Hector S, Balz K. Radiation-induced loss of endothelial alkaline phosphatase activity and development of myocardial degeneration. An ultrastructural study. Lab Invest 1994;71(2):252–60.

10. Yusuf SW, Howell RM, Gomez D, et al. Radiation-related heart and vascular disease. Future Oncol 2015;11(14):2067–76.

11. Yusuf SW. Radiation related cardiovascular disease. In: Yusuf SW, Banchs Jose, editors. Cancer and cardiovascular disease: a concise clinical atlas. Cham (Switzerland): Springer International Publishing; 2018. p. 71–80.

12. Al-Kindi SG, Oliveira GH. Incidence and trends of cardiovascular mortality after common cancers in young adults: analysis of surveillance, epidemiology and end-results program. World J Cardiol 2016;8(6): 368–74.

13. Underberg RW, Lagerwaard FJ, Slotman BJ, et al. Benefit of respiration-gated stereotactic radiotherapy for stage I lung cancer: an analysis of 4DCT datasets. Int J Radiat Oncol Biol Phys 2005; 62(2):554–60.

14. Gayed IW, Liu HH, Yusuf SW, et al. The prevalence of myocardial ischemia after concurrent chemoradiation therapy as detected by gated myocardial perfusion imaging in patients with esophageal cancer. J Nucl Med 2006;47(11):1756–62.

15. Gayed IW, Liu HH, Wei X, et al. Patterns of cardiac perfusion abnormalities after chemoradiotherapy in patients with lung cancer. J Thorac Oncol 2009; 4(2):179–84.

16. Darby SC, Cutter DJ, Boerma M, et al. Radiation-related heart disease: current knowledge and future prospects. Int J Radiat Oncol Biol Phys 2010;76(3): 656–65.

17. Hancock SL, Tucker MA, Hoppe RT. Factors affecting late mortality from heart disease after treatment of Hodgkin's disease. JAMA 1993; 270(16):1949–55.

18. Hooning MJ, Botma A, Aleman BM, et al. Long-term risk of cardiovascular disease in 10-year survivors of breast cancer. J Natl Cancer Inst 2007;99(5):365–75.

19. Lancellotti P, Nkomo VT, Badano LP, et al. Expert consensus for multi-modality imaging evaluation of cardiovascular complications of radiotherapy in adults: a report from the European Association of Cardiovascular Imaging and the American Society of Echocardiography. J Am Soc Echocardiogr 2013;26(9):1013–32.

20. van Nimwegen FA, Schaapveld M, Janus CP, et al. Cardiovascular disease after Hodgkin lymphoma treatment: 40-year disease risk. JAMA Intern Med 2015;175(6):1007–17.

21. Marks LB, Yu X, Prosnitz RG, et al. The incidence and functional consequences of RT-associated cardiac perfusion defects. Int J Radiat Oncol Biol Phys 2005;63(1):214–23.

22. Upadhaya BR, Chakravarti RN, Wahi PL. Post-irradiation vascular injury and accelerated development of experimental atherosclerosis. Indian J Med Res 1972;60(3):403–8.

23. Ebrahimian TG, Beugnies L, Surette J, et al. Chronic exposure to external low-dose gamma radiation induces an increase in anti-inflammatory and anti-oxidative parameters resulting in atherosclerotic plaque size reduction in ApoE(-/-) Mice. Radiat Res 2018;189(2):187–96.

24. Lamberts HB, de BW. Contributions to the study of immediate and early x-ray reactions with regard to chemo-protection. VII. X-ray-induced atheromatous lesions in the arterial wall of hypercholesterolaemic rabbits. Int J Radiat Biol Relat Stud Phys Chem Med 1963;6:343–50.

25. Sams A. Histological changes in the larger blood vessels of the hind limb of the mouse after X-irradiation. Int J Radiat Biol Relat Stud Phys Chem Med 1965;9:165–74.

26. Shimizu Y, Kodama K, Nishi N, et al. Radiation exposure and circulatory disease risk: Hiroshima and Nagasaki atomic bomb survivor data, 1950-2003. BMJ 2010;340:b5349.

27. Tribble DL, Barcellos-Hoff MH, Chu BM, et al. Ionizing radiation accelerates aortic lesion formation in fat-fed mice via SOD-inhibitable processes. Arterioscler Thromb Vasc Biol 1999; 19(6):1387–92.

28. Weintraub NL, Jones WK, Manka D. Understanding radiation-induced vascular disease. J Am Coll Cardiol 2010;55(12):1237–9.

29. Orzan F, Brusca A, Conte MR, et al. Severe coronary artery disease after radiation therapy of the chest and mediastinum: clinical presentation and treatment. Br Heart J 1993;69(6):496.

30. Brosius FC, Waller BF, Roberts WC. Radiation heart disease: analysis of 16 young (aged 15 to 33 years) necropsy patients who received over 3,500 rads to the heart. Am J Med 1981;70(3):519–30.

31. Raghunathan D, Khilji MI, Hassan SA, et al. Radiation-induced cardiovascular disease. Curr Atheroscler Rep 2017;19(5):22.

32. van Nimwegen FA, Schaapveld M, Janus CPM, et al. Cardiovascular disease after Hodgkin lymphoma treatment: 40-year disease risk of cardiovascular disease after Hodgkin lymphoma treatment for cardiovascular disease after Hodgkin lymphoma treatment. JAMA Intern Med 2015;175(6):1007–17.

33. Hull MC, Morris CG, Pepine CJ, et al. Valvular dysfunction and carotid, subclavian, and coronary

artery disease in survivors of Hodgkin lymphoma treated with radiation therapy. JAMA 2003;290(21): 2831–7.

34. Heidenreich PA, Hancock SL, Lee BK, et al. Asymptomatic cardiac disease following mediastinal irradiation. J Am Coll Cardiol 2003;42(4): 743–9.

35. Gujral DM, Lloyd G, Bhattacharyya S. Radiation-induced valvular heart disease. Heart 2016;102(4): 269–76.

36. Cutter DJ, Schaapveld M, Darby SC, et al. Risk of valvular heart disease after treatment for Hodgkin lymphoma. J Natl Cancer Inst 2015;107(4) [pii: djv008].

37. Veinot JP, Edwards WD. Pathology of radiation-induced heart disease: a surgical and autopsy study of 27 cases. Hum Pathol 1996;27(8):766–73.

38. Yarnold J, Brotons MC. Pathogenetic mechanisms in radiation fibrosis. Radiother Oncol 2010;97(1): 149–61.

39. Nadlonek NA, Weyant MJ, Yu JA, et al. Radiation induces osteogenesis in human aortic valve interstitial cells. J Thorac Cardiovasc Surg 2012;144(6): 1466–70.

40. Perrault DJ, Levy M, Herman JD, et al. Echocardiographic abnormalities following cardiac radiation. J Clin Oncol 1985;3(4):546–51.

41. Brand MD, Abadi CA, Aurigemma GP, et al. Radiation-associated valvular heart disease in Hodgkin's disease is associated with characteristic thickening and fibrosis of the aortic-mitral curtain. J Heart Valve Dis 2001;10(5):681–5.

42. Hering D, Faber L, Horstkotte D. Echocardiographic features of radiation-associated valvular disease. Am J Cardiol 2003;92(2):226–30.

43. Botma A, Aleman BMP, Taylor CW, et al. Long-term risk of cardiovascular disease in 10-year survivors of breast cancer. J Natl Cancer Inst 2007;99(5): 365–75.

44. Rodemann HP, Bamberg M. Cellular basis of radiation-induced fibrosis. Radiother Oncol 1995; 35(2):83–90.

45. Yusuf SW, Sami S, Daher IN. Radiation-induced heart disease: a clinical update. Cardiol Res Pract 2011;2011:317659.

46. Robert Stewart J, Fajardo LF. Radiation-induced heart disease: an update. Prog Cardiovasc Dis 1984;27(3):173–94.

47. Taunk NK, Haffty BG, Kostis JB, et al. Radiation-induced heart disease: pathologic abnormalities and putative mechanisms. Front Oncol 2015;5:39.

48. Hancock SL, Donaldson SS, Hoppe RT. Cardiac disease following treatment of Hodgkin's disease in children and adolescents. J Clin Oncol 1993;11(7): 1208–15.

49. Carmel RJ, Kaplan HS. Mantle irradiation in Hodgkin's disease. An analysis of technique, tumor

eradication, and complications. Cancer 1976;37(6): 2813–25.

50. Wei X, Liu HH, Tucker SL, et al. Risk factors for pericardial effusion in inoperable esophageal cancer patients treated with definitive chemoradiation therapy. Int J Radiat Oncol Biol Phys 2008;70(3): 707–14.

51. Fukada J, Shigematsu N, Ohashi T, et al. Pericardial and pleural effusions after definitive radiotherapy for esophageal cancer. J Radiat Res 2012;53(3):447–53.

52. Yusuf SW, Venkatesulu BP, Mahadevan LS, et al. Radiation-induced cardiovascular disease: a clinical perspective. Front Cardiovasc Med 2017;4:66.

53. Kumawat M, Lahiri TK, Agarwal D. Constrictive pericarditis: retrospective study of 109 patients. Asian Cardiovasc Thorac Ann 2018;26(5):347–52.

54. Bertog SC, Thambidorai SK, Parakh K, et al. Constrictive pericarditis: etiology and cause-specific survival after pericardiectomy. J Am Coll Cardiol 2004;43(8):1445–52.

55. Ling LH, Oh JK, Schaff HV, et al. Constrictive pericarditis in the modern era: evolving clinical spectrum and impact on outcome after pericardiectomy. Circulation 1999;100(13):1380–6.

56. Adams MJ, Lipshultz SE, Schwartz C, et al. Radiation-associated cardiovascular disease: manifestations and management. Semin Radiat Oncol 2003; 13(3):346–56.

57. Orzan F, Brusca A, Gaita F, et al. Associated cardiac lesions in patients with radiation-induced complete heart block. Int J Cardiol 1993;39(2):151–6.

58. Slama MS, Le Guludec D, Sebag C, et al. Complete atrioventricular block following mediastinal irradiation: a report of six cases. Pacing Clin Electrophysiol 1991;14(7):1112–8.

59. Donnellan E, Phelan D, McCarthy CP, et al. Radiation-induced heart disease: a practical guide to diagnosis and management. Cleve Clin J Med 2016;83(12):914–22.

60. Larsen RL, Jakacki RI, Vetter VL, et al. Electrocardiographic changes and arrhythmias after cancer therapy in children and young adults. Am J Cardiol 1992;70(1):73–7.

61. Abouegylah M, Braunstein LZ, Alm El-Din MA, et al. Evaluation of radiation-induced cardiac toxicity in breast cancer patients treated with Trastuzumab-based chemotherapy. Breast Cancer Res Treat 2019;174(1):179–85.

62. Chello M, Mastroroberto P, Romano R, et al. Changes in the proportion of types I and III collagen in the left ventricular wall of patients with post-irradiative pericarditis. Cardiovasc Surg 1996;4(2):222–6.

63. van der Pal HJ, van Dalen EC, van Delden E, et al. High risk of symptomatic cardiac events in childhood cancer survivors. J Clin Oncol 2012;30(13):1429–37.

64. Guldner L, Haddy N, Pein F, et al. Radiation dose and long term risk of cardiac pathology following

radiotherapy and anthracyclin for a childhood cancer. Radiother Oncol 2006;81(1):47–56.

65. van Nimwegen FA, Ntentas G, Darby SC, et al. Risk of heart failure in survivors of Hodgkin lymphoma: effects of cardiac exposure to radiation and anthracyclines. Blood 2017;129(16): 2257–65.

66. Gomez DR, Yusuf SW, Munsell MF, et al. Prospective exploratory analysis of cardiac biomarkers and electrocardiogram abnormalities in patients receiving thoracic radiation therapy with high-dose heart exposure. J Thorac Oncol 2014;9(10): 1554–60.

67. Lund MB, Ihlen H, Voss BM, et al. Increased risk of heart valve regurgitation after mediastinal radiation for Hodgkin's disease: an echocardiographic study. Heart 1996;75(6):591.

68. Yeh ET, Tong AT, Lenihan DJ, et al. Cardiovascular complications of cancer therapy: diagnosis, pathogenesis, and management. Circulation 2004; 109(25):3122–31.

69. Jurcut R, Ector J, Erven K, et al. Radiotherapy effects on systolic myocardial function detected by strain rate imaging in a left-breast cancer patient. Eur Heart J 2007;28(24):2966.

70. Tsai H-R, Gjesdal O, Wethal T, et al. Left ventricular function assessed by two-dimensional speckle tracking echocardiography in long-term survivors of Hodgkin's lymphoma treated by mediastinal radiotherapy with or without anthracycline therapy. Am J Cardiol 2011;107(3): 472–7.

71. European Association of Echocardiography, Sicari R, Nihoyannopoulos P, Evangelista A, et al. Stress echocardiography expert consensus statement: European Association of Echocardiography (EAE) (a registered branch of the ESC). Eur J Echocardiogr 2008;9(4):415–37.

Arrhythmogenic Anticancer Drugs in Cardio-Oncology

Isaac Rhea, MD[a,b], Paula Hernandez Burgos, MD[b,c], Michael G. Fradley, MD[a,b],*

KEYWORDS

- Arrhythmia • Cardio-oncology • Chemotherapy • Heart block • Ventricular tachycardia
- Atrial fibrillation

KEY POINTS

- Multiple cancer therapies are associated with cardiac arrhythmias through a variety of pathophysiologic mechanisms.
- Atrial fibrillation and atrial flutter are common during cancer therapy but should rarely limit continued delivery of therapy.
- Ventricular arrhythmias are not common during cancer therapy and are more often secondary to other cardiac pathologies.
- QT interval monitoring is recommended for some agents, although it is often not a reliable predictor of ventricular arrhythmias.
- Bradyarrhythmias are common and rarely require intervention, but special attention must be paid to heart block in checkpoint inhibitor therapy.

INTRODUCTION

Over the past several decades, the landscape of anticancer therapy has rapidly evolved and produced innovative, efficacious treatment options. As a result, there are projected to be 16.9 million cancer survivors in the United States this year, which is approximately 5% of the total US population.[1] In cancer survivors, there are emerging data suggesting increased cardiovascular morbidity and mortality when compared with the general population.[2] Although most attention in cardio-oncology is focused on systolic dysfunction and vascular occlusions, some of the most common cardiac abnormalities in patients with cancer are arrhythmias.[3] We discuss the agents most frequently associated with common atrial and ventricular rhythm abnormalities and their impact on the clinical care of patients with cancer.

ATRIAL ARRHYTHMIAS

Atrial arrhythmias are extremely common in patients with cancer, and it is often difficult to distinguish causality, because factors such as anticancer agent, type of surgery, and even presence of cancer, have all been associated with the development of arrhythmias.[4–6] Evaluation and management of atrial fibrillation (AF) and atrial flutter (AFL) is among the most common reason for inpatient cardiology consultations on patients with cancer.[7] Incident AF/AFL in patients with cancer is associated with an increased risk of heart failure and

Disclosure: The authors have nothing to disclose.
[a] Division of Cardiovascular Medicine, Morsani College of Medicine, University of South Florida, 2 Tampa General Circle, Tampa, FL 33606, USA; [b] Cardio-Oncology Program, Moffitt Cancer Center, Tampa, FL 33612, USA; [c] Department of Internal Medicine, Morsani College of Medicine, University of South Florida, 2 Tampa General Circle, Tampa, FL 33606, USA
* Corresponding author. 12902 USF Magnolia Drive, MCB-CPT, Tampa, FL 33612-9416.
E-mail address: mfradley@health.usf.edu

thromboembolism.[8] A large portion of new AF/AFL are encountered in the context of recent surgery, but many anticancer medications are also independently associated with the development of these arrhythmias. Management of these rhythm disturbances often requires a nuanced approach which may differ from the typical treatments offered to patients without cancer with similar arrhythmias.[5,9]

Anthracyclines

Doxorubicin and other anthracyclines are well known for causing systolic dysfunction; however, they also are associated with a higher incidence of AF, even in the case of normal left ventricular (LV) function.[10] However, previous work by Kilickap and colleagues[11] noted that, on 48-h Holter monitoring following first infusion of doxorubicin, the rate of paroxysmal AF was 10.3%. In a prospective series by Amioka and colleagues[12] with patients undergoing anthracycline therapy having electrocardiograms (ECGs) performed during clinic visits, the rate was at 6%. The arrhythmic mechanisms are widely disputed and include impaired intracellular signaling, the buildup of toxic metabolites and reactive oxygen species, or direct myocardial toxicity.[13] Atrial and ventricular arrhythmias are also frequently encountered in the setting of anthracycline-induced cardiomyopathy. In a study by Mazur and colleagues[14] looking at interrogation reports from implantable cardioverter-defibrillator (ICDs) placed in patients with chemotherapy-associated cardiac dysfunction, the rate of AF was 56.6%, with similar results reported by Fradley and colleagues.[15] In general, the rates of arrhythmias in patients with chemotherapy-induced LV dysfunction seem to be equivalent to those with other forms of nonischemic cardiomyopathy.[15]

Melphalan and Hematopoietic Stem Cell Transplantation

Melphalan is a nitrogen mustard-class chemotherapy agent used primarily in preconditioning regimens before hematopoietic stem cell transplantation (HSCT). In 1 series by Arun and colleagues[16] of 91 patients with amyloid light-chain amyloidosis undergoing high-dose melphalan before autologous HSCT, the authors noted the incidence of peritransplant AF/AFL to be 13.1%. In another series at Moffitt Cancer Center, of 438 patients who received melphalan before HSCT, 11% developed supraventricular arrhythmias, including AF, which was substantially higher than in patients who received non-melphalan-containing regimens.[17]

There also seems to be an increased incidence of AF in the setting of HSCT regardless of the precondition regimen. For example, in a study of 278 multiple myeloma patients receiving autologous HSCT, the incidence of new AF/AFL following HSCT was 27%.[18] Factors associated with new AF in this study also included renal failure, hypertension, fluid retention, and amyloidosis.[18] In addition, new AF/AFL post-HSCT is associated with worse outcomes. In a study by Tonorezos and colleagues[19] of 1177 consecutive patients receiving HSCT from 1999 to 2009, posttransplant arrhythmias (predominantly AF/AFL) were associated with longer median hospital stay, higher likelihood of in-hospital death, and higher likelihood of death within 1 year of transplant. Moreover, on multivariable analysis, the development of posttransplant arrhythmias was found to be an independent predictor of death.[19]

Carfilzomib

Multiple myeloma patients have a remarkably high prevalence of AF/AFL (14.6%), and a portion of this is likely related to the use of proteasome inhibitors, especially carfilzomib.[20] Although carfilzomib is most commonly associated with LV dysfunction and heart failure, AF/AFL is also frequently observed, at rates significantly higher than with use of other proteasome inhibitors.[21,22] In the Endeavor Trial, the incidence of carfilzomib-induced AF/AFL was 3.2% compared with 2.2% in patients treated with bortezomib.[23] In another retrospective review of 130 clinical trial patients treated with carfilzomib, the incidence of AF/AFL was 3.8%.[24]

Tyrosine Kinase Inhibitors

Tyrosine kinase inhibitors (TKIs) target various intracellular signaling pathways necessary for cellular growth. There are several categories of TKIs that are known to have arrhythmogenic effects. Vascular endothelial growth factor receptor (VEGFR) inhibitors target the intracellular signaling needed for angiogenesis. Such agents are known to be associated with increased hypertension and systolic dysfunction, and there are also data suggesting that VEGFR inhibitors are associated with increased AF/AFL.[25,26] In a phase II trial of 39 patients with hepatocellular carcinoma treated with sorafenib and 5-fluorouacil (5-FU), the incidence of AF/AFL was 5%.[27]

Bcr-Abl TKIs are a subgroup of TKIs that target the region of the Philadelphia chromosome responsible for uncontrolled cellular division. These agents have drastically altered the approach to management of chronic myelogenous leukemia (CML). Ponatinib, an agent frequently used in CML that also possesses anti-VEGFR activity is well known for its association with arterial thrombi noted in the EPIC study.[28] In that same study, however, there was a 3% incidence of AF/AFL in the ponatinib arm compared with 0% in the imatinib arm.[28] Bosutinib seems to have a modest association with AF (2%), and nilotinib likely has a low incidence of AF/AFL.[29–31] In such agents, the proposed mechanism for arrhythmias is the inhibition of the phosphoinositide 3-kinase (PI3K) signaling pathway, leading to prolonged repolarization and increasing the risk of multiple arrhythmias.[32]

Ibrutinib

Ibrutinib is a Bruton's tyrosine kinase (BTK) inhibitor used for the treatment of multiple B-cell hematologic malignancies, such as chronic lymphocytic leukemia and mantle cell lymphoma (MCL).[33,34] Multiple studies have reported a surprisingly increased incidence of AF/AFL (2% to 16%).[35] A meta-analysis by Yun and colleagues[36] of 4 randomized trials determined the incidence of new AF/AFL to be 8.18%, with a relative risk (RR) of 8.81 compared with alternative agents/placebo. The incidence increases with prolonged use and higher dose.[35] The arrhythmic mechanism is hypothesized to be related to the on-target inhibition of BTK and TEC protein leading to inhibition of the PI3K/AKT pathways.[37,38]

Although the increased rate of AF is significant, ibrutinib's inherent antiplatelet effects leading to increased bleeding complications is also pertinent. In 1 of the initial phase II studies in patients with MCL, 4 out of 111 patients on ibrutinib therapy were diagnosed with new subdural hematomas while on therapy following episodes of trauma, yet all of these patients were also on either aspirin and/or warfarin at the time of the event.[34] Following this, the use of warfarin in ibrutinib patients has been heavily discouraged, and many subsequent cancer trials excluded patients taking warfarin.[39] Thus, therapeutic warfarin for AF/AFL prophylaxis is generally avoided.[40,41] Fortunately, direct oral anticoagulants (DOACs) appear to be safe alternatives despite the potential for cytochrome P450 and P-glycoprotein interactions, although dedicated studies are lacking.[42,43]

Management of Atrial Fibrillation/Atrial Flutter

Management strategies for cancer treatment-related AF/AFL are largely similar to those for the general population. A rhythm-control or rate-control strategy is first considered to avoid tachycardia-mediated cardiomyopathy. Multiple trials, including the original AFFIRM trial and the more recent ORBIT-AF Registry confirmed that a rhythm-control strategy is generally not superior to a rate-control strategy.[44] The CHA2DS2-VASc score is still the predominant methodology of determining the risk of stroke associated with AF and possesses the best data and associated guidelines, although there are some data to suggest that the score may underestimate risk at lower scores and yet overestimate risk at higher scores, especially in patients with cancer.[45–47] The 2019 update to the guidelines encourages starting therapeutic anticoagulation with vitamin K antagonists, heparin analogs, or DOACs when the CVASC score is ≥2 for men or ≥3 for women, provided the bleeding risk is not excessive and the cause of AF is not related to mitral stenosis or prosthetic heart valves.[46] DOACs are gaining favor in treatment of patients with cancer because they require significantly less monitoring compared with alternative agents, and have been used successfully for deep vein thrombosis treatment in patients with cancer.[48] However, all major guidelines still recommend heparin products over DOACs for venous thromboembolism.[49,50] No guidelines address anticoagulant choice for stroke prophylaxis in AF/AFL patients with cancer, although there are some subanalyses of major trials, such as ARISTOLTE, that are encouraging.[51] A subanalysis of the ENGAGE-AF with edoxaban, which included 1153 AF/AFL patients with newly diagnosed cancer or recurrence of remote cancer, found that these patients had a lower incidence of composite stroke/myocardial infarction/embolism compared with patients without cancer.[52]

However, anticoagulation in patients with cancer can be challenging because of increased bleeding diatheses and drug-drug interactions. For example, a major exception to standard AF/AFL anticoagulation regimens in patients with cancer is the aforementioned ibrutinib/warfarin combination. Many of the agents used for rate/rhythm control and anticoagulation can have interactions with the anticancer agents, which can lead to antiarrhythmic toxicity or increased bleeding from intensification of the anticoagulant effects. For example, all DOACs are metabolized via P-glycoprotein to varying degrees, and the factor Xa inhibitors including apixaban and rivaroxaban use CYP3A4.[53,54] Moreover, many of these patients have thrombocytopenia. Although anticoagulation in patients with platelet counts above 50,000 seems to be safe, the risk of bleeding likely outweighs the prophylactic benefit at values below 50,000.[55]

There are several nonpharmacologic approaches for treating AF/AFL that may be options for patients with cancer. Cardioversion is often recommended for new-onset AF/AFL, although strict adherence to anticoagulation is required after the procedure.[56] Ablation of atrial arrhythmias is a possibility in select cases; however, studies have yet to demonstrate the procedure decreases the risk of thrombosis.[57] Specifically, current guidelines recommend anticoagulating all patients postablation indefinitely, as dictated by the CHA2DS2-VASc score, regardless of the perceived success or failure of the procedure.[58] The WATCHMAN left atrial appendage occlusion device is an option for patients who cannot tolerate long-term anticoagulation; however, the postprocedural requirement of 3 to 6 months of concomitant dual antiplatelet therapy with therapeutic anticoagulation makes the procedure challenging in many patients with cancer because many of them have a higher bleeding tendency.[59]

VENTRICULAR ARRHYTHMIAS AND QT PROLONGATION

Although less common than atrial arrhythmias, ventricular arrhythmias (VA) are also a potential electrophysiologic complication of cancer therapies and can lead to serious adverse events including sudden cardiac death (SCD). Multiple risk factors contribute to this phenomenon, including electrolytic disturbances, systemic inflammation, or primary toxicity from antineoplastic agents through QT prolongation, direct cardiac injury, or ischemia.[60] In cancer trials, SCD is presumed to be related to drug-induced QT prolongation more so than undiagnosed coronary disease, although in the general population undiagnosed high-grade coronary disease is diagnosed in up to 80% of cases.[61] Nevertheless, the evidence of SCD for nearly all modern cancer agents including TKIs is minimal because of the low prevalence and also the difficulty diagnosing a primary arrhythmic event in patients who often have advanced malignancies.[62–64] QT prolongation corrected for heart rate (QTc) greater than 500 ms increases the risk of SCD through torsades de pointes (TdP), a form of polymorphic ventricular tachycardia. It should be noted that, whereas the QT interval is easily measured from a standard 12-lead electrocardiogram, it is actually a relatively poor predictor of SCD. Generally speaking, in patients with QTc less than 500 ms and an active malignancy, it is extremely rare for the risk of drug-induced malignant arrhythmia to exceed the potential life-prolonging benefits of an anticancer therapy.[65]

5-Flourouracil

5-FU, an antimetabolite primarily used with gastrointestinal cancers, is associated with coronary ischemia largely from coronary vasospasm, which can lead to VA.[66] A study by Yilmaz and colleagues[67] evaluating the cardiac rhythm of patients receiving a 5-FU regimen found a significant increase in ventricular premature complexes (VPC) per hour before and during the first 24-h of treatment (12.7 ± 29.6 vs 38.1 ± 42.1, $P = .002$). Although increased VPCs can suggest a higher risk of sustained VA, there is equivocal evidence in the case of 5-FU. One study from Pakistan shows a rate of combined nonsustained ventricular tachycardia (NSVT) and sustained ventricular tachycardia (VT) with 5-FU of 3.7%,[68] and yet a meta-analysis by Abdel-Rahman[69] of 3223 patients from 5 randomized trials showed the incidence of ventricular tachycardia to be 0.16%. There are also some case reports suggesting that capecitabine, a 5-FU precursor, may be associated with ventricular fibrillation (VF).[70] The incidence of coronary vasospasm and the associated VA has prompted some studies at telemetry monitoring during infusion, but the actual incidence of ischemic events or arrhythmias is too small to make this practical for a general population with cancer.[71]

Anthracyclines

There is a significant risk of VA with use of anthracyclines, but this seems to be present when there is significant chemotherapy-induced systolic dysfunction rather than direct arrhythmic or QT-prolonging effects. For example, a meta-analysis by Porta-Sánchez and colleagues[72] noted that anthracyclines as a class have a <1% risk of causing prolongation of QT. In the previously mentioned study by Mazur and colleagues,[14] of 23 patients with ICDs for anthracycline-related cardiomyopathy, the incidence of NSVT and sustained VT/VF over 5.5 ± 3.0 years was 73.9% and 30.4%, respectively, which was not significantly different from the control group of nonanthracycline-related nonischemic cardiomyopathy. A similar study by Fradley and colleagues[15] of 9 patients with anthracycline cardiomyopathy showed similar results, with an incidence of NSVT and combined VT/VF at 44.4%, which again was similar to nonischemic cardiomyopathy controls. Overall, it seems that anthracyclines have little direct influence on the electrical system, and nearly all cases of VA including TdP following use of anthracyclines can be attributed to either LV dysfunction or other triggers.[73]

Arsenic trioxide

Arsenic trioxide is a chemotherapy agent that is known to be associated with classic HERG channel-mediated QT prolongation, as well as TdP and sudden death.[74] In a series of 99 patients with advanced malignancies, arsenic prolonged the QTc in 38 patients, with 26 developing a QTc ≥500 ms. In this series, the prolongation was transient, and asymptomatic TdP developed briefly in 1 patient with hypokalemia, but did not recur after potassium repletion.[75] In another series of 10 patients in a phase I/II trial to determine the optimal dosing of arsenic, 3 patients died suddenly, although only 1 death occurred while on telemetry and it occurred following abrupt asystole rather than TdP.[76] Finally, an analysis of over 3000 electrocardiograms from 113 patients treated with arsenic reported a Fridericia-corrected QT interval of greater than 500 ms in 26% without the occurrence of clinically significant adverse cardiac events.[77] Fortunately, in modern doses the incidence of TdP is very rare, but ECG screening and regular electrolyte optimization is recommended before and during therapy by the National Comprehensive Cancer Center guidelines.[78]

Tyrosine kinase inhibitors

Sunitinib, a VEGFR inhibitor, is a first-line treatment for metastatic renal cell carcinoma.[79,80] In earlier trials, 2.3% of patients had QT prolongation greater than 500 ms, and TdP occurred in less than 0.1%.[13,81] Monitoring with ECG is suggested at baseline and every 3 months thereafter regardless of previous cardiac history.[82]

Nilotinib, another BCR-Abl TKI used in CML, also has a known association with QT prolongation.[81] It has a black box warning for QT prolongation, and SCD has been reported in 0.3% of patients, but increased risk of TdP has not been reported.[32,81] Phase I clinical trials revealed a 5- to 15-ms QT prolongation, but during the ENESTnd trial there were no events of QTc prolongation more than 500 ms and no TdP or malignant arrhythmias identified after long-term follow-up.[83]

Vandetanib, commonly used for refractory medullary thyroid carcinoma, also carries a black box warning for increased risk of QTc prolongation, TdP, and SCD.[84] A meta-analysis compared the overall risk of hypertension and QTc prolongation in patients with non-small-cell lung cancer treated with vandetanib alone or with chemotherapy to control groups and found vandetanib significantly increased the risk of QT prolongation (RR = 7.90, 95% CI 4.03–15.50, P<.00001).[85]

Vemurafenib is a TKI effective against unresectable or metastatic melanoma with BRAF V600 E mutation. It was initially shown to be a QT-prolonging medication in the BRIM-2 trial, and subsequently the Expanded Access Program revealed that 7% of patients had an increased

QTc of more than 480 ms, and 3% of more than 500 ms.[86] This therapy requires periodic ECGs for QT monitoring.[87]

A review and meta-analysis by Porta-Sánchez and colleagues[72] evaluated the QT-prolonging effect of various TKIs and found that, whereas sunitinib, nilotinib, and vandetanib had a considerable effect in the QT interval, this effect was not immediately harmful and was not predictive of an increased risk of life-threatening arrhythmias.[88] Similarly, Ghatalia and colleagues[89] performed a meta-analysis of randomized phase II and III clinical trials comparing VEGFR TKIs against placebo to evaluate the RR of QTc prolongation and serious arrhythmias. The RR of QTc prolongation in the TKI arm was 8.66 (95% CI 4.92–15.2, P = .001) compared with 2.69 in the placebo arm (95% CI 1.33–5.44, P = .006), with most events being asymptomatic. Although sunitinib and vandetanib were associated with a statistically significant risk of QTc prolongation, there was no consequent increase in the rate of serious arrhythmias. General considerations for monitoring and prevention of QT prolongation in patients taking TKIs include the avoidance of concomitant treatment with QT-prolonging agents, serial ECG monitoring, electrolytic replacement, and renal and hepatic dose adjustment.[63]

Ibrutinib

A major study evaluated the incidence of VA in patients taking ibrutinib and revealed a weighted average incidence of 678 events per 100,000 person-years. Among patients without coronary artery disease and congestive heart failure taking ibrutinib, the incidence was 669 per 100,000 person-years, significantly higher in comparison with the reported incidence of 51.9 per 100,000 person-years among patients not taking ibrutinib (RR = 12.9, P<.001; adverse event rate = 11.9, P<.001).[90] Another, more recent, study used the Federal Drug Administration Adverse Event Reporting System to evaluate VA in ibrutinib-treated patients, and identified 7 episodes of VT/VF and 6 cases of SCD.[91] Interestingly, despite the increased risk of arrhythmia, ibrutinib does not prolong the QT interval significantly and may even shorten it.[92]

Cyclin-dependent kinase 4/6 inhibitors

A newer class of anticancer drugs called cyclin-dependent kinase 4/6 inhibitors induce replication arrest by blocking the retinoblastoma protein. One of these agents, ribociclib, was approved for patients with metastatic hormone receptor-positive, HER2-negative breast cancer. Within the first 4 weeks of treatment, 3.3% of patients had prolongation of the QTc interval to more than 480 ms when treated at the 600-mg dose, with normalization following dose reduction or cessation.[93] ECG monitoring at baseline, day 14 in cycle 1 and day 1 in cycle 2 is recommended.[94]

BRADYCARDIA

Bradycardia, defined as a hazard ratio <60, is common regardless of cancer status. In the Baltimore Longitudinal Study of Aging, sinus bradycardia was present in approximately 4% of the general population over 40 years old.[95] Most bradycardia encountered in patients with cancer is unrelated to cancer therapy, but in some instances specific anticancer drugs can be responsible.

Anaplastic Lymphoma Kinase Inhibitors

Anaplastic lymphoma kinase inhibitors are agents primarily used in the treatment of non-small-cell lung cancer. Among their adverse effects, sinus bradycardia is frequently reported. Although it is not widely used, ceritinib has a rate of bradycardia of approximately 3%.[96] Crizotinib, however, has a much higher incidence of bradycardia. On a recent large retrospective analysis of 2 large-scale trials, 42% of 1053 patients experienced at least 1 episode of sinus bradycardia, although only 9 patients were symptomatic to the point of needing a dose change.[97] The largest determining factor of posttreatment sinus bradycardia was a lower baseline heart rate.[97] Case reports note the heart rate can at times drop asymptomatically to less than 45 bpm and, on rare occasions, can be symptomatic.[98,99] In another retrospective review of 42 patients, there was an average decrease in heart rate by 26.1 bpm, with 69% of patients experiencing sinus bradycardia at some point.[100] Of note, there was greater tumor response in those patients who developed bradycardia.[100]

In instances in which symptomatic bradycardia does develop, the first step would be discontinuation of other atrioventricular (AV) nodal blocking agents including β-blockers, nondihydropyridine calcium channel blockers, and α-2 agonists.

Taxanes

Taxanes, particularly paclitaxel, are known to cause bradycardia; however, this is rarely clinically significant. One phase II study of paclitaxel in ovarian cancer noted an incidence of bradycardia of 29%.[101] In a study by Rowinsky and colleagues,[102] 2 of 140 patients treated with paclitaxel experienced higher degree AV block, including 1 with transient heart block that eventually required a pacemaker. Despite these findings, telemetry monitoring during infusion is generally not indicated.

Immune Checkpoint Inhibitors

These new agents have revolutionized the treatment of many cancers such as melanoma and lung cancer and are slowly finding utility in other malignancies.[103,104] They are also known to cause complete heart block, usually in the context of myocarditis. It is important to note that, unlike some other forms of myocarditis which are chiefly characterized by heart failure symptoms, checkpoint inhibitor myocarditis can present largely with conduction changes including complete heart block.[105,106] In a recent study by Mahmood and colleagues,[107] a multicenter registry of patients with suspected immune checkpoint inhibitor myocarditis was created with special attention to major adverse cardiac events (MACE) including cardiovascular death, cardiac arrest, cardiogenic shock, and hemodynamically significant complete heart block. In this group, an abnormal ECG and abnormal troponin were the most common findings associated with the development of MACE. Complete heart block due to checkpoint inhibitor myocarditis can be fatal and should be approached with great caution and it may be reasonable to have a lower threshold for pacemaker placement in these patients once they develop complete heart block.

SUMMARY

Multiple anticancer therapies have clinically pertinent electrophysiologic consequences. Atrial arrhythmias are common encountered during cancer treatment and should be treated accordingly but rarely require cessation of cancer therapy. Although some agents are associated with malignant VA, this is most often as a secondary manifestation of cardiac injury either through systolic dysfunction or coronary ischemia. Primary QT prolongation is rarely a cause for treatment discontinuation and as it is not especially predictive of VA especially if the QTc remains below 500 ms. Although bradyarrhythmias in patients with cancer are extremely common, they are frequently asymptomatic and rarely require intervention.

REFERENCES

1. Bluethmann SM, Mariotto AB, Rowland JH. Anticipating the "silver tsunami": prevalence trajectories and comorbidity burden among older cancer

survivors in the United States. Cancer Epidemiol Biomarkers Prev 2016;25(7):1029–36.

2. Bradshaw PT, Stevens J, Khankari N, et al. Cardiovascular disease mortality among breast cancer survivors. Epidemiology 2016;27(1):6–13.

3. Nickel AC, Patel A, Saba NF, et al. Incidence of cancer treatment-induced arrhythmia associated with novel targeted chemotherapeutic agents. J Am Heart Assoc 2018;7(20):e010101.

4. Farmakis D, Parissis J, Filippatos G. Insights into onco-cardiology: atrial fibrillation in cancer. J Am Coll Cardiol 2014;63(10):945–53.

5. Erichsen R, Christiansen CF, Mehnert F, et al. Colorectal cancer and risk of atrial fibrillation and flutter: a population-based case-control study. Intern Emerg Med 2012;7(5):431–8.

6. Guzzetti S, Costantino G, Vernocchi A, et al. First diagnosis of colorectal or breast cancer and prevalence of atrial fibrillation. Intern Emerg Med 2008; 3(3):227–31.

7. Fradley MG, Brown AC, Shields B, et al. Developing a comprehensive cardio-oncology program at a Cancer Institute: the Moffitt Cancer Center experience. Oncol Rev 2017;11(2):340.

8. Hu YF, Liu CJ, Chang PM, et al. Incident thromboembolism and heart failure associated with new-onset atrial fibrillation in cancer patients. Int J Cardiol 2013;165(2):355–7.

9. Mc Cormack O, Zaborowski A, King S, et al. New-onset atrial fibrillation post-surgery for esophageal and junctional cancer: incidence, management, and impact on short- and long-term outcomes. Ann Surg 2014;260(5):772–8 [discussion: 778].

10. Cardinale D, Colombo A, Bacchiani G, et al. Early detection of anthracycline cardiotoxicity and improvement with heart failure therapy. Circulation 2015;131(22):1981–8.

11. Kilickap S, Barista I, Akgul E, et al. Early and late arrhythmogenic effects of doxorubicin. South Med J 2007;100(3):262–5.

12. Amioka M, Sairaku A, Ochi T, et al. Prognostic significance of new-onset atrial fibrillation in patients with non-Hodgkin's lymphoma treated with anthracyclines. Am J Cardiol 2016;118(9): 1386–9.

13. Tamargo J, Caballero R, Delpon E. Cancer chemotherapy and cardiac arrhythmias: a review. Drug Saf 2015;38(2):129–52.

14. Mazur M, Wang F, Hodge DO, et al. Burden of cardiac arrhythmias in patients with anthracycline-related cardiomyopathy. JACC Clin Electrophysiol 2017;3(2):139–50.

15. Fradley MG, Viganego F, Kip K, et al. Rates and risk of arrhythmias in cancer survivors with chemotherapy-induced cardiomyopathy compared with patients with other cardiomyopathies. Open Heart 2017;4(2):e000701.

16. Arun M, Brauneis D, Doros G, et al. The incidence of atrial fibrillation among patients with AL amyloidosis undergoing high-dose melphalan and stem cell transplantation: experience at a single institution. Bone Marrow Transplant 2017;52(9):1349–51.

17. Feliz V, Saiyad S, Ramarao SM, et al. Melphalan-induced supraventricular tachycardia: incidence and risk factors. Clin Cardiol 2011;34(6):356–9.

18. Sureddi RK, Amani F, Hebbar P, et al. Atrial fibrillation following autologous stem cell transplantation in patients with multiple myeloma: incidence and risk factors. Ther Adv Cardiovasc Dis 2012;6(6): 229–36.

19. Tonorezos ES, Stillwell EE, Calloway JJ, et al. Arrhythmias in the setting of hematopoietic cell transplants. Bone Marrow Transplant 2015;50(9): 1212–6.

20. Shah N, Rochlani Y, Pothineni NV, et al. Burden of arrhythmias in patients with multiple myeloma. Int J Cardiol 2016;203:305–6.

21. Iannaccone A, Bruno G, Ravera A, et al. Evaluation of cardiovascular toxicity associated with treatments containing proteasome inhibitors in multiple myeloma therapy. High Blood Press Cardiovasc Prev 2018;25(2):209–18.

22. Chen JH, Lenihan DJ, Phillips SE, et al. Cardiac events during treatment with proteasome inhibitor therapy for multiple myeloma. Cardio Oncol 2017; 3(1). https://doi.org/10.1186/s40959-017-0023-9.

23. Dimopoulos MA, Goldschmidt H, Niesvizky R, et al. Carfilzomib or bortezomib in relapsed or refractory multiple myeloma (ENDEAVOR): an interim overall survival analysis of an open-label, randomised, phase 3 trial. Lancet Oncol 2017;18(10):1327–37.

24. Atrash S, Tullos A, Panozzo S, et al. Cardiac complications in relapsed and refractory multiple myeloma patients treated with carfilzomib. Blood Cancer J 2015;5:e272.

25. Nazer B, Humphreys BD, Moslehi J. Effects of novel angiogenesis inhibitors for the treatment of cancer on the cardiovascular system: focus on hypertension. Circulation 2011;124(15):1687–91.

26. Mego M, Reckova M, Obertova J, et al. Increased cardiotoxicity of sorafenib in sunitinib-pretreated patients with metastatic renal cell carcinoma. Ann Oncol 2007;18(11):1906–7.

27. Petrini I, Lencioni M, Ricasoli M, et al. Phase II trial of sorafenib in combination with 5-fluorouracil infusion in advanced hepatocellular carcinoma. Cancer Chemother Pharmacol 2012;69(3):773–80.

28. Lipton JH, Chuah C, Guerci-Bresler A, et al. Ponatinib versus imatinib for newly diagnosed chronic myeloid leukaemia: an international, randomised, open-label, phase 3 trial. Lancet Oncol 2016; 17(5):612–21.

29. Kantarjian HM, Cortes JE, Kim DW, et al. Bosutinib safety and management of toxicity in leukemia

patients with resistance or intolerance to imatinib and other tyrosine kinase inhibitors. Blood 2014; 123(9):1309–18.

30. Kim TD, le Coutre P, Schwarz M, et al. Clinical cardiac safety profile of nilotinib. Haematologica 2012; 97(6):883–9.

31. Ishikawa J, Matsumura I, Kawaguchi T, et al. Efficacy and safety of switching to nilotinib in patients with CML-CP in major molecular response to imatinib: results of a multicenter phase II trial (NILSw trial). Int J Hematol 2018;107(5):535–40.

32. Fradley MG, Moslehi J. QT prolongation and oncology drug development. Card Electrophysiol Clin 2015;7(2):341–55.

33. Byrd JC, Furman RR, Coutre SE, et al. Targeting BTK with ibrutinib in relapsed chronic lymphocytic leukemia. N Engl J Med 2013;369(1):32–42.

34. Wang ML, Rule S, Martin P, et al. Targeting BTK with ibrutinib in relapsed or refractory mantle-cell lymphoma. N Engl J Med 2013;369(6):507–16.

35. Wiczer TE, Levine LB, Brumbaugh J, et al. Cumulative incidence, risk factors, and management of atrial fibrillation in patients receiving ibrutinib. Blood Adv 2017;1(20):1739–48.

36. Yun S, Vincelette ND, Acharya U, et al. Risk of atrial fibrillation and bleeding diathesis associated with ibrutinib treatment: a systematic review and pooled analysis of four randomized controlled trials. Clin Lymphoma Myeloma Leuk 2017;17(1):31–7.e13.

37. Pretorius L, Du XJ, Woodcock EA, et al. Reduced phosphoinositide 3-kinase (p110alpha) activation increases the susceptibility to atrial fibrillation. Am J Pathol 2009;175(3):998–1009.

38. McMullen JR, Boey EJ, Ooi JY, et al. Ibrutinib increases the risk of atrial fibrillation, potentially through inhibition of cardiac PI3K-Akt signaling. Blood 2014;124(25):3829–30.

39. Wang ML, Blum KA, Martin P, et al. Long-term follow-up of MCL patients treated with single-agent ibrutinib: updated safety and efficacy results. Blood 2015;126(6):739–45.

40. Imbruvica (ibrutinib) [package insert]. Sunnyvale (CA): Pharmacyclics LLC; 2018.

41. Imbruvica: EPAR- product information [package insert]. Beerse (Belgium): Janssen Pharmaceutica NV; 2018.

42. Burger JA, Tedeschi A, Barr PM, et al. Ibrutinib as initial therapy for patients with chronic lymphocytic leukemia. N Engl J Med 2015;373(25):2425–37.

43. Byrd JC, Furman RR, Coutre SE, et al. Three-year follow-up of treatment-naive and previously treated patients with CLL and SLL receiving single-agent ibrutinib. Blood 2015;125(16):2497–506.

44. Wyse DG, Waldo AL, DiMarco JP, et al. A comparison of rate control and rhythm control in patients with atrial fibrillation. N Engl J Med 2002;347(23):1825–33.

45. January CT, Wann LS, Alpert JS, et al. 2014 AHA/ACC/HRS guideline for the management of patients with atrial fibrillation: a report of the American College of Cardiology/American Heart Association Task Force on Practice Guidelines and the Heart Rhythm Society. J Am Coll Cardiol 2014;64(21): e1–76.

46. January CT, Wann LS, Calkins H, et al. 2019 AHA/ACC/HRS focused update of the 2014 AHA/ACC/HRS guideline for the management of patients with atrial fibrillation: a report of the American College of Cardiology/American Heart Association Task Force on Clinical Practice Guidelines and the Heart Rhythm Society. J Am Coll Cardiol 2019. https://doi.org/10.1016/j.jacc.2019.01.011.

47. D'Souza M, Carlson N, Fosbol E, et al. CHA2DS2-VASc score and risk of thromboembolism and bleeding in patients with atrial fibrillation and recent cancer. Eur J Prev Cardiol 2018;25(6): 651–8.

48. Young AM, Marshall A, Thirlwall J, et al. Comparison of an oral factor Xa inhibitor with low molecular weight heparin in patients with cancer with venous thromboembolism: results of a randomized trial (SELECT-D). J Clin Oncol 2018;36(20): 2017–23.

49. National Comprehesive Cancer Network. Cancer-associated venous thromboembolic disease (version 2.2018). Available at: https://www.nccn.org/professionals/physician_gls/pdf/vte.pdf. Accessed May 13, 2019.

50. Kearon C, Akl EA, Ornelas J, et al. Antithrombotic therapy for VTE disease: CHEST guideline and expert panel report. Chest 2016;149(2):315–52.

51. Melloni C, Dunning A, Granger CB, et al. Efficacy and safety of apixaban versus warfarin in patients with atrial fibrillation and a history of cancer: insights from the ARISTOTLE trial. Am J Med 2017; 130(12):1440–8.e1.

52. Fanola CL, Ruff CT, Murphy SA, et al. Efficacy and safety of edoxaban in patients with active malignancy and atrial fibrillation: analysis of the ENGAGE AF - TIMI 48 trial. J Am Heart Assoc 2018;7(16):e008987.

53. Rhea IB, Lyon AR, Fradley MG. Anticoagulation of cardiovascular conditions in the cancer patient: review of old and new therapies. Curr Oncol Rep 2019;21(5):45.

54. Ganatra S, Sharma A, Shah S, et al. Ibrutinib-associated atrial fibrillation. JACC Clin Electrophysiol 2018;4(12):1491–500.

55. Janion-Sadowska A, Papuga-Szela E, Lukaszuk R, et al. Non-vitamin K antagonist oral anticoagulants in patients with atrial fibrillation and thrombocytopenia. J Cardiovasc Pharmacol 2018;72(3):153–60.

56. Kirchhof P, Benussi S, Kotecha D, et al. 2016 ESC Guidelines for the management of atrial fibrillation

developed in collaboration with EACTS. Eur Heart J 2016;37(38):2893–962.

57. Da Costa A, Thevenin J, Roche F, et al. Results from the Loire-Ardeche-Drome-Isere-Puy-de-Dome (LADIP) trial on atrial flutter, a multicentric prospective randomized study comparing amiodarone and radiofrequency ablation after the first episode of symptomatic atrial flutter. Circulation 2006;114(16):1676–81.

58. Calkins H, Hindricks G, Cappato R, et al. 2017 HRS/EHRA/ECAS/APHRS/SOLAECE expert consensus statement on catheter and surgical ablation of atrial fibrillation. Heart Rhythm 2017;14(10):e275–444.

59. Masoudi FA, Calkins H, Kavinsky CJ, et al. 2015 ACC/HRS/SCAI left atrial appendage occlusion device societal overview. J Am Coll Cardiol 2015; 66(13):1497–513.

60. Enriquez A, Biagi J, Redfearn D, et al. Increased incidence of ventricular arrhythmias in patients with advanced cancer and implantable cardioverter-defibrillators. JACC Clin Electrophysiol 2017;3(1):50–6.

61. Adabag AS, Peterson G, Apple FS, et al. Etiology of sudden death in the community: results of anatomical, metabolic, and genetic evaluation. Am Heart J 2010;159(1):33–9.

62. Stancampiano FF, Palmer WC, Getz TW, et al. Rare incidence of ventricular tachycardia and torsades de Pointes in hospitalized patients with prolonged QT who later received levofloxacin: a retrospective study. Mayo Clin Proc 2015;90(5): 606–12.

63. Lenihan DJ, Kowey PR. Overview and management of cardiac adverse events associated with tyrosine kinase inhibitors. Oncologist 2013;18(8): 900–8.

64. Lenihan DJ, Oliva S, Chow EJ, et al. Cardiac toxicity in cancer survivors. Cancer 2013;119(Suppl 11): 2131–42.

65. Menna P, Salvatorelli E, Minotti G. Cancer drugs and QT prolongation: weighing risk against benefit. Expert Opin Drug Saf 2017;16(10):1099–102.

66. Armanious MA, Mishra S, Fradley MG. Electrophysiologic toxicity of chemoradiation. Curr Oncol Rep 2018;20(6):45.

67. Yilmaz U, Oztop I, Ciloglu A, et al. 5-Fluorouracil increases the number and complexity of premature complexes in the heart: a prospective study using ambulatory ECG monitoring. Int J Clin Pract 2007; 61(5):795–801.

68. Khan MA, Masood N, Husain N, et al. A retrospective study of cardiotoxicities induced by 5-fluouracil (5-FU) and 5-FU based chemotherapy regimens in Pakistani adult cancer patients at Shaukat Khanum Memorial Cancer Hospital & Research Center. J Pak Med Assoc 2012;62(5): 430–4.

69. Abdel-Rahman O. 5-Fluorouracil-related cardiotoxicity; findings from five randomized studies of 5-fluorouracil-based regimens in metastatic colorectal cancer. Clin Colorectal Cancer 2019;18(1): 58–63.

70. Kido K, Adams VR, Morehead RS, et al. Capecitabine-induced ventricular fibrillation arrest: possible Kounis syndrome. J Oncol Pharm Pract 2016;22(2): 335–40.

71. Pizzolato JF, Baum MS, Steingart RM, et al. Cardiac toxicity of 5FU: does prophylactic telemetry monitoring of patients at increased risk for cardiac toxicity improve safety? A 10-year experience. J Clin Oncol 2004;22(14_suppl):8107.

72. Porta-Sánchez A, Gilbert C, Spears D, et al. Incidence, diagnosis, and management of QT prolongation induced by cancer therapies: a systematic review. J Am Heart Assoc 2017;6(12). https://doi.org/10.1161/JAHA.117.007724.

73. Arbel Y, Swartzon M, Justo D. QT prolongation and Torsades de Pointes in patients previously treated with anthracyclines. Anticancer Drugs 2007;18(4): 493–8.

74. Ficker E, Kuryshev YA, Dennis AT, et al. Mechanisms of arsenic-induced prolongation of cardiac repolarization. Mol Pharmacol 2004;66(1):33–44.

75. Barbey JT, Pezzullo JC, Soignet SL. Effect of arsenic trioxide on QT interval in patients with advanced malignancies. J Clin Oncol 2003; 21(19):3609–15.

76. Westervelt P, Brown AB, Adkins DR, et al. Sudden death among patients with acute promyelocytic leukemia treated with arsenic trioxide. Blood 2001;98(2):266–71.

77. Roboz GJ, Ritchie EK, Carlin RF, et al. Prevalence, management, and clinical consequences of QT interval prolongation during treatment with arsenic trioxide. J Clin Oncol 2014;32(33):3723–8.

78. National Comprehensive Cancer Network. Acute myeloid leukemia guidelines version 3-2019. Available at: https://www.nccn.org/professionals/physician_gls/pdf/aml.pdf. Accessed May 10, 2019.

79. Kerkela R, Woulfe KC, Durand JB, et al. Sunitinib-induced cardiotoxicity is mediated by off-target inhibition of AMP-activated protein kinase. Clin Transl Sci 2009;2(1):15–25.

80. Chen MH, Kerkela R, Force T. Mechanisms of cardiac dysfunction associated with tyrosine kinase inhibitor cancer therapeutics. Circulation 2008; 118(1):84–95.

81. Viganego F, Singh R, Fradley MG. Arrhythmias and other electrophysiology issues in cancer patients receiving chemotherapy or radiation. Curr Cardiol Rep 2016;18(6):52.

82. Choi BS. Risks associated with sunitinib use and monitoring to improve patient outcomes. Korean J Intern Med 2014;29(1):23–6.

83. Aghel N, Delgado DH, Lipton JH. Cardiovascular toxicities of BCR-ABL tyrosine kinase inhibitors in chronic myeloid leukemia: preventive strategies and cardiovascular surveillance. Vasc Health Risk Manag 2017;13:293–303.

84. Buza V, Rajagopalan B, Curtis AB. Cancer treatment-induced arrhythmias: focus on chemotherapy and targeted therapies. Circ Arrhythm Electrophysiol 2017;10(8). https://doi.org/10.1161/CIRCEP.117.005443.

85. Zhou Y, Zhang Y, Zou H, et al. The multi-targeted tyrosine kinase inhibitor vandetanib plays a bifunctional role in non-small cell lung cancer cells. Sci Rep 2015;5:8629.

86. Bronte E, Bronte G, Novo G, et al. What links BRAF to the heart function? New insights from the cardiotoxicity of BRAF inhibitors in cancer treatment. Oncotarget 2015;6(34):35589–601.

87. Zelboraf (vemurafenib) [package insert]. South San Francisco (CA): Genentech USA Inc.; 2011. Available at: https://www.accessdata.fda.gov/drugsatfda_docs/label/2017/202429s012lbl.pdf.

88. Shah RR, Morganroth J, Shah DR. Cardiovascular safety of tyrosine kinase inhibitors: with a special focus on cardiac repolarisation (QT interval). Drug Saf 2013;36(5):295–316.

89. Ghatalia P, Je Y, Kaymakcalan MD, et al. QTc interval prolongation with vascular endothelial growth factor receptor tyrosine kinase inhibitors. Br J Cancer 2015;112(2):296–305.

90. Guha A, Derbala MH, Zhao Q, et al. Ventricular arrhythmias following ibrutinib initiation for lymphoid malignancies. J Am Coll Cardiol 2018;72(6):697–8.

91. Lampson BL, Yu L, Glynn RJ, et al. Ventricular arrhythmias and sudden death in patients taking ibrutinib. Blood 2017;129(18):2581–4.

92. de Jong J, Hellemans P, Jiao JJ, et al. Ibrutinib does not prolong the corrected QT interval in healthy subjects: results from a thorough QT study. Cancer Chemother Pharmacol 2017;80(6):1227–37.

93. Hortobagyi GN, Stemmer SM, Burris HA, et al. Ribociclib as first-line therapy for HR-positive, advanced breast cancer. N Engl J Med 2016;375(18):1738–48.

94. Spring LM, Zangardi ML, Moy B, et al. Clinical management of potential toxicities and drug interactions related to cyclin-dependent kinase 4/6 inhibitors in breast cancer: practical considerations and recommendations. Oncologist 2017;22(9):1039–48.

95. Tresch DD, Fleg JL. Unexplained sinus bradycardia: clinical significance and long-term prognosis in apparently healthy persons older than 40 years. Am J Cardiol 1986;58(10):1009–13.

96. Khozin S, Blumenthal GM, Zhang L, et al. FDA approval: ceritinib for the treatment of metastatic anaplastic lymphoma kinase-positive non-small cell lung cancer. Clin Cancer Res 2015;21(11):2436–9.

97. Ou SH, Tang Y, Polli A, et al. Factors associated with sinus bradycardia during crizotinib treatment: a retrospective analysis of two large-scale multinational trials (PROFILE 1005 and 1007). Cancer Med 2016;5(4):617–22.

98. Ou SH, Azada M, Dy J, et al. Asymptomatic profound sinus bradycardia (heart rate </=45) in non-small cell lung cancer patients treated with crizotinib. J Thorac Oncol 2011;6(12):2135–7.

99. Gallucci G, Tartarone A, Lombardi L, et al. When crizotinib-induced bradycardia becomes symptomatic: role of concomitant drugs. Expert Rev Anticancer Ther 2015;15(7):761–3.

100. Ou SH, Tong WP, Azada M, et al. Heart rate decrease during crizotinib treatment and potential correlation to clinical response. Cancer 2013;119(11):1969–75.

101. McGuire WP, Rowinsky EK, Rosenshein NB, et al. Taxol: a unique antineoplastic agent with significant activity in advanced ovarian epithelial neoplasms. Ann Intern Med 1989;111(4):273–9.

102. Rowinsky EK, McGuire WP, Guarnieri T, et al. Cardiac disturbances during the administration of taxol. J Clin Oncol 1991;9(9):1704–12.

103. Hodi FS, O'Day SJ, McDermott DF, et al. Improved survival with ipilimumab in patients with metastatic melanoma. N Engl J Med 2010;363(8):711–23.

104. Topalian SL, Hodi FS, Brahmer JR, et al. Safety, activity, and immune correlates of anti-PD-1 antibody in cancer. N Engl J Med 2012;366(26):2443–54.

105. Heinzerling L, Ott PA, Hodi FS, et al. Cardiotoxicity associated with CTLA4 and PD1 blocking immunotherapy. J Immunother Cancer 2016;4:50.

106. Johnson DB, Balko JM, Compton ML, et al. Fulminant myocarditis with combination immune checkpoint blockade. N Engl J Med 2016;375(18):1749–55.

107. Mahmood SS, Fradley MG, Cohen JV, et al. Myocarditis in patients treated with immune checkpoint inhibitors. J Am Coll Cardiol 2018;71(16):1755–64.

Cardiac Interventional Procedures in Cardio-Oncology Patients

Teodora Donisan, MD[a], Dinu Valentin Balanescu, MD[a],
Nicolas Palaskas, MD[a], Juan Lopez-Mattei, MD[a], Kaveh Karimzad, MD[a],
Peter Kim, MD[a], Konstantinos Charitakis, MD[b], Mehmet Cilingiroglu, MD[c],
Konstantinos Marmagkiolis, MD[d], Cezar Iliescu, MD[a],*

KEYWORDS

- Acute coronary syndrome • Cardio-oncology • Coronary artery disease
- Interventional oncocardiology • Percutaneous coronary intervention
- Transcatheter aortic valve replacement

KEY POINTS

- Interventional cardio-oncology is an emerging field. Modern tools are available for the safe and effective treatment of patients with cancer requiring invasive therapies.
- Patients with cancer are less likely to be treated according to societal guidelines because of perceived high risk, especially in cases of acute coronary syndrome.
- Most patients with cancer can be treated with minimally invasive therapies when clinically indicated, such as percutaneous coronary intervention or transcatheter valve replacements.
- Pericardial disease is frequent in the cancer population. The treatment of pericardial effusions depends on the acuity and cause. They can be effectively managed with medical therapy, simple pericardiocentesis, extended catheter drainage, pericardial sclerotherapy and intrapericardial treatments, percutaneous balloon pericardiotomy, or surgical window.
- Endomyocardial biopsies are essential for the modern diagnosis of cardiac tumors, myocarditis, or infiltrative diseases.

INTRODUCTION

Comorbidities specific to the cardio-oncology population contribute to the challenges in the interventional management of patients with cancer with cardiovascular disease (CVD). Patients with cancer have generally been excluded from cardiovascular randomized clinical trials, particularly those assessing invasive approaches. However, endovascular procedures may represent a valid option in patients with cancer with a range of CVDs because of their minimally invasive nature. This article presents the specific challenges that interventional cardiologists face when caring for patients with cancer and the modern tools to optimize care.

Disclosure: The authors have nothing to disclose.
[a] Department of Cardiology, The University of Texas MD Anderson Cancer Center, 1400 Pressler Street, Unit 1451, Houston, TX 77030, USA; [b] Department of Cardiology, McGovern Medical School at The University of Texas Health Science Center at Houston, 6431 Fannin Street, Houston, TX 77030, USA; [c] Department of Cardiology, Arkansas Heart Hospital, 1701 South Shackleford Road, Little Rock, AR 72211, USA; [d] Florida Hospital, Pepin Heart Institute, 3100 East Fletcher Avenue, Tampa, FL 33613, USA
* Corresponding author.
E-mail address: ciliescu@mdanderson.org
twitter: @TDonisan (T.D.); @dinubalanescu (D.V.B.); @cezar_ciliescu (C.I.)

Cardiol Clin 37 (2019) 469–486
https://doi.org/10.1016/j.ccl.2019.07.012

CORONARY ARTERY DISEASE AND ACUTE CORONARY SYNDROME
Causes, Pathophysiology, Epidemiology

Shared risk factors between cancer and CVD predispose to the coexistence of these conditions.[1] As modern cancer therapies are becoming more effective, the mean age of cancer survivors is increasing, and, with it, the risk for CVD.[2] Recent data suggest that cancer survivorship status is in itself an independent risk factor for CVD.[3]

Although a direct causative relationship has not been definitively proved between cancer and coronary artery disease (CAD), several pathogenic mechanisms in malignancies increase the risk for CAD. These mechanisms also differentiate CAD in patients with cancer from the general cardiovascular population. Prothrombotic, procoagulative, and proinflammatory factors all lead to endothelial damage and atherosclerosis progression.[4,5] This effect seems to be stage dependent, with advanced cancers being linked to a higher risk of arterial thromboembolism.[6] Furthermore, ruptured coronary atherosclerotic plaques promote thrombosis and lead to acute coronary syndromes (ACSs). Approximately 15% of patients with ACSs have active cancer or a malignancy history.[7]

Several chemotherapeutic agents have been linked with vascular toxicities and CAD. Increased vasoreactivity, vasospasm, and ischemic events have been observed following administration of 5-fluorouracil, paclitaxel, docetaxel, cyclophosphamide, or cisplatin.[8–10] Tyrosine kinase inhibitors (TKIs) are notoriously associated with vascular events, particularly ponatinib (6.2% prevalence),[11] followed by nilotinib, dasatinib, and imatinib.[12] Small molecule TKIs (such as sorafenib and erlotinib) have also been linked to cardiovascular events in ∼3% of patients.[9] Anti–vascular endothelial growth factor TKIs (eg, bevacizumab) may lead to hypertension and arterial thrombotic events,[13] possibly caused by decreased nitric oxide synthesis.[14] Severe cases of myocardial infarction have been described following treatment with all-trans-retinoic acid.[15] Immune checkpoint inhibitors such as nivolumab and atezolizumab may trigger ACS through coronary vasospasm.[16]

Radiation-induced CAD (RI-CAD) is a particularly aggressive form of CAD specific to the cancer population that develops secondary to direct endothelial damage rather than vasospasm.[17] The risk for RI-CAD is directly proportional to the cumulative dose of mediastinal radiation administered.[18] The most important risk factors are younger age at the time of treatment and cumulative doses greater than 30 Gy.[18] CAD in these patients generally manifests 5 to 10 years following chest radiation therapy.[5] Although there no current guidelines for screening or managing RI-CAD, the authors recommend regular assessment for ischemic burden and aggressive control of the traditional cardiovascular risk factors.[5] Patients with RI-CAD are at increased risk for in-stent restenosis and may require more interventions compared with the general population.[19] They also present with angina or heart failure (HF) less frequently than the general cardiovascular population, and are at a higher risk for fatal cardiovascular events.[20]

Clinical Features and Diagnostic Challenges

Clinicians should be aware of the special considerations for the diagnosis and management of CAD or ACS in patients with cancer.[21] Patients with cancer with CAD or ACS are less likely than the general population to present with angina, possibly because of ongoing use of analgesics for their malignancy.[22] The most common presenting symptom of ACS in patients with cancer is dyspnea in 44% of patients, whereas chest pain was seen in only 30%.[22] Atypical presentations are frequent, whereas ACS may be confounded by other malignancy-related symptoms. Suspicion for ACS should be raised in cases of new-onset hypotension, arrhythmias, HF, syncope, altered mental status, or sudden cardiac death, with special attention in patients undergoing active chemotherapy.

Rapid recognition of ACS in patients with cancer is essential to improve outcomes. Once ACS suspicion is established, rapid measurement of cardiac biomarkers (troponin I, creatinine kinase-MB [muscle/brain]) should be performed with repeat measurements every 6 to 8 hours until either 2 or 3 normal measurements or observation of a downward trend are obtained. Concurrently, coagulation studies and serial electrocardiograms (ECGs) should be performed. If available, these should be compared with previous ECGs to aid in acute diagnosis. Non-ST elevation myocardial infarction (NSTEMI) is more frequent than ST elevation myocardial infarction (STEMI). An echocardiographic assessment may be useful, because it may show new-onset HF in the setting of ACS. Other imaging modalities, such as myocardial perfusion imaging, cardiac MRI, cardiac computed tomography angiography, and cardiac PET have a limited role in the setting of ACS, but may offer important information for assessment of CAD and cardiovascular risk.

Despite advances in noninvasive imaging, coronary angiography remains the gold standard for

CAD assessment. It provides physiologic coronary lesion evaluation, measurement of intracardiac pressures, and percutaneous coronary intervention (PCI) when indicated. Approximately 10% of patients undergoing PCI have either active cancer or a history of cancer.[23] These patients are at an increased risk for bleeding, target lesion revascularization, and cardiovascular adverse events compared with patients without cancer.[23–27] However, PCI improves outcomes in most patients with cancer with ACS compared with no PCI.[22,28,29] However, in patients with metastatic cancer, data suggest no benefit of PCI versus optimal medical therapy.[30] A particularly challenging situation in patients with cancer with CAD or ACS is the presence of chronic thrombocytopenia. Thrombocytopenia in patients with cancer may be the result of anticancer treatments or the malignancy. Concerns for bleeding may prompt interventional cardiologists to defer invasive approaches or PCI because of the need for dual antiplatelet therapy (DAPT). However, recent data suggest that cardiac catheterization and PCI are safe in thrombocytopenic patients with meticulous vascular access and use of vascular closure devices, and improve cardiovascular outcomes.[31–34]

Physiologic assessment of coronary lesions with fractional flow reserve (FFR) or instantaneous wave-free ratio (iFR) is particularly useful for revascularization decision, particularly in intermediate lesions (40%–70%) based on percentage diameter stenosis or quantitative coronary angiography.[35,36] FFR is a measurement of flow across stenotic lesions, which may account for the myocardial mass supplied by a specific coronary vessel and myocardial viability. FFR assessment is crucial for assessing left main coronary artery and ostial lesions, which are difficult to interpret angiographically and are frequent in patients with cancer.[37] In the general population, an FFR greater than 0.8 suggests no hemodynamic significance. In patients with cancer, an FFR threshold of less than or equal to 0.75 has been documented to be safe and to provide a reasonable compromise between revascularizing significant lesions and deferring some unnecessary procedures.[38,39] iFR has been shown to be noninferior to FFR with regard to lesion assessment, decreases procedural time, and does not require adenosine administration.[40,41] An iFR cutoff point of 0.89 seems to be safe. Recent evidence suggests that noninvasive physiologic assessment with coronary computed tomography angiography–derived FFR may be superior to invasive FFR[42]; however, these results have not yet been validated in the cancer population.

Intracoronary imaging may provide important anatomic information regarding coronary lesion stability.[19] Intravascular ultrasonography (IVUS) and optical coherence tomography have been shown to be noninferior to FFR for identifying lesions that may be safely deferred from revascularization.[43–46] Stenosis of the left main coronary artery should be assessed by IVUS.[47]

Management of Acute Coronary Syndrome

Interventional cardio-oncology teams face the challenge of offering optimal care to all patients while avoiding unnecessary invasive procedures in this inherently high-risk population. Cancer treatment should be temporarily suspended if ACS is suspected.[48] Because of comorbidities and perceived risks, management of ACS according to societal guidelines is significantly underused in the oncology population.[49–52] Current data suggest that the American Heart Association (AHA)/ American College of Cardiology (ACC) guidelines for ACS management[53] should be used in most patients, regardless of cancer status or treatment. Early angiography (within 24 hours) should be performed if the initial TIMI (Thrombolysis in Myocardial Infarction) score is greater than or equal to 3. The authors recommend using a modified TIMI score, with the addition of 1 point for each of the following: history of chest radiation therapy or known prothrombotic or phase I chemotherapies. If revascularization is indicated, either bare metal stents (BMSs) or new-generation drug-eluting stents (DESs) may be used. Traditionally, BMS have been used in patients with cancer because of shorter need for DAPT. However, newer-generation DESs may allow for DAPT duration as short as 4 weeks, similar to BMS.[54] In thrombocytopenic patients with stents, aspirin (as a single antiplatelet treatment) should be considered if platelet counts are greater than 10,000/µL, with the addition of a P2Y12 inhibitor if platelet counts are greater than 30,000/µL, although there are case series that report stenting and DAPT in patients with platelet counts less than 30,000/µL. If platelet counts are less than 50,000/µL, prasugrel, ticagrelor, or GPIIb-IIIa inhibitors should be avoided.

Takotsubo Syndrome

Special considerations apply to patients with cancer presenting with Takotsubo syndrome (TS). TS is an acute HF syndrome that may present similarly to NSTEMI or STEMI. It was traditionally considered a benign condition; however, recent data suggest that outcomes may be similar to ACS.[55–57] The prevalence of TS in patients with cancer presenting with ACS suspicion is between 10% and 20%, much higher than in the noncancer population.[58] TS may be triggered by emotional or physical stressors (eg, invasive procedures) or by cancer treatment (chemotherapy, radiation therapy). Several chemotherapeutic agents have been linked with TS, including 5-fluorouracil (most common), paclitaxel, sunitinib, rituximab, bevacizumab, cytarabine, capecitabine.[59,60] Chemotherapy-induced TS is associated with higher risks for complications and mortality.[56] Differentiating between TS and ACS may prove difficult, especially because TS may also present with high serum troponin level, signs of myocardial ischemia, and evidence of CAD.[61] On TS resolution, chemotherapy may be promptly resumed.

STRUCTURAL VALVE DISEASE

Patients with cancer have a high risk of developing valvular disease because of their exposure to cardiotoxic anticancer agents and chest radiation.[62–64]

Transcatheter Aortic Valve Replacement

Aortic stenosis (AS) is an important cardiovascular comorbidity in patients with cancer, because of the frequent co-occurrence of these two conditions.[65,66] AS is an independent predictor of increased cardiovascular mortality in patients with cancer, irrespective of whether the cancer is active or not.[67,68] AS management in patients with cancer is challenging because surgical aortic valve replacement (SAVR) is often deemed prohibitive or high risk while maximal cancer treatments are held or postponed because of the advert events associated with severe symptomatic AS.

Although AS has traditionally been treated via SAVR, modern approaches include an emphasis on the interventional management via transcatheter aortic valve replacement (TAVR). TAVR was initially recommended for nonoperable or high-risk patients,[69] but nowadays it is approved for intermediate-risk and low-risk patients[70]; ongoing studies have been investigating its role even in asymptomatic patients.[71] Cancer was considered as a contraindication for SAVR.[72] Cardiac surgery is associated with high morbidity in patients with a history of cancer,[73] especially with previous mediastinal radiation therapy.[74] TAVR seems to be an acceptable-risk intervention for the treatment of AS and may allow patients to undergo cancer treatment as indicated.[75,76] Although TAVR can overcome the technical difficulties typically associated with SAVR,[77] major comorbidities similarly influence postprocedural prognosis after TAVR and SAVR.[78] There is evidence in favor of aortic valve replacement in patients with cancer regardless of the cancer type or treatment,[79] with TAVR yielding the best results on survival.[76]

The appropriate timing for TAVR depends on the clinical scenario. TAVR is considered in patients with cancers in remission and in those with a prognosis of more than 1 year.[80,81] It could be appropriate for TAVR to be performed in early-stage cancers after remissive therapy, and in later-stage cancers before more aggressive treatments.[82–84] Patients with active, advanced, untreated cancers have a worse prognosis after TAVR than patients in remission.[65,81,85] In patients with final stages of disease (eg, advanced, metastatic disease, severe anemia, symptomatic HF), and an estimated survival of less than 1 year, a more conservative approach focusing on improving quality of life during palliative treatment should be preferred. In those cases, balloon valvuloplasty can be considered.[21,86]

Other Interventional Valvular Procedures

Transcatheter mitral valve repair with MitraClip offers good results in high-risk patients,[87,88] even in cardiac amyloid-light chain (AL) amyloidosis.[89] There are concerns that, in patients with a history of malignancy, MitraClip could be associated with increased mortality.[90]

The use of transcatheter mitral valve replacement has been reported in a series of 18 valve-in-valve procedures in high-risk patients, including a lung cancer case, with good clinical and hemodynamic results, suggesting its feasibility in the cancer population.[91]

Patients with chemotherapy-induced cardiomyopathy (CCMP) have a higher incidence of severe tricuspid regurgitation requiring tricuspid valve repair.[92] Unlike the treatment goals for TAVR and transcatheter mitral valve replacement, which can be curative, transcatheter tricuspid valve interventions (TTVIs) are considered in the context of multilevel HF therapy.[93] At the moment, there are no clear guidelines to define the patient profile that could benefit from TTVI, although there is a correlation between significant tricuspid valve regurgitation and increased mortality.[94] There have been few successful cases of valve-in-valve transcatheter tricuspid valve replacements reported.[95,96]

Carcinoid heart disease (CHD) is a rare complication of carcinoid syndrome that more commonly involves the right side of the heart.[97] Although the tricuspid and pulmonary valves are most commonly involved, the mitral and aortic valves can be affected as well.[98] Valvular surgery can improve outcomes in CHD, with acceptable risks.[99] Transcatheter valve replacements on native or bioprosthetic tricuspid and pulmonary valves (ie, valve-in-valve procedures) have been reported.[99–103]

DEVICE-BASED THERAPIES FOR ADVANCED HEART FAILURE

HF from CCMP and radiotherapy-induced cardiomyopathy (RCMP) greatly influence survival and morbidity in cancer survivors.[104–106] CCMP and RCMP typically present in younger patients, most likely female, with fewer traditional comorbidities, and are biventricular cardiomyopathies, often with significant right ventricular dysfunction. CCMP has worse outcomes than other HF causes,[107] potentially leading to end-stage HF requiring advanced therapies.[108,109] Because of concerns related to survival in patients with cancer, unlike other populations with advanced HF, patients with CCMP do not benefit from implantable cardiac defibrillators (ICDs), left ventricular assist devices (LVADs), or transplant as frequently as patients without cancer.[110–112] There is also a concern that the immunosuppressive therapy required after transplant could accelerate malignancy recurrence. However, some investigators suggest that, despite the higher incidence of malignancy and infection in patients with CCMP receiving heart transplants, their survival is comparable with those receiving transplants for other cardiomyopathies.[108,113]

Implantable Defibrillators and Cardiac Resynchronization Therapy

ICDs and cardiac resynchronization therapy (CRT) significantly decrease mortality and are recommended in specific cases of systolic HF, regardless of the cause.[114] The utility of CRT and ICD has been documented in CCMP, leading to clinical, echocardiographic, and functional improvements.[115–118] However, patients with HF caused by CCMP or RCMP are less likely to receive ICDs and CRT than those with other HF causes.[115,119] The appropriate use of these advanced HF treatments could potentially affect cancer care as well, allowing the continuation of therapies that prolong survival.[115]

Patients with cardiovascular implantable electronic devices such as pacemakers and ICDs who require neutron-producing radiotherapy can experience device malfunction (eg, pacing or sensing threshold changes, rapid battery depletion, signal interference, loss of stored events, parameter or programming events).[120,121] These events are rare, nearly always software based, and transient when they do occur. Data suggest that high beam energy is the cause for the malfunction and not the total radiation dose.[120–122]

Durable Mechanical Circulatory Support

Mechanical circulatory support (MCS) is an alternative mode of advanced therapy for CCMP as a bridge to heart transplant or as destination therapy.[123–125] It has been used to improve survival and functional capacity in patients with CCMP, although they have increased bleeding risks.[119,126–128] There have also been reports stating that the presence of LVAD can significantly change cancer management.[129] Although in most cardiomyopathies the dysfunction mainly affects the left ventricle and ~90% of MCS patients can be treated with LVAD alone,[130] patients with CCMP experience right ventricular failure more often and could benefit from a right ventricular assist device or the use of a total artificial heart.[119] Patients with CCMP require biventricular support more often than patients with other nonischemic cardiomyopathies who receive heart transplants.[108] The need for biventricular support is associated with a poorer prognosis.[119,130] The implication of MCS in patients with RCMP, especially with a restrictive physiology, is less understood and further studies are required.[131,132]

Pulmonary Artery Pressure Telemonitoring

CardioMEMS is an implantable wireless device used for the remote monitoring of pulmonary artery pressures in patients with chronic HF.[133] It can significantly influence HF management by providing daily hemodynamic information, allowing prompt and personalized management.[134] The CardioMEMS system can safely be used, with only 1% device-related complication, mainly consisting of easily manageable puncture site bleeding.[133] Its use has not yet been documented in patients with cancer.

PERICARDIAL INTERVENTIONS

Pericardial disease is an important comorbidity in patients with cancer. Although in the general population pericarditis is usually a benign and self-limiting disease,[135] in patients with cancer it is associated with increased short-term and long-term mortality.[136] Pericarditis can be a marker of occult cancer when it occurs as an isolated finding,[136] but even more so when it is associated with pericardial effusion.[137,138]

Pericardial effusions in patients with cancer can be either malignant or nonmalignant. The pericardium can be affected directly through malignant infiltration from adjacent structures, pericardial hemorrhage, or hematogenous or lymphatic dissemination of cancer cells.[139] The most common cancers associated with pericardial disease are breast cancer, lung cancer, leukemia, and lymphoma.[140–142] Primary pericardial cancers are very rare and include pericardial mesothelioma (most commonly), sarcomas, and lymphomas.[143] The pericardium can be affected indirectly as part of the paraneoplastic syndrome, by cancer treatments, or from opportunistic infections.[144] The anticancer treatments associated with pericardial effusions include chemotherapy (eg, anthracyclines, cyclophosphamide, cytarabine, imatinib, dasatinib, interferon, arsenic trioxide, docetaxel, and 5-fluorouracil), bone marrow transplant, and mediastinal radiotherapy.[64]

Small and moderate pericardial effusions are often asymptomatic, but patients can present with dyspnea, cough, tachycardia, pulsus paradoxus, and hypotension, depending on the fluid volume and whether it developed acutely. Although ECG can be useful in the diagnosis of acute pericarditis and cardiac MRI (CMR) is best at visualizing pericardial inflammation and thickening, transthoracic echocardiography (TTE) is the imaging modality of choice.[64] TTE can be used to immediately and fully assess the hemodynamic effects of the effusion and for serial monitoring before and after treatment.

The treatment of pericardial effusion depends on the acuity and cause, varying between medical management (eg, chemotherapy, corticotherapy), simple pericardiocentesis, extended catheter drainage, pericardial sclerotherapy and intrapericardial treatments, percutaneous balloon pericardiotomy, or surgical window.[145]

Pericardiocentesis and Extended Catheter Drainage

Pericardiocentesis is a minimally invasive approach that can be performed under local anesthesia. It requires a needle to be placed in the pericardial space, most commonly through the subxiphoid or apical-intercostal area, usually under echocardiographic or fluoroscopic guidance.[146–150] In case of suboptimal image quality on echocardiography or for patients in the postoperative period, computed tomography guidance can be a useful alternative.[151] Although blind pericardiocentesis can be performed in emergencies, this technique has a very high complication rate.[152] The most serious complications of pericardiocentesis are laceration and perforation of the myocardium or the coronaries, but other complications can also arise: pneumothorax, arrhythmias, air embolisms, or peritoneal cavity or abdominal viscera puncture.[149,153]

Pericardiocentesis is performed for 3 main indications: cardiac tamponade, large pericardial effusions (≥2 cm), or for diagnostic purposes.[154] Pericardiocentesis can be an isolated

intervention, but an intrapericardial catheter is often kept for prolonged fluid evacuation.[155] In severe pericardial effusions, brain natriuretic peptide levels are suppressed and may increase after pericardiocentesis.[156] Rapid pericardial fluid drainage of more than 1 L should be avoided and prolonged pericardial drainage favored because of the risks of acute pulmonary edema.

Prolonged catheter drainage is an effective means to prevent pericardial fluid reaccumulation probably not only because of fluid drainage itself but also because of the obliteration of the pericardial space after the inflammation provoked by the catheter. The optimal duration to keep the pericardial drain tube is 3 to 5 days, a shorter duration being associated with increased recurrence and a longer duration with increased infection rates.[154,157] A pericardial window should be considered if the output is still high 6 to 7 days after the pericardiocentesis.

Although an International Normalized Ratio greater than 1.5 and thrombocytopenia less than 50.000/μL are relative contraindications to the procedure and should be corrected before the procedure,[158] pericardiocentesis and pericardial drainage are deemed safe even in thrombocytopenic patients with cancer.[147,154,159] Factors associated with increased mortality in patients with malignant effusions are older age (>65 years), severe thrombocytopenia (platelet counts <20.000/μL), lung cancer, pericardial fluid cytology positive for malignancy, and drainage duration.[154]

Right heart catheterization can be performed simultaneously with the pericardiocentesis in order to monitor the hemodynamic improvement as the effusion is drained and to identify anomalies persisting in the case of effusive-constrictive pericarditis.[160]

The successful management of pericardial effusions does not only imply relief of immediate symptoms and hemodynamic instability but it also prevents fluid reacummulation.[155] The latter issue is particularly problematic in patients with cancer, who can have up to 5 times more reinterventions than patients with nonneoplastic effusions.[161] The recurrence rate for pericardial effusions is higher for percutaneous pericardiocentesis than for pericardiotomy, although the length of stay and intensive care unit admissions are similar between the two approaches.[162] A systematic review found that extended pericardial drainage, pericardial sclerosis, and balloon pericardiotomy were all associated with significantly lower recurrence rates that plain pericardiocentesis.[163]

Pericardial Sclerotherapy and Intrapericardial Treatments

Although the preferred management for recurrent pericardial effusion is surgery, intrapericardial injection of chemotherapeutic (eg, cisplatin, thiotepa, bleomycin, bevacizumab) or sclerosing (eg, doxycycline, tetracycline) agents can be attempted.[149] These agents can be used for their ability to induce fibrosis and promote intrapericardial adhesions but also as a synergistic antineoplastic treatment strategy. Local intrapericardial chemotherapy for the treatment of neoplastic pericardial disease can be an effective way to control pericardial effusion and masses immediately, but the recurrence rate makes the therapeutic advantage to pericardial drainage modest.[157,164–168]

Pericardial Windows

Surgical decompression of the pericardium, also known as pericardiotomy, pericardiostomy, and window pericardiectomy, by either conventional heart surgery or video-assisted thoracoscopy, is an alternative to minimally invasive percutaneous procedures.[169,170] Although the surgical treatment of malignant effusions may offer a more definitive solution,[162,169,171] it is associated with significant complications.[172,173] At the same time, patients with cancer are poor surgical candidates with significant perioperative risks.[174]

Because malignant effusions have high recurrence rates[175] and the definitive treatment via surgery is not an ideal option for patients with cancer, alternative options have been sought. Percutaneous balloon pericardiotomy (PBP) is especially used as a palliative measure for patients with a reduced life expectancy to improve quality of life.[158] PBP is a transcutaneous approach involving the inflation of a balloon catheter through the pericardial space to create a pericardial window.[176] This technique creates a communication with the mediastinal, pleural, or peritoneal space, where resorptive capacity is greater.[177] It is a safe and effective therapeutic alternative to surgery, even in high-risk patients,[176,178] but its success rate is low in malignant mesothelioma.[179] A major concern for this procedure is the spread of neoplastic cells to the pleural or peritoneal cavity.[149] Contraindications include major coagulation disorders, effusive-constrictive pericarditis, loculated pericardial effusions, large left pleural effusion, advanced respiratory insufficiency, and pneumectomy.[180]

Pericardioscopy, and pericardial and epicardial biopsies

Pericardioscopy allows the visualization of the pericardial space and biopsies from the pericardial and epicardial layers with more accuracy, avoiding epicardial vessels and increasing the probability of uncovering the underlying cause.[181] Establishing a definitive diagnosis was thought to be an additional argument for the surgical approach as well, which allows pericardial tissue sampling.[155] More recent studies have shown that there is no additional diagnostic yield from direct surgical observation, cytologic analysis, and pericardial histopathology in patients with negative pericardial fluid cytology.[141,169,172,182]

ENDOMYOCARDIAL BIOPSY

Endomyocardial biopsy (EMB) is commonly used for the surveillance of cardiac allograft rejection and, to a lesser extent, for the diagnosis of unexplained ventricular dysfunction.[183] The latter indication is patient specific, because other modern diagnostic tools (eg, TTE, CMR, nuclear studies) can often help narrow down the diagnosis noninvasively. EMB is essential in a small number of situations: to monitor cardiac transplant rejection status, to diagnose suspected myocarditis or infiltrative cardiomyopathy, to diagnose cardiac tumors, to detect suspected drug toxicity, or to diagnose secondary cardiac involvement by systemic disease.[183–186]

EMB is frequently performed through the femoral or jugular veins.[187] Biopsy samples should be obtained from the interventricular septum, because sampling the thin right ventricular free wall is dangerous.[188] A minimum of 5 right ventricular samples should be obtained, although this number has a lower diagnostic yield for myocarditis than for transplant rejection.[189] Left-sided biopsies are thought to be more complicated and are seldom required, in cases of specific left ventricular masses, lesions, or regions of interest.[190] Although it is considered that the diagnostic yield from left ventricular biopsies could be higher,[191] more recent data indicate that right and left ventricular EMB are similar when inflammation of viral genome is assessed.[192] The most important factor influencing the diagnostic yield of EMB is the number of samples obtained.[192] The tissue samples obtained should be analyzed using histology, immunohistochemistry, and viral genomes.[193] Similar to the guidance used in other interventional procedures (eg, pericardiocentesis), echocardiography and fluoroscopy are most commonly used, although they both have limitations mainly stemming from their two-dimensional nature.[184,194,195] Fluoroscopy cannot visualize soft tissue and the directionality of the bioptome is difficult to determine in individual projections, whereas echocardiography may miss the tip of the bioptome and the chordae tendineae are not well visualized and can be damaged.[196] Three-dimensional imaging could provide an alternative to better visualize cardiac structures and to guide biopsy instrumentation.[197,198]

Although a safe procedure, EMB is associated with procedural complications and long-term sequelae. More commonly reported complications include access site hematoma, transient blocks and arrhythmias, tricuspid insufficiency, and occult pulmonary embolism.[183,196,199] Current flexible bioptomes reduced the life-threatening complication rate to less than 1%.[92,200] The risk of clinically relevant perforation is lower in cardiac transplant recipients after 3 months and in patients with prior pericardial instrumentation than in patients with no previous cardiac procedures, because of the fibrosis and near obliteration of the pericardial space, causing any right ventricular perforation to be immediately contained by the pericardium.[196] Only patients who require repeated EMB, such as heart transplant recipients, are at risk of long-term complications, such as coronary artery to right ventricular fistula and severe tricuspid valve regurgitation.[201,202] EMB tricuspid valve regurgitation is important because of the frequent occurrence in patients undergoing multiple procedures and can lead to increased mortalities even in asymptomatic individuals.[202,203] Potential measures to limit damage to the tricuspid valve and supporting structures would be to use longer sheaths allowing the bioptome to pass through the valve with minimal contact with the valve apparatus.[154]

MYOCARDITIS AND CARDIOMYOPATHY

Myocarditis is a polymorphic disease with a variable clinical presentation ranging from fulminant to acute, subacute, or chronic arrhythmia, or HF, to asymptomatic biventricular dysfunction.[193,204] It is an inflammatory disease with infectious, autoimmune, toxic, or idiopathic causes. Prognosis is mainly related to the cause and severity of biventricular dysfunction at presentation, although risk stratification is uncertain, especially because of a lack of diagnosis confirmation by EMB.[193,204] CMR can identify edema and gadolinium enhancement, making it a valid noninvasive option to aid in the diagnosis of myocarditis alongside EMB, but it cannot replace EMB, which is still considered the gold standard for diagnosis.[193,205]

EMB is essential in guiding the therapeutic approach because it can detect giant cell or eosinophilic myocarditis and it can exclude infectious agents in patients who may be candidates for immunosuppressive treatments.[190,193,206,207] Giant cell myocarditis and necrotizing eosinophilic myocarditis have poor prognoses, but they can respond to corticosteroid therapy.[208,209] Lymphocytic myocarditis and hypersensitivity myocarditis have better prognoses,[208] can be treated with corticosteroid therapy as well, but a drug reaction can also be considered and certain medications can be modified or discontinued.[210] EMB can thus be instrumental in deciding the therapeutic action and discussing prognosis.

Among the toxins incriminated in the cause of inflammatory cardiomyopathies are chemotherapeutic drugs (especially anthracyclines), catecholamines, cytokines, cocaine, and alcohol.[211] In patients with suspected anthracycline-induced cardiomyopathy, the purpose of EMB in cases in which the cause of the cardiac dysfunction is unclear is to determine whether anthracycline doses can be increased, or for research purposes.[184] An emerging role for EMB could be to help better understand and develop more appropriate therapies for the cardiac toxicities of novel anticancer treatments, such as immune checkpoint inhibitors or chimeric antigen receptor T-cell therapy,[212,213] although there are no specific guidelines in this regard. EMB can be useful in the management of arrhythmia of uncertain cause, because it can diagnose occult myocardial disease (cardiomyopathy, myocarditis, arrhythmogenic cardiomyopathy, or amyloidosis).[214,215]

Infiltrative Diseases

EMB can be used to diagnose cardiac sarcoidosis and amyloidosis. Cardiac sarcoidosis is a rare but potentially fatal condition.[216,217] It can present in various ways, from minimally symptomatic or asymptomatic, to congestive HF, conduction abnormalities, and sudden death.[217] All patients diagnosed with sarcoidosis should be screened for cardiac involvement because of the potential life-threatening complications and because it responds to corticotherapy. Initial work-up includes ECG and TTE, but further imaging can be required (ie, CMR, PET, single-photon emission CT).[217,218] EMB can confirm the presence of granulomas or scaring, but it also serves a prognostic purpose, because a positive EMB for sarcoidosis is associated with a shorter median survival time, possibly reflecting a more widespread granulomatous inflammation.[216] EMB is insensitive in sarcoidosis because of the patchy myocardial involvement and because sarcoid tends to involve the base of the heart (an area not usually biopsied),[190,219] so treatment is recommended in cases of strongly suspected sarcoidosis despite negative EMB.[220]

Sarcoidosis is associated with systolic dysfunction, but other infiltrative diseases, such as amyloidosis or Fabry disease, cause restrictive cardiomyopathies with thickened ventricular walls that may resemble hypertrophic cardiomyopathy. Although EMB has no role for the diagnosis of hypertrophic cardiomyopathy, it is recommended in cases of highly suspected amyloidosis or Fabry disease, because of its prognostic and therapeutic implications.[184,221] However, multimodality modern imaging is starting to provide more and more information to aid in the diagnosis of infiltrative diseases.[218,222,223] Amyloid may be diagnosed and immunotyped, with management implications. Note that amyloid can deposit only in the heart, so a negative extracardiac biopsy does not necessarily exclude cardiac amyloidosis.[190] AL amyloid is seen in primary amyloidosis and plasma cell dyscrasia, including myeloma. These patients have worse prognoses than patients with senile or familial forms,[224,225] but they can respond to chemotherapy or stem cell transplant.[226] An accurate diagnosis of Fabry disease is also important because enzyme replacement therapy (eg, recombinant alpha-galactosidase A, galactose) may improve cardiac dysfunction.[227,228]

Patients with cancer are at risk from iron overload because of their need for repeated transfusions. This condition could lead to cardiac hemochromatosis, a reversible cause of cardiomyopathy.[229] Hemochromatosis is most commonly quantified with hepatic biopsies, but there is no association between liver and myocardial iron deposition. EMB can confirm the diagnosis of cardiac hemochromatosis and speed up the initiation of appropriate therapy.

CARDIAC TUMORS

Although cardiac tumors are very rare, their accurate diagnosis is an essential issue for cardio-oncologists, because they can significantly alter management. Multimodality imaging is often needed to determine the cause, providing useful information both independently and in corroboration with EMB.[230,231] EMB can be used for the diagnosis of cardiac tumors, be they benign or malignant (primary or secondary), if the diagnosis cannot be made in any other way, if the result can alter the therapeutic approach, if it has a high likelihood of being successful, and if it can be performed by an experienced operator.[184] Right-sided tumors can easily be biopsied through transvenous biopsy and left-sided tumors can be accessed via transseptal puncture or retrograde via arterial access.[232] If imaging features are suggestive for atrial myxoma, EMB is contraindicated, because this tumor has a high likelihood of embolization.[184] Although the heart is more commonly

affected by metastatic disease, when there usually are other more accessible metastasis locations present, there are certain cancers with an affinity toward the heart, such as melanoma.[190] In such cases, EMB may be the most accessible tissue and allow treatment or palliation, as appropriate.

SUMMARY

Interventional oncocardiology is an emerging field. As an ancillary diagnostic modality it provides invaluable information for complex clinical scenarios. Moreover, it offers minimally invasive therapeutic options in this frail patient subgroup with cancer and heart disease. Modern tools are available for the safe and effective treatment of patients with cancer requiring invasive procedures. Larger studies are needed to confirm the value and expand the role of interventional oncocardiology.

REFERENCES

1. Whitlock MC, Yeboah J, Burke GL, et al. Cancer and its association with the development of coronary artery calcification: an assessment from the multi-ethnic study of atherosclerosis. J Am Heart Assoc 2015;4(11) [pii:e002533].
2. Barac A, Murtagh G, Carver JR, et al. Cardiovascular health of patients with cancer and cancer survivors: a roadmap to the next level. J Am Coll Cardiol 2015;65(25):2739–46.
3. Winther JF, Bhatia S, Cederkvist L, et al. Risk of cardiovascular disease among Nordic childhood cancer survivors with diabetes mellitus: a report from adult life after childhood cancer in Scandinavia. Cancer 2018;124(22):4393–400.
4. Oren O, Herrmann J. Arterial events in cancer patients-the case of acute coronary thrombosis. J Thorac Dis 2018;10(Suppl 35):S4367–85.
5. Giza DE, Iliescu G, Hassan S, et al. Cancer as a risk factor for cardiovascular disease. Curr Oncol Rep 2017;19(6):39.
6. Navi BB, Reiner AS, Kamel H, et al. Risk of arterial thromboembolism in patients with cancer. J Am Coll Cardiol 2017;70(8):926–38.
7. Banasiak W, Zymlinski R, Undas A. Optimal management of cancer patients with acute coronary syndrome. Pol Arch Intern Med 2018;128(4):244–53.
8. Meyer CC, Calis KA, Burke LB, et al. Symptomatic cardiotoxicity associated with 5-fluorouracil. Pharmacotherapy 1997;17(4):729–36.
9. Yeh ET, Bickford CL. Cardiovascular complications of cancer therapy: incidence, pathogenesis, diagnosis, and management. J Am Coll Cardiol 2009; 53(24):2231–47.
10. Czaykowski PM, Moore MJ, Tannock IF. High risk of vascular events in patients with urothelial

transitional cell carcinoma treated with cisplatin based chemotherapy. J Urol 1998;160(6 Pt 1): 2021–4.

11. Cortes JE, Kantarjian H, Shah NP, et al. Ponatinib in refractory Philadelphia chromosome-positive leukemias. N Engl J Med 2012;367(22):2075–88.

12. Caldemeyer L, Dugan M, Edwards J, et al. Long-term side effects of tyrosine kinase inhibitors in chronic myeloid leukemia. Curr Hematol Malig Rep 2016;11(2):71–9.

13. Schutz FA, Je Y, Azzi GR, et al. Bevacizumab increases the risk of arterial ischemia: a large study in cancer patients with a focus on different subgroup outcomes. Ann Oncol 2011;22(6):1404–12.

14. Syrigos KN, Karapanagiotou E, Boura P, et al. Bevacizumab-induced hypertension: pathogenesis and management. BioDrugs 2011;25(3):159–69.

15. Escudier SM, Kantarjian HM, Estey EH. Thrombosis in patients with acute promyelocytic leukemia treated with and without all-trans retinoic acid. Leuk Lymphoma 1996;20(5–6):435–9.

16. Ferreira M, Pichon E, Carmier D, et al. Coronary toxicities of Anti-PD-1 and Anti-PD-L1 immunotherapies: a case report and review of the literature and international registries. Target Oncol 2018;13(4): 509–15.

17. Paszat LF, Mackillop WJ, Groome PA, et al. Mortality from myocardial infarction after adjuvant radiotherapy for breast cancer in the surveillance, epidemiology, and end-results cancer registries. J Clin Oncol 1998;16(8):2625–31.

18. Darby SC, Ewertz M, McGale P, et al. Risk of ischemic heart disease in women after radiotherapy for breast cancer. N Engl J Med 2013; 368(11):987–98.

19. Balanescu DV, Donisan T, Dayah T, et al. Refractory radiation-induced coronary artery disease: mapping the path and guiding treatment with optical coherence tomography 2019;35(5):759–60.

20. Hancock SL, Tucker MA, Hoppe RT. Factors affecting late mortality from heart disease after treatment of Hodgkin's disease. JAMA 1993; 270(16):1949–55.

21. Iliescu CA, Grines CL, Herrmann J, et al. SCAI Expert consensus statement: evaluation, management, and special considerations of cardio-oncology patients in the cardiac catheterization laboratory (endorsed by the cardiological society of India, and sociedad Latino Americana de Cardiologia intervencionista). Catheter Cardiovasc Interv 2016;87(5):E202–23.

22. Yusuf SW, Daraban N, Abbasi N, et al. Treatment and outcomes of acute coronary syndrome in the cancer population. Clin Cardiol 2012;35(7): 443–50.

23. Potts JE, Iliescu CA, Lopez Mattei JC, et al. Percutaneous coronary intervention in cancer patients: a report of the prevalence and outcomes in the United States. Eur Heart J 2019; 40(22):1790–800.

24. Tabata N, Sueta D, Yamamoto E, et al. Outcome of current and history of cancer on the risk of cardiovascular events following percutaneous coronary intervention: a Kumamoto University Malignancy and Atherosclerosis (KUMA) study. Eur Heart J Qual Care Clin Outcomes 2018;4(4):290–300.

25. Landes U, Kornowski R, Bental T, et al. Long-term outcomes after percutaneous coronary interventions in cancer survivors. Coron Artery Dis 2017; 28(1):5–10.

26. Shivaraju A, Patel V, Fonarow GC, et al. Temporal trends in gastrointestinal bleeding associated with percutaneous coronary intervention: analysis of the 1998-2006 Nationwide Inpatient Sample (NIS) database. Am Heart J 2011;162(6):1062–8.e5.

27. Velders MA, Boden H, Hofma SH, et al. Outcome after ST elevation myocardial infarction in patients with cancer treated with primary percutaneous coronary intervention. Am J Cardiol 2013;112(12): 1867–72.

28. Kurisu S, Iwasaki T, Ishibashi K, et al. Comparison of treatment and outcome of acute myocardial infarction between cancer patients and non-cancer patients. Int J Cardiol 2013;167(5):2335–7.

29. Goloshchapov-Aksenov RS, Lebedev AV, Mirzonov VA. Primary percutaneous coronary angioplasty in patients with acute coronary syndrome and concomitant cancer. Vestn Rentgenol Radiol 2012;1:17–20 [in Russian].

30. Guddati AK, Joy PS, Kumar G. Analysis of outcomes of percutaneous coronary intervention in metastatic cancer patients with acute coronary syndrome over a 10-year period. J Cancer Res Clin Oncol 2016;142(2):471–9.

31. Vaitkus PT, Dickens C, McGrath MK. Low bleeding risk from cardiac catheterization in patients with advanced liver disease. Catheter Cardiovasc Interv 2005;65(4):510–2.

32. Raphael CE, Spoon DB, Bell MR, et al. Effect of preprocedural thrombocytopenia on prognosis after percutaneous coronary intervention. Mayo Clin Proc 2016;91(8):1035–44.

33. Iliescu C, Balanescu DV, Donisan T, et al. Safety of diagnostic and therapeutic cardiac catheterization in cancer patients with acute coronary syndrome and chronic thrombocytopenia. Am J Cardiol 2018;122(9):1465–70.

34. Iliescu C, Durand JB, Kroll M. Cardiovascular interventions in thrombocytopenic cancer patients. Tex Heart Inst J 2011;38(3):259–60.

35. Van Belle E, Rioufol G, Pouillot C, et al. Outcome impact of coronary revascularization strategy reclassification with fractional flow reserve at time of diagnostic angiography: insights from a large

French multicenter fractional flow reserve registry. Circulation 2014;129(2):173–85.

36. Li J, Elrashidi MY, Flammer AJ, et al. Long-term outcomes of fractional flow reserve-guided vs. angiography-guided percutaneous coronary intervention in contemporary practice. Eur Heart J 2013;34(18):1375–83.

37. Courtis J, Rodes-Cabau J, Larose E, et al. Usefulness of coronary fractional flow reserve measurements in guiding clinical decisions in intermediate or equivocal left main coronary stenoses. Am J Cardiol 2009;103(7):943–9.

38. Bech GJ, De Bruyne B, Pijls NH, et al. Fractional flow reserve to determine the appropriateness of angioplasty in moderate coronary stenosis: a randomized trial. Circulation 2001;103(24):2928–34.

39. Pijls NH, van Schaardenburgh P, Manoharan G, et al. Percutaneous coronary intervention of functionally nonsignificant stenosis: 5-year follow-up of the DEFER Study. J Am Coll Cardiol 2007;49(21):2105–11.

40. Gotberg M, Christiansen EH, Gudmundsdottir IJ, et al. Instantaneous wave-free ratio versus fractional flow reserve to guide PCI. N Engl J Med 2017;376(19):1813–23.

41. Davies JE, Sen S, Dehbi HM, et al. Use of the instantaneous wave-free ratio or fractional flow reserve in PCI. N Engl J Med 2017;376(19):1824–34.

42. Lu MT, Ferencik M, Roberts RS, et al. Noninvasive FFR derived from coronary CT angiography: management and outcomes in the PROMISE trial. JACC Cardiovasc Imaging 2017;10(11):1350–8.

43. Waksman R, Legutko J, Singh J, et al. FIRST: fractional flow reserve and intravascular ultrasound relationship study. J Am Coll Cardiol 2013;61(9):917–23.

44. Johnson NP, Kirkeeide RL, Gould KL. Coronary anatomy to predict physiology: fundamental limits. Circ Cardiovasc Imaging 2013;6(5):817–32.

45. Gonzalo N, Escaned J, Alfonso F, et al. Morphometric assessment of coronary stenosis relevance with optical coherence tomography: a comparison with fractional flow reserve and intravascular ultrasound. J Am Coll Cardiol 2012;59(12):1080–9.

46. Iliescu C, LeBeau JT, Silva G, et al. Optical coherence tomography-guided antiplatelet therapy in patients with coronary artery disease and cancer: the protect-oct registry. J Am Coll Cardiol 2013;61(10_S):E1128.

47. Park SJ, Ahn JM, Kang SJ, et al. Intravascular ultrasound-derived minimal lumen area criteria for functionally significant left main coronary artery stenosis. JACC Cardiovasc Interv 2014;7(8):868–74.

48. Al-Hawwas M, Tsitlakidou D, Gupta N, et al. Acute coronary syndrome management in cancer patients. Curr Oncol Rep 2018;20(10):78.

49. Iannaccone M, D Ascenzo F, De Filippo O, et al. Optimal medical therapy in patients with malignancy undergoing percutaneous coronary intervention for acute coronary syndrome: a BleeMACS substudy. Am J Cardiovasc Drugs 2017;17(1):61–71.

50. Gong IY, Yan AT, Ko DT, et al. Temporal changes in treatments and outcomes after acute myocardial infarction among cancer survivors and patients without cancer, 1995 to 2013. Cancer 2018;124(6):1269–78.

51. Rohrmann S, Witassek F, Erne P, et al. Treatment of patients with myocardial infarction depends on history of cancer. Eur Heart J Acute Cardiovasc Care 2018;7(7):639–45.

52. Iannaccone M, D'Ascenzo F, Vadala P, et al. Prevalence and outcome of patients with cancer and acute coronary syndrome undergoing percutaneous coronary intervention: a BleeMACS substudy. Eur Heart J Acute Cardiovasc Care 2018;7(7):631–8.

53. Amsterdam EA, Wenger NK, Brindis RG, et al. 2014 AHA/ACC guideline for the management of patients with non-ST-elevation acute coronary syndromes: executive summary: a report of the American College of Cardiology/American Heart Association Task Force on Practice Guidelines. Circulation 2014;130(25):2354–94.

54. Levine GN, Bates ER, Bittl JA, et al. 2016 ACC/AHA guideline focused update on duration of dual antiplatelet therapy in patients with coronary artery disease: a report of the American College of Cardiology/American Heart Association Task Force on clinical practice guidelines: an update of the 2011 ACCF/AHA/SCAI guideline for percutaneous coronary intervention, 2011 ACCF/AHA guideline for coronary artery bypass graft surgery, 2012 ACC/AHA/ACP/AATS/PCNA/SCAI/STS guideline for the diagnosis and management of patients with stable ischemic heart disease, 2013 accf/aha guideline for the management of st-elevation myocardial infarction, 2014 AHA/ACC guideline for the management of patients with non-ST-elevation acute coronary syndromes, and 2014 ACC/AHA guideline on perioperative cardiovascular evaluation and management of patients undergoing noncardiac surgery. Circulation 2016;134(10):e123–55.

55. Stiermaier T, Moeller C, Oehler K, et al. Long-term excess mortality in takotsubo cardiomyopathy: predictors, causes and clinical consequences. Eur J Heart Fail 2016;18(6):650–6.

56. Tornvall P, Collste O, Ehrenborg E, et al. A case-control study of risk markers and mortality in takotsubo stress cardiomyopathy. J Am Coll Cardiol 2016;67(16):1931–6.

57. Munoz E, Iliescu G, Vejpongsa P, et al. Takotsubo stress cardiomyopathy: "Good News" in cancer patients? J Am Coll Cardiol 2016;68(10):1143–4.

58. Prasad A, Lerman A, Rihal CS. Apical ballooning syndrome (Tako-Tsubo or stress cardiomyopathy): a mimic of acute myocardial infarction. Am Heart J 2008;155(3):408–17.

59. Iliescu CA, Grines CL, Herrmann J, et al. SCAI expert consensus statement: evaluation, management, and special considerations of cardio-oncology patients in the cardiac catheterization laboratory (endorsed by the cardiological society of India, and sociedad Latino Americana de Cardiologia intervencionista). Catheter Cardiovasc Interv 2016;87(5):895–9.

60. Giza DE, Lopez-Mattei J, Vejpongsa P, et al. Stress-induced cardiomyopathy in cancer patients. Am J Cardiol 2017;120(12):2284–8.

61. Templin C, Ghadri JR, Diekmann J, et al. Clinical features and outcomes of takotsubo (Stress) cardiomyopathy. N Engl J Med 2015;373(10):929–38.

62. Gujral DM, Lloyd G, Bhattacharyya S. Radiation-induced valvular heart disease. Heart 2016; 102(4):269–76.

63. Taylor CW, Wang Z, Macaulay E, et al. Exposure of the heart in breast cancer radiation therapy: a systematic review of heart doses published during 2003 to 2013. Int J Radiat Oncol Biol Phys 2015; 93(4):845–53.

64. Chang HM, Okwuosa TM, Scarabelli T, et al. Cardiovascular complications of cancer therapy: best practices in diagnosis, prevention, and management: part 2. J Am Coll Cardiol 2017;70(20): 2552–65.

65. Mangner N, Woitek FJ, Haussig S, et al. Impact of active cancer disease on the outcome of patients undergoing transcatheter aortic valve replacement. J Interv Cardiol 2018;31(2):188–96.

66. Faggiano P, Frattini S, Zilioli V, et al. Prevalence of comorbidities and associated cardiac diseases in patients with valve aortic stenosis. Potential implications for the decision-making process. Int J Cardiol 2012;159(2):94–9.

67. Okura Y, Ishigaki S, Sakakibara S, et al. Prognosis of cancer patients with aortic stenosis under optimal cancer therapies and conservative cardiac treatments. Int Heart J 2018;59(4):750–8.

68. Minamino-Muta E, Kato T, Morimoto T, et al. Malignant disease as a comorbidity in patients with severe aortic stenosis: clinical presentation, outcomes, and management. Eur Heart J Qual Care Clin Outcomes 2018;4(3):180–8.

69. Leon M, Smith C, Mack M, et al. Transcatheter aortic-valve implantation for aortic stenosis in patient who cannot undergo surgery. N Engl J Med 2010;363:1597–607.

70. Mack MJ, Leon MB, Thourani VH, et al. Transcatheter aortic-valve replacement with a balloon-expandable valve in low-risk patients. N Engl J Med 2019;380(18):1695–705.

71. Campo J, Tsoris A, Kruse J, et al. Prognosis of severe asymptomatic aortic stenosis with and without surgery. Ann Thorac Surg 2019;108(1):74–9.

72. Watanabe Y, Kozuma K, Hioki H, et al. Comparison of results of transcatheter aortic valve implantation in patients with versus without active cancer. Am J Cardiol 2016;118(4):572–7.

73. Lorusso R, Vizzardi E, Johnson DM, et al. Cardiac surgery in adult patients with remitted or active malignancies: a review of preoperative screening, surgical management and short- and long-term postoperative results. Eur J Cardiothorac Surg 2018;54(1):10–8.

74. Donnellan E, Masri A, Johnston DR, et al. Long-term outcomes of patients with mediastinal radiation-associated severe aortic stenosis and subsequent surgical aortic valve replacement: a matched cohort study. J Am Heart Assoc 2017; 6(5) [pii:e005396].

75. Liu VY, Agha AM, Lopez-Mattei J, et al. Interventional cardio-oncology: adding a new dimension to the cardio-oncology field. Front Cardiovasc Med 2018;5:48.

76. Schechter M, Balanescu DV, Donisan T, et al. An update on the management and outcomes of cancer patients with severe aortic stenosis. Catheter Cardiovasc Interv 2018. [Epub ahead of print].

77. Latib A, Montorfano M, Figini F, et al. Percutaneous valve replacement in a young adult for radiation-induced aortic stenosis. J Cardiovasc Med (Hagerstown) 2012;13(6):397–8.

78. Szeto WY, Svensson LG, Rajeswaran J, et al. Appropriate patient selection or health care rationing? Lessons from surgical aortic valve replacement in the Placement of Aortic Transcatheter Valves I trial. J Thorac Cardiovasc Surg 2015;150(3):557–68.e11.

79. Yusuf SW, Sarfaraz A, Durand JB, et al. Management and outcomes of severe aortic stenosis in cancer patients. Am Heart J 2011;161(6):1125–32.

80. Mrak M, Ambrozic J, Music S, et al. Transcatheter aortic valve implantation in a cancer patient denied for surgical aortic valve replacement-a case report. Wien Klin Wochenschr 2016;128(13–14):516–20.

81. Berkovitch A, Guetta V, Barbash IM, et al. Favorable short-term and long-term outcomes among patients with prior history of malignancy undergoing transcatheter aortic valve implantation. J Invasive Cardiol 2018;30(3):105–9.

82. Komatsu H, Izumi N, Tsukioka T, et al. Pulmonary resection for lung cancer following transcatheter aortic valve implantation for severe aortic valve stenosis: a case report. Ann Thorac Cardiovasc Surg 2018. https://doi.org/10.5761/atcs.cr.5718-00028.

83. Drevet G, Maury JM, Farhat F, et al. Transcatheter aortic valve implantation: a safe and efficient procedure to treat an aortic valve stenosis before

lung cancer resection. Gen Thorac Cardiovasc Surg 2019;67(3):321–3.

84. Sakai T, Yahagi K, Miura S, et al. Transcatheter aortic valve implantation for patients with lung cancer and aortic valve stenosis. J Thorac Dis 2018; 10(5):E387–90.

85. Landes U, Iakobishvili Z, Vronsky D, et al. Transcatheter aortic valve replacement in oncology patients with severe aortic stenosis. JACC Cardiovasc Interv 2019;12(1):78–86.

86. Kogoj P, Devjak R, Bunc M. Balloon aortic valvuloplasty (BAV) as a bridge to aortic valve replacement in cancer patients who require urgent noncardiac surgery. Radiol Oncol 2014;48(1):62–6.

87. Lim DS, Reynolds MR, Feldman T, et al. Improved functional status and quality of life in prohibitive surgical risk patients with degenerative mitral regurgitation after transcatheter mitral valve repair. J Am Coll Cardiol 2014;64(2):182–92.

88. Marmagkiolis K, Hakeem A, Ebersole DG, et al. Clinical outcomes of percutaneous mitral valve repair with MitraClip for the management of functional mitral regurgitation. Catheter Cardiovasc Interv 2019;1–7. [Epub ahead of print].

89. Krishnaswamy A, Hanna M, Goodman A, et al. First reported case of MitraClip placement due to mitral valve flail in the setting of cardiac amyloidosis. Circ Heart Fail 2016;9(8) [pii:e003069].

90. Oner A, Ince H, Paranskaya L, et al. Previous malignancy is an independent predictor of follow-up mortality after percutaneous treatment of mitral valve regurgitation by means of MitraClip. Cardiovasc Ther 2017;35(2):e12239.

91. Cerillo AG, Gasbarri T, Celi S, et al. Transapical transcatheter valve-in-valve implantation for failed mitral bioprostheses: gradient, symptoms, and functional status in 18 high-risk patients up to 5 years. Ann Thorac Surg 2016;102(4):1289–95.

92. Drury JH, Labovitz AJ, Miller LW. Echocardiographic guidance for endomyocardial biopsy. Echocardiography 1997;14(5):469–74.

93. Taramasso M, Maisano F. Transcatheter tricuspid valve intervention: state of the art. EuroIntervention 2017;13(Aa):Aa40–50.

94. Krishnaswamy A, Navia J, Kapadia SR. Transcatheter tricuspid valve replacement. Interv Cardiol Clin 2018;7(1):65–70.

95. Aboulhosn J, Cabalka AK, Levi DS, et al. Transcatheter valve-in-ring implantation for the treatment of residual or recurrent tricuspid valve dysfunction after prior surgical repair. JACC Cardiovasc Interv 2017;10(1):53–63.

96. McElhinney DB, Cabalka AK, Aboulhosn JA, et al. Transcatheter tricuspid valve-in-valve implantation for the treatment of dysfunctional surgical bioprosthetic valves: an international, multicenter registry study. Circulation 2016;133(16):1582–93.

97. Hassan SA, Banchs J, Iliescu C, et al. Carcinoid heart disease. Heart 2017;103(19):1488–95.

98. Balanescu DV, Donisan T, Lopez-Mattei J, et al. The 1, 2, 3, 4 of carcinoid heart disease: comprehensive cardiovascular imaging is the mainstay of complex surgical treatment. Oncol Lett 2019; 17(5):4126–32.

99. Conradi L, Schaefer A, Mueller GC, et al. Carcinoid heart valve disease: transcatheter pulmonary valve-in-valve implantation in failing biological xenografts. J Heart Valve Dis 2015;24(1):110–4.

100. Loyalka P, Schechter M, Nascimbene A, et al. Transcatheter pulmonary valve replacement in a carcinoid heart. Tex Heart Inst J 2016;43(4):341–4.

101. Khan JN, Doshi SN, Rooney SJ, et al. Transcatheter pulmonary and tricuspid valve-in-valve replacement for bioprosthesis degeneration in carcinoid heart disease. Eur Heart J Cardiovasc Imaging 2016;17(1):114.

102. Kesarwani M, Ports TA, Rao RK, et al. First-in-human transcatheter pulmonic valve implantation through a tricuspid valve bioprosthesis to treat native pulmonary valve regurgitation caused by carcinoid syndrome. JACC Cardiovasc Interv 2015;8(10):e161–3.

103. Mortazavi A, Reul RM, Cannizzaro L, et al. Transvenous transcatheter valve-in-valve implantation after bioprosthetic tricuspid valve failure. Tex Heart Inst J 2014;41(5):507–10.

104. Chen J, Long JB, Hurria A, et al. Incidence of heart failure or cardiomyopathy after adjuvant trastuzumab therapy for breast cancer. J Am Coll Cardiol 2012;60(24):2504–12.

105. Romond EH, Jeong JH, Rastogi P, et al. Seven-year follow-up assessment of cardiac function in NSABP B-31, a randomized trial comparing doxorubicin and cyclophosphamide followed by paclitaxel (ACP) with ACP plus trastuzumab as adjuvant therapy for patients with node-positive, human epidermal growth factor receptor 2-positive breast cancer. J Clin Oncol 2012;30(31):3792–9.

106. Mulrooney DA, Yeazel MW, Kawashima T, et al. Cardiac outcomes in a cohort of adult survivors of childhood and adolescent cancer: retrospective analysis of the Childhood Cancer Survivor Study cohort. BMJ 2009;339:b4606.

107. Felker GM, Thompson RE, Hare JM, et al. Underlying causes and long-term survival in patients with initially unexplained cardiomyopathy. N Engl J Med 2000;342(15):1077–84.

108. Oliveira GH, Hardaway BW, Kucheryavaya AY, et al. Characteristics and survival of patients with chemotherapy-induced cardiomyopathy undergoing heart transplantation. J Heart Lung Transplant 2012;31(8):805–10.

109. Bianco CM, Al-Kindi SG, Oliveira GH. Advanced heart failure therapies for cancer therapeutics-

related cardiac dysfunction. Heart Fail Clin 2017; 13(2):327–36.

110. Costanzo MR, Dipchand A, Starling R, et al. The international society of heart and lung transplantation guidelines for the care of heart transplant recipients. J Heart Lung Transplant 2010;29(8):914–56.

111. Ponikowski P, Voors AA, Anker SD, et al. 2016 ESC guidelines for the diagnosis and treatment of acute and chronic heart failure: the Task Force for the diagnosis and treatment of acute and chronic heart failure of the European Society of Cardiology (ESC). Developed with the special contribution of the Heart Failure Association (HFA) of the ESC. Eur J Heart Fail 2016;18(8):891–975.

112. Feldman D, Pamboukian SV, Teuteberg JJ, et al. The 2013 international society for heart and lung transplantation guidelines for mechanical circulatory support: executive summary. J Heart Lung Transpl 2013;32(2):157–87.

113. Thomas GR, McDonald MA, Day J, et al. A matched cohort study of patients with end-stage heart failure from anthracycline-induced cardiomyopathy requiring advanced cardiac support. Am J Cardiol 2016;118(10):1539–44.

114. Russo AM, Stainback RF, Bailey SR, et al. ACCF/HRS/AHA/ASE/HFSA/SCAI/SCCT/SCMR 2013 appropriate use criteria for implantable cardioverter-defibrillators and cardiac resynchronization therapy: a report of the American College of cardiology Foundation appropriate use criteria task force, Heart Rhythm Society, American Heart Association, American Society of Echocardiography, Heart Failure Society of America, Society for Cardiovascular Angiography and Interventions, Society of Cardiovascular Computed Tomography, and Society for Cardiovascular Magnetic Resonance. Heart Rhythm 2013;10(4):e11–58.

115. Fadol AP, Mouhayar E, Reyes-Gibby CC. The use of cardiac resynchronization therapy in cancer patients with heart failure. J Clin Exp Res Cardiol 2017;3(1).

116. Ajijola OA, Nandigam KV, Chabner BA, et al. Usefulness of cardiac resynchronization therapy in the management of Doxorubicin-induced cardiomyopathy. Am J Cardiol 2008;101(9):1371–2.

117. Rickard J, Kumbhani DJ, Baranowski B, et al. Usefulness of cardiac resynchronization therapy in patients with Adriamycin-induced cardiomyopathy. Am J Cardiol 2010;105(4):522–6.

118. Moss AJ, Hall WJ, Cannom DS, et al. Cardiac-resynchronization therapy for the prevention of heart-failure events. N Engl J Med 2009;361(14):1329–38.

119. Oliveira GH, Dupont M, Naftel D, et al. Increased need for right ventricular support in patients with chemotherapy-induced cardiomyopathy undergoing mechanical circulatory support: outcomes from the INTERMACS Registry (Interagency Registry for Mechanically Assisted Circulatory Support). J Am Coll Cardiol 2014;63(3):240–8.

120. Grant JD, Jensen GL, Tang C, et al. Radiotherapy-induced malfunction in contemporary cardiovascular implantable electronic devices: clinical incidence and predictors. JAMA Oncol 2015;1(5):624–32.

121. Zaremba T, Jakobsen AR, Sogaard M, et al. Risk of device malfunction in cancer patients with implantable cardiac device undergoing radiotherapy: a population-based cohort study. Pacing Clin Electrophysiol 2015;38(3):343–56.

122. Elders J, Kunze-Busch M, Smeenk RJ, et al. High incidence of implantable cardioverter defibrillator malfunctions during radiation therapy: neutrons as a probable cause of soft errors. Europace 2013;15(1):60–5.

123. Kirklin JK, Naftel DC, Pagani FD, et al. Long-term mechanical circulatory support (destination therapy): on track to compete with heart transplantation? J Thorac Cardiovasc Surg 2012;144(3):584–603 [discussion: 597–8].

124. Slaughter MS, Rogers JG, Milano CA, et al. Advanced heart failure treated with continuous-flow left ventricular assist device. N Engl J Med 2009;361(23):2241–51.

125. Deo SV, Al-Kindi SG, Oliveira GH. Management of advanced heart failure due to cancer therapy: the present role of mechanical circulatory support and cardiac transplantation. Curr Treat Options Cardiovasc Med 2015;17(6):388.

126. Freilich M, Stub D, Esmore D, et al. Recovery from anthracycline cardiomyopathy after long-term support with a continuous flow left ventricular assist device. J Heart Lung Transplant 2009;28(1):101–3.

127. Simsir SA, Lin SS, Blue LJ, et al. Left ventricular assist device as destination therapy in doxorubicin-induced cardiomyopathy. Ann Thorac Surg 2005;80(2):717–9.

128. Sayin OA, Ozpeker C, Schoenbrodt M, et al. Ventricular assist devices in patients with chemotherapy-induced cardiomyopathy: new modalities. Acta Cardiol 2015;70(4):430–4.

129. Loyaga-Rendon RY, Inampudi C, Tallaj JA, et al. Cancer in end-stage heart failure patients supported by left ventricular assist devices. ASAIO J 2014;60(5):609–12.

130. Cleveland JC Jr, Naftel DC, Reece TB, et al. Survival after biventricular assist device implantation: an analysis of the Interagency registry for Mechanically assisted circulatory support database. J Heart Lung Transplant 2011;30(8):862–9.

131. DePasquale EC, Nasir K, Jacoby DL. Outcomes of adults with restrictive cardiomyopathy after heart transplantation. J Heart Lung Transplant 2012; 31(12):1269–75.

132. Mukku RB, Fonarow GC, Watson KE, et al. Heart failure therapies for end-stage chemotherapy-induced cardiomyopathy. J Card Fail 2016;22(6):439–48.

133. Abraham WT, Stevenson LW, Bourge RC, et al. Sustained efficacy of pulmonary artery pressure to guide adjustment of chronic heart failure therapy: complete follow-up results from the CHAMPION randomised trial. Lancet 2016;387(10017):453–61.

134. Adamson PB, Abraham WT, Stevenson LW, et al. Pulmonary artery pressure-guided heart failure management reduces 30-day readmissions. Circ Heart Fail 2016;9(6) [pii:e002600].

135. Imazio M, Brucato A, Barbieri A, et al. Good prognosis for pericarditis with and without myocardial involvement: results from a multicenter, prospective cohort study. Circulation 2013;128(1):42–9.

136. Sogaard KK, Farkas DK, Ehrenstein V, et al. Pericarditis as a marker of occult cancer and a prognostic factor for cancer mortality. Circulation 2017;136(11):996–1006.

137. Imazio M, Spodick DH, Brucato A, et al. Controversial issues in the management of pericardial diseases. Circulation 2010;121(7):916–28.

138. Ben-Horin S, Bank I, Guetta V, et al. Large symptomatic pericardial effusion as the presentation of unrecognized cancer: a study in 173 consecutive patients undergoing pericardiocentesis. Medicine (Baltimore) 2006;85(1):49–53.

139. Quint LE. Thoracic complications and emergencies in oncologic patients. Cancer Imaging 2009;9(Special issue A):S75–82.

140. Kyto V, Sipila J, Rautava P. Clinical profile and influences on outcomes in patients hospitalized for acute pericarditis. Circulation 2014;130(18):1601–6.

141. Pawlak Cieslik A, Szturmowicz M, Fijalkowska A, et al. Diagnosis of malignant pericarditis: a single centre experience. Kardiol Pol 2012;70(11):1147–53.

142. Kim SH, Kwak MH, Park S, et al. Clinical characteristics of malignant pericardial effusion associated with recurrence and survival. Cancer Res Treat 2010;42(4):210–6.

143. Restrepo CS, Vargas D, Ocazionez D, et al. Primary pericardial tumors. Radiographics 2013;33(6):1613–30.

144. Mainzer G, Zaidman I, Hatib I, et al. Intrapericardial steroid treatment for recurrent pericardial effusion in a patient with acute lymphoblastic Leukaemia. Hematol Oncol 2011;29(4):220–1.

145. Ghosh AK, Crake T, Manisty C, et al. Pericardial disease in cancer patients. Curr Treat Options Cardiovasc Med 2018;20(7):60.

146. Maisch B, Ristic AD, Seferovic PM, et al. Interventional pericardiology: pericardiocentesis, pericardioscopy, pericardial biopsy, balloon pericardiotomy, and intrapericardial therapy. Heidelberg (Germany): Springer Science & Business Media; 2011.

147. Iliescu C, Khair T, Marmagkiolis K, et al. Echocardiography and fluoroscopy-guided pericardiocentesis for cancer patients with cardiac tamponade and thrombocytopenia. J Am Coll Cardiol 2016;68(7):771–3.

148. Tsang TS, Enriquez-Sarano M, Freeman WK, et al. Consecutive 1127 therapeutic echocardiographically guided pericardioceneses: clinical profile, practice patterns, and outcomes spanning 21 years. Mayo Clin Proc 2002;77(5):429–36.

149. Maisch B, Ristic AD, Pankuweit S, et al. Percutaneous therapy in pericardial diseases. Cardiol Clin 2017;35(4):567–88.

150. Lekhakul A, Assawakawintip C, Fenstad ER, et al. Safety and outcome of percutaneous drainage of pericardial effusions in patients with cancer. Am J Cardiol 2018;122(6):1091–4.

151. Vilela EM, Ruivo C, Guerreiro CE, et al. Computed tomography-guided pericardiocentesis: a systematic review concerning contemporary evidence and future perspectives. Ther Adv Cardiovasc Dis 2018;12(11):299–307.

152. Wong B, Murphy J, Chang CJ, et al. The risk of pericardiocentesis. Am J Cardiol 1979;44(6):1110–4.

153. Maggiolini S, De Carlini CC, Imazio M. Evolution of the pericardiocentesis technique. J Cardiovasc Med (Hagerstown) 2018;19(6):267–73.

154. El Haddad D, Iliescu C, Yusuf SW, et al. Outcomes of cancer patients undergoing percutaneous pericardiocentesis for pericardial effusion. J Am Coll Cardiol 2015;66(10):1119–28.

155. Vaitkus PT, Herrmann HC, LeWinter MM. Treatment of malignant pericardial effusion. Jama 1994;272(1):59–64.

156. Lauri G, Rossi C, Rubino M, et al. B-type natriuretic peptide levels in patients with pericardial effusion undergoing pericardiocentesis. Int J Cardiol 2016;212:318–23.

157. Maisch B, Ristic AD, Pankuweit S, et al. Neoplastic pericardial effusion. Efficacy and safety of intrapericardial treatment with cisplatin. Eur Heart J 2002;23(20):1625–31.

158. Adler Y, Charron P, Imazio M, et al. 2015 ESC guidelines for the diagnosis and management of pericardial diseases: the task force for the diagnosis and management of pericardial diseases of the European Society of Cardiology (ESC) Endorsed by: The European Association for Cardio-Thoracic Surgery (EACTS). Eur Heart J 2015;36(42):2921–64.

159. Kepez A, Sari I, Cincin A, et al. Pericardiocentesis in patients with thrombocytopenia and high international normalized ratio: case report and review of the literature. Platelets 2014;25(2):140–1.

160. Sagrista-Sauleda J, Angel J, Permanyer-Miralda G, et al. Long-term follow-up of idiopathic chronic

pericardial effusion. N Engl J Med 1999;341(27): 2054–9.

161. Gornik HL, Gerhard-Herman M, Beckman JA. Abnormal cytology predicts poor prognosis in cancer patients with pericardial effusion. J Clin Oncol 2005;23(22):5211–6.

162. Labbe C, Tremblay L, Lacasse Y. Pericardiocentesis versus pericardiotomy for malignant pericardial effusion: a retrospective comparison. Curr Oncol 2015;22(6):412–6.

163. Virk SA, Chandrakumar D, Villanueva C, et al. Systematic review of percutaneous interventions for malignant pericardial effusion. Heart 2015; 101(20):1619–26.

164. Kunitoh H, Tamura T, Shibata T, et al. A randomised trial of intrapericardial bleomycin for malignant pericardial effusion with lung cancer (JCOG9811). Br J Cancer 2009;100(3):464–9.

165. Lestuzzi C, Bearz A, Lafaras C, et al. Neoplastic pericardial disease in lung cancer: impact on outcomes of different treatment strategies. A multicenter study. Lung Cancer 2011;72(3):340–7.

166. Bishiniotis TS, Antoniadou S, Katseas G, et al. Malignant cardiac tamponade in women with breast cancer treated by pericardiocentesis and intrapericardial administration of triethylenethiophosphoramide (thiotepa). Am J Cardiol 2000;86(3):362–4.

167. Colleoni M, Martinelli G, Beretta F, et al. Intracavitary chemotherapy with thiotepa in malignant pericardial effusions: an active and well-tolerated regimen. J Clin Oncol 1998;16(7):2371–6.

168. Chen D, Zhang Y, Shi F, et al. Intrapericardial bevacizumab safely and effectively treats malignant pericardial effusion in advanced cancer patients. Oncotarget 2016;7(32):52436–41.

169. McDonald JM, Meyers BF, Guthrie TJ, et al. Comparison of open subxiphoid pericardial drainage with percutaneous catheter drainage for symptomatic pericardial effusion. Ann Thorac Surg 2003; 76(3):811–5 [discussion: 816].

170. Park JS, Rentschler R, Wilbur D. Surgical management of pericardial effusion in patients with malignancies. Comparison of subxiphoid window versus pericardiectomy. Cancer 1991;67(1):76–80.

171. Celik S, Lestuzzi C, Cervesato E, et al. Systemic chemotherapy in combination with pericardial window has better outcomes in malignant pericardial effusions. J Thorac Cardiovasc Surg 2014;148(5): 2288–93.

172. Patel N, Rafique AM, Eshaghian S, et al. Retrospective comparison of outcomes, diagnostic value, and complications of percutaneous prolonged drainage versus surgical pericardiotomy of pericardial effusion associated with malignancy. Am J Cardiol 2013;112(8):1235–9.

173. Saltzman AJ, Paz YE, Rene AG, et al. Comparison of surgical pericardial drainage with percutaneous catheter drainage for pericardial effusion. J Invasive Cardiol 2012;24(11):590–3.

174. Horowitz M, Neeman E, Sharon E, et al. Exploiting the critical perioperative period to improve long-term cancer outcomes. Nat Rev Clin Oncol 2015; 12(4):213–26.

175. Rafique AM, Patel N, Biner S, et al. Frequency of recurrence of pericardial tamponade in patients with extended versus nonextended pericardial catheter drainage. Am J Cardiol 2011;108(12): 1820–5.

176. Bhardwaj R, Gharib W, Gharib W, et al. Evaluation of safety and feasibility of percutaneous balloon pericardiotomy in hemodynamically significant pericardial effusion (review of 10-years experience in single center). J Interv Cardiol 2015;28(5): 409–14.

177. Navarro Del Amo LF, Cordoba Polo M, Orejas Orejas M, et al. Percutaneous balloon pericardiotomy in patients with recurrent pericardial effusion. Rev Esp Cardiol 2002;55(1):25–8.

178. Swanson N, Mirza I, Wijesinghe N, et al. Primary percutaneous balloon pericardiotomy for malignant pericardial effusion. Catheter Cardiovasc Interv 2008;71(4):504–7.

179. Ovunc K, Aytemir K, Ozer N, et al. Percutaneous balloon pericardiotomy for patients with malignant pericardial effusion including three malignant pleural mesotheliomas. Angiology 2001;52(5): 323–9.

180. Ziskind AA, Pearce AC, Lemmon CC, et al. Percutaneous balloon pericardiotomy for the treatment of cardiac tamponade and large pericardial effusions: description of technique and report of the first 50 cases. J Am Coll Cardiol 1993;21(1):1–5.

181. Maisch B, Rupp H, Ristic A, et al. Pericardioscopy and epi- and pericardial biopsy - a new window to the heart improving etiological diagnoses and permitting targeted intrapericardial therapy. Heart Fail Rev 2013;18(3):317–28.

182. Cullinane CA, Paz IB, Smith D, et al. Prognostic factors in the surgical management of pericardial effusion in the patient with concurrent malignancy. Chest 2004;125(4):1328–34.

183. Singh V, Mendirichaga R, Savani GT, et al. Comparison of utilization trends, indications, and complications of endomyocardial biopsy in native versus donor hearts (from the Nationwide Inpatient Sample 2002 to 2014). Am J Cardiol 2018;121(3): 356–63.

184. Cooper LT, Baughman KL, Feldman AM, et al. The role of endomyocardial biopsy in the management of cardiovascular disease: a scientific statement from the American Heart Association, the American College of Cardiology, and the European Society of Cardiology. Circulation 2007;116(19):2216–33.

185. Ishibashi-Ueda H, Matsuyama TA, Ohta-Ogo K, et al. Significance and value of endomyocardial biopsy based on our own experience. Circ J 2017; 81(4):417–26.

186. Francis R, Lewis C. Myocardial biopsy: techniques and indications. Heart 2018;104(11):950–8.

187. Anderson JL, Marshall HW. The femoral venous approach to endomyocardial biopsy: comparison with internal jugular and transarterial approaches. Am J Cardiol 1984;53(6):833–7.

188. Ardehali H, Kasper EK, Baughman KL. Diagnostic approach to the patient with cardiomyopathy: whom to biopsy. Am Heart J 2005;149(1):7–12.

189. Hauck AJ, Kearney DL, Edwards WD. Evaluation of postmortem endomyocardial biopsy specimens from 38 patients with lymphocytic myocarditis: implications for role of sampling error. Mayo Clin Proc 1989;64(10):1235–45.

190. Veinot JP. Endomyocardial biopsy–when and how? Cardiovasc Pathol 2011;20(5):291–6.

191. Chimenti C, Frustaci A. Contribution and risks of left ventricular endomyocardial biopsy in patients with cardiomyopathies: a retrospective study over a 28-year period. Circulation 2013;128(14): 1531–41.

192. Escher F, Lassner D, Kuhl U, et al. Analysis of endomyocardial biopsies in suspected myocarditis–diagnostic value of left versus right ventricular biopsy. Int J Cardiol 2014;177(1):76–8.

193. Caforio AL, Pankuweit S, Arbustini E, et al. Current state of knowledge on aetiology, diagnosis, management, and therapy of myocarditis: a position statement of the European Society of Cardiology Working Group on Myocardial and Pericardial Diseases. Eur Heart J 2013;34(33):2636–48, 2648a-2648d.

194. Miller LW, Labovitz AJ, McBride LA, et al. Echocardiography-guided endomyocardial biopsy. A 5-year experience. Circulation 1988;78(5 Pt 2): Iii99–102.

195. Blomstrom-Lundqvist C, Noor AM, Eskilsson J, et al. Safety of transvenous right ventricular endomyocardial biopsy guided by two-dimensional echocardiography. Clin Cardiol 1993;16(6):487–92.

196. From AM, Maleszewski JJ, Rihal CS. Current status of endomyocardial biopsy. Mayo Clin Proc 2011; 86(11):1095–102.

197. Amitai ME, Schnittger I, Popp RL, et al. Comparison of three-dimensional echocardiography to two-dimensional echocardiography and fluoroscopy for monitoring of endomyocardial biopsy. Am J Cardiol 2007;99(6):864–6.

198. Platts D, Brown M, Javorsky G, et al. Comparison of fluoroscopic versus real-time three-dimensional transthoracic echocardiographic guidance of endomyocardial biopsies. Eur J Echocardiogr 2010; 11(7):637–43.

199. Kreher SK, Ulstad VK, Dick CD, et al. Frequent occurrence of occult pulmonary embolism from venous sheaths during endomyocardial biopsy. J Am Coll Cardiol 1992;19(3):581–5.

200. Sloan KP, Bruce CJ, Oh JK, et al. Complications of echocardiography-guided endomyocardial biopsy. J Am Soc Echocardiogr 2009;22(3):324.e1-4.

201. Sandhu JS, Uretsky BF, Zerbe TR, et al. Coronary artery fistula in the heart transplant patient. A potential complication of endomyocardial biopsy. Circulation 1989;79(2):350–6.

202. Wong RC, Abrahams Z, Hanna M, et al. Tricuspid regurgitation after cardiac transplantation: an old problem revisited. J Heart Lung Transplant 2008; 27(3):247–52.

203. Burgess MI, Aziz T, Yonan N. Clinical relevance of subclinical tricuspid regurgitation after orthotopic cardiac transplantation. J Am Soc Echocardiogr 1999;12(2):164.

204. Kindermann I, Kindermann M, Kandolf R, et al. Predictors of outcome in patients with suspected myocarditis. Circulation 2008;118(6):639–48.

205. Baccouche H, Mahrholdt H, Meinhardt G, et al. Diagnostic synergy of non-invasive cardiovascular magnetic resonance and invasive endomyocardial biopsy in troponin-positive patients without coronary artery disease. Eur Heart J 2009;30(23): 2869–79.

206. Leone O, Veinot JP, Angelini A, et al. 2011 consensus statement on endomyocardial biopsy from the association for European cardiovascular Pathology and the society for cardiovascular Pathology. Cardiovasc Pathol 2012;21(4):245–74.

207. Caforio ALP, Cheng C, Perazzolo Marra M, et al. How to improve therapy in myocarditis: role of cardiovascular magnetic resonance and of endomyocardial biopsy. Eur Heart J Suppl 2019;21(Suppl B):B19–22.

208. Cooper LT Jr, Berry GJ, Shabetai R. Idiopathic giant-cell myocarditis–natural history and treatment. Multicenter giant cell myocarditis study Group Investigators. N Engl J Med 1997;336(26): 1860–6.

209. deMello DE, Liapis H, Jureidini S, et al. Cardiac localization of eosinophil-granule major basic protein in acute necrotizing myocarditis. N Engl J Med 1990;323(22):1542–5.

210. Taliercio CP, Olney BA, Lie JT. Myocarditis related to drug hypersensitivity. Mayo Clin Proc 1985; 60(7):463–8.

211. Dominguez F, Kuhl U, Pieske B, et al. Update on myocarditis and inflammatory cardiomyopathy: re-emergence of endomyocardial biopsy. Rev Esp Cardiol (Engl Ed) 2016;69(2):178–87.

212. Lyon AR, Yousaf N, Battisti NML, et al. Immune checkpoint inhibitors and cardiovascular toxicity. Lancet Oncol 2018;19(9):e447–58.

213. Burstein DS, Maude S, Grupp S, et al. Cardiac profile of chimeric antigen receptor T cell therapy in children: a single-institution experience. Biol Blood Marrow Transplant 2018;24(8):1590–5.

214. d'Amati G, Factor SM. Endomyocardial biopsy findings in patients with ventricular arrhythmias of unknown origin. Cardiovasc Pathol 1996;5(3): 139–44.

215. Strain JE, Grose RM, Factor SM, et al. Results of endomyocardial biopsy in patients with spontaneous ventricular tachycardia but without apparent structural heart disease. Circulation 1983;68(6): 1171–81.

216. Ardehali H, Howard DL, Hariri A, et al. A positive endomyocardial biopsy result for sarcoid is associated with poor prognosis in patients with initially unexplained cardiomyopathy. Am Heart J 2005; 150(3):459–63.

217. Kim JS, Judson MA, Donnino R, et al. Cardiac sarcoidosis. Am Heart J 2009;157(1):9–21.

218. Tadamura E, Yamamuro M, Kubo S, et al. Images in cardiovascular medicine. Multimodality imaging of cardiac sarcoidosis before and after steroid therapy. Circulation 2006;113(20):e771–3.

219. Tadamura E, Yamamuro M, Kubo S, et al. Effectiveness of delayed enhanced MRI for identification of cardiac sarcoidosis: comparison with radionuclide imaging. AJR Am J Roentgenol 2005;185(1):110–5.

220. Uemura A, Morimoto S, Hiramitsu S, et al. Histologic diagnostic rate of cardiac sarcoidosis: evaluation of endomyocardial biopsies. Am Heart J 1999;138(2 Pt 1):299–302.

221. Falk RH, Skinner M. The systemic amyloidoses: an overview. Adv Intern Med 2000;45:107–37.

222. Militaru S, Ginghina C, Popescu BA, et al. Multimodality imaging in Fabry cardiomyopathy: from early diagnosis to therapeutic targets. Eur Heart J Cardiovasc Imaging 2018;19(12):1313–22.

223. Maceira AM, Joshi J, Prasad SK, et al. Cardiovascular magnetic resonance in cardiac amyloidosis. Circulation 2005;111(2):186–93.

224. Dubrey SW, Cha K, Skinner M, et al. Familial and primary (AL) cardiac amyloidosis: echocardiographically similar diseases with distinctly different clinical outcomes. Heart 1997;78(1):74–82.

225. Nakahashi T, Arita T, Yamaji K, et al. Impact of clinical and echocardiographic characteristics on occurrence of cardiac events in cardiac amyloidosis as proven by endomyocardial biopsy. Int J Cardiol 2014;176(3):753–9.

226. Skinner M, Sanchorawala V, Seldin DC, et al. High-dose melphalan and autologous stem-cell transplantation in patients with AL amyloidosis: an 8-year study. Ann Intern Med 2004;140(2):85–93.

227. Eng CM, Guffon N, Wilcox WR, et al. Safety and efficacy of recombinant human alpha-galactosidase A replacement therapy in Fabry's disease. N Engl J Med 2001;345(1):9–16.

228. Frustaci A, Chimenti C, Ricci R, et al. Improvement in cardiac function in the cardiac variant of Fabry's disease with galactose-infusion therapy. N Engl J Med 2001;345(1):25–32.

229. Aronow WS. Management of cardiac hemochromatosis. Arch Med Sci 2018;14(3):560–8.

230. Palaskas N, Thompson K, Gladish G, et al. Evaluation and management of cardiac tumors. Curr Treat Options Cardiovasc Med 2018;20(4):29.

231. Donisan T, Balanescu DV, Lopez-Mattei JC, et al. In search of a less invasive approach to cardiac tumor diagnosis: multimodality imaging assessment and biopsy. JACC Cardiovasc Imaging 2018; 11(8):1191–5.

232. Chan KL, Veinot J, Leach A, et al. Diagnosis of left atrial sarcoma by transvenous endocardial biopsy. Can J Cardiol 2001;17(2):206–8.

Diagnosis and Treatment of Cardiac Amyloidosis Related to Plasma Cell Dyscrasias

Kevin M. Alexander, MD[a,b,c], Alessandro Evangelisti, BS[b,d],
Ronald M. Witteles, MD[e,*]

KEYWORDS

- Amyloidosis • Immunoglobulin light chain • Cardiomyopathy • Myeloma • Chemotherapy

KEY POINTS

- Light chain amyloidosis is a plasma cell dyscrasia that is characterized by the production of misfolded free light chains that deposit as amyloid fibrils in different organs.
- The disease course in immunoglobulin light chains (AL) amyloidosis is defined by the pattern of organ involvement, with severe cardiac infiltration being associated with the poorest survival.
- Early diagnosis and treatment are imperative to minimize end-organ damage and improve survival.
- The diagnosis of AL amyloidosis consists of identification of a monoclonal gammopathy and tissue biopsy evidence of AL amyloid deposits.
- Management of AL cardiac amyloidosis focuses on administering targeted anti-plasma cell therapies to eliminate the production of amyloidogenic light chains and using supportive heart failure therapies.

INTRODUCTION

Amyloidosis refers to a family of protein-misfolding diseases. Through a variety of mechanisms, precursor proteins misfold and ultimately form rigid, insoluble amyloid fibrils that deposit in one or more organs. The pattern of organ involvement is specific to the particular amyloidogenic precursor protein. Of the amyloid diseases, those that affect the heart lead to the greatest morbidity and mortality through restrictive cardiomyopathy, arrhythmia, and sudden death. In the past, cardiac amyloidosis was considered to be a rare disease. However, recent observational studies and autopsy series suggest that cardiac amyloidosis is markedly underdiagnosed and is a major cause of heart failure.[1,2] The 2 most common forms of cardiac amyloidosis are caused by immunoglobulin light chains (AL), usually produced by plasma cells, or transthyretin (ATTR), a carrier protein

Conflict of Interest: Dr K.M. Alexander has received an investigator-initiated research grant from Pfizer. Dr R. M. Witteles has received consulting fees (modest) from Pfizer and Alnylam and has received clinical trial support from Pfizer, Alnylam, and Eidos. Mr A. Evangelisti does not have any conflict of interest to declare.
^a Division of Cardiovascular Medicine, Stanford Amyloid Center, Stanford University School of Medicine, Stanford, CA, USA; ^b Stanford Cardiovascular Institute, Stanford University School of Medicine, Stanford, CA, USA; ^c Advanced Heart Failure and Transplant Cardiology, Stanford University School of Medicine, 1651 Page Mill Road, Room 2300, Palo Alto, CA 94305, USA; ^d Stanford University School of Medicine, 1651 Page Mill Road, Room 2300, Palo Alto, CA 94305, USA; ^e Division of Cardiovascular Medicine, Stanford Amyloid Center, Stanford University School of Medicine, 300 Pasteur Drive, Lane #158, Stanford, CA 94305, USA
* Corresponding author.
E-mail address: witteles@stanford.edu
Twitter: @KMAlexanderMD (K.M.A.); @Ron_Witteles (R.M.W.)

Cardiol Clin 37 (2019) 487–495
https://doi.org/10.1016/j.ccl.2019.07.013

synthesized by the liver. AL cardiac amyloidosis, in particular, is a deadly disease, which if not treated is associated with a median survival of 6 months.[3] In the last decade, significant advancements have been made for treating AL amyloidosis. These therapies, which target the light chain-producing plasma dyscrasias, are the most effective when the disease is diagnosed early and before profound end-organ damage has occurred. This review discusses a current approach to the diagnosis and treatment of AL amyloidosis.

DIAGNOSIS
Clinical Features

AL amyloidosis is a lymphoproliferative disorder, in which a clonal population produces an amyloidogenic light chain. AL amyloidosis most commonly arises because of an abnormal clonal plasma cell, but it can more rarely occur because of clonal light chain production by lymphoma or chronic lymphocytic leukemia. Importantly, AL amyloidosis is a distinct entity from another plasma cell disorder, myeloma (Fig. 1). The pathogenesis in AL amyloidosis is driven by the plasma cell clone's secretion of an amyloidogenic light chain, which causes amyloid fibril formation and subsequent tissue damage. Myeloma is characterized by complications of the clonal plasma cell proliferation itself. In myeloma, plasma cells replace other cellular components of the bone marrow, potentially leading to anemia, hypercalcemia, bony lesions, and renal impairment (typically because of aggregation of normally folded light chains in renal tubules, causing cast nephropathy and renal impairment).

Thus, myeloma patients most commonly have ≥20% plasma cell on bone marrow biopsy, whereas those with AL amyloidosis alone often have a lower plasma cell burden. Although AL amyloidosis and myeloma are separate disorders, approximately 10% of patients with AL amyloidosis have evidence of concomitant myeloma.

Systemic AL amyloidosis often affects multiple organ systems. Renal involvement is very common and most commonly manifests as nephrotic syndrome. Cardiac infiltration is also prevalent and is associated with a progressive restrictive cardiomyopathy, atrial and ventricular arrhythmias, and conduction disease. Other commonly affected organ systems include the nervous system (eg, peripheral neuropathy, autonomic dysfunction) and gastrointestinal tract (eg, dysphagia, hepatic dysfunction, gastroparesis, malabsorption).

Clinical Signs

On clinical examination, patients with AL amyloidosis may have periorbital purpura or other ecchymoses. Macroglossia may be seen in up to 10% of patients.[4] There may be signs of hypervolemia or hypoalbuminemia (eg, elevated jugular venous pressure, hepatomegaly, lower extremity edema). Signs of peripheral neuropathy may be subtle, but often first present as numbness and tingling in the feet. Symptoms of carpal tunnel syndrome, usually bilateral, are also common.

Noninvasive Testing for Cardiac Involvement

Noninvasive cardiac testing can reveal features suggestive of cardiac amyloidosis and should

Clinical Observations
1. Abnormal plasma cells proliferate and occupy a percentage of the bone marrow.
2. Abnormal plasma cells produce monoclonal antibodies (M spike).
3. Abnormal plasma cells produce excess monoclonal free light chain (kappa or lambda).

Monoclonal Gammopathy of Undetermined Significance	Multiple Myeloma	Light Chain Amyloidosis
➤ <10% plasma cells in the bone marrow	➤ ≥10% plasma cells in the bone marrow	➤ Can occur with any plasma cell % clone
➤ Monoclonal spike of immunoglobulin or light chains in the serum and/or urine	➤ Monoclonal spike of immunoglobulin or light chains in the serum and/or urine	➤ Monoclonal spike of immunoglobulin or light chains in the serum and/or urine
➤ Abnormal κ/λ ratio <0.26 or >1.65	➤ Abnormal κ/λ ratio <0.26 or >1.65	➤ Abnormal κ/λ ratio <0.26 or >1.65
➤ No organ or tissue damage	➤ Organ and tissue damage	➤ Circulating light chains form amyloid fibrils and deposit in tissues

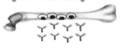

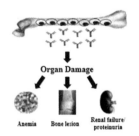

Organ Damage

Anemia   Bone lesion   Renal failure/ proteinuria

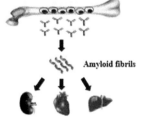

Amyloid fibrils

Fig. 1. Plasma cell dyscrasias.

encourage the pursuit of confirmatory testing (ie, biopsy). An electrocardiogram may reveal low voltage or atrioventricular or interventricular conduction delays.[5,6] A transthoracic echocardiogram often will reveal concentric left ventricular hypertrophy, left and right atrial enlargement, and occasionally, right ventricular hypertrophy. Transmitral Doppler frequently will show a diminished or absent A-wave, likely reflective of left atrial dysfunction in the setting of amyloid infiltration. Tissue Doppler imaging is usually consistent with diastolic dysfunction. Longitudinal strain imaging has been used with increasing frequency. Cardiac amyloidosis has a unique strain pattern, in which longitudinal strain in the basal left ventricular wall segments is significantly impaired, whereas apical strain is relatively preserved.[7] Because of this relatively specific finding, longitudinal strain imaging may be a potential tool to assist in early disease diagnosis and to monitor treatment response in cardiac amyloid patients.[8]

Cardiac magnetic resonance can identify many of the morphologic features of cardiac amyloidosis detected by transthoracic echocardiography. In addition, cardiac amyloidosis may be associated with difficulty nulling the myocardium after gadolinium administration.[9] Some degree of late gadolinium enhancement, in a noncoronary distribution, is usually seen.[10] Cardiac amyloidosis is also associated with a significantly elevated extracellular volume by T1 mapping.[11]

Cardiac PET is actively being explored as a diagnostic tool for AL cardiac amyloidosis. Several radionuclide tracers, including ^{18}F-florbetapir, ^{11}C-Pittsburgh compound B, and ^{18}F-florbetaben, which have been used to detect β-amyloid in Alzheimer disease, also have binding specificity for cardiac amyloid.[12–15] Clinical studies are underway to test the diagnostic value of these tracers in amyloid cardiomyopathy.[16]

Confirmatory Testing and Risk Stratification for Immunoglobulin Light Chains Cardiac Amyloidosis

Despite the significant advancements made in the noninvasive assessment of AL cardiac amyloidosis, the gold standard for diagnosis remains tissue biopsy evidence of AL amyloid fibrils and identification of a monoclonal plasma cell disorder. To evaluate for the presence of a plasma cell dyscrasia, serum and urine protein electrophoresis with immunofixation and serum free light chains analysis (ie, kappa and lambda levels and ratio) should be performed. These tests have a high sensitivity for detecting an abnormal monoclonal paraprotein. The absence of a monoclonal

band and a normal serum free light chain kappa/lambda ratio make the diagnosis of systemic AL amyloidosis unlikely. However, these results do not rule out other forms of systemic amyloidosis (eg, ATTR). In addition to serum free light chain analysis and protein electrophoresis with immunofixation, patients with suspected AL amyloidosis should undergo a bone marrow biopsy to assess plasma cell percentage and to further characterize any clonal population.

To establish the presence of amyloid deposition in cases of suspected cardiac amyloidosis, the authors favor obtaining an endomyocardial biopsy, which is a relatively safe procedure at experienced centers.[17,18] Another affected organ (eg, liver, kidney) may be biopsied instead to confirm the presence of AL amyloid deposits if it is the predominant organ of clinical involvement. These solid organ biopsy sites are preferable to an abdominal fat pad biopsy, which has a lower sensitivity.[19] It is critical that the amyloid deposits are subtyped (eg, AL, ATTR) and not assumed to be AL amyloidosis if a patient has a plasma cell dyscrasia and biopsy-proven amyloid deposits. Particularly in the older population, monoclonal gammopathy of undetermined significance and ATTR amyloidosis are both relatively common.[20,21] Therefore, amyloid deposits must be subtyped, even if they are found in the bone marrow (where ATTR deposits can occur in blood vessels). Subtyping is ideally performed by mass spectrometry, but in experienced hands can also be performed with immunohistochemistry.[22]

Patients with a confirmed diagnosis of AL amyloidosis should undergo disease stratification for prognostication and treatment planning. The revised staging system from the Mayo Clinic is most frequently used (**Table 1**). This score assesses disease severity based on markers of cardiac injury (troponin T- and N-terminal pro-B-type natriuretic peptide levels) and the difference

Table 1
Revised Mayo prognostic staging for immunoglobulin light chains amyloidosis

Stage	Median Survival (mo)	5-y Survival (%)
I	94.1	59
II	40.3	42
III	14	20
IV	5.8	14

Assign 1 point for each of the following: N-terminal pro-B-type natriuretic peptide ≥1800 pg/mL; troponin T ≥0.025 ng/mL; free light chain difference ≥18 mg/dL. A score range of 0 to 3 correlates with stages I to IV, respectively.

between involved and uninvolved serum free light chain levels.

HEART FAILURE MANAGEMENT FOR IMMUNOGLOBULIN LIGHT CHAINS CARDIOMYOPATHY

Diuretics are a cornerstone of symptomatic heart failure management. Given that right-sided heart failure and bowel edema are frequently present, choosing a diuretic with greater bioavailability (ie, torsemide or bumetanide) should be considered. A loop diuretic in combination with a potassium-sparing aldosterone antagonist can be an effective combination. Titration of other standard heart failure medications is often limited by hypotension. Because of severe diastolic dysfunction, cardiac amyloid patients often have a very limited stroke volume and rely on a higher heart rate to achieve an adequate cardiac output. Moreover, many patients develop orthostatic hypotension related to autonomic dysfunction. For these reasons, afterload-reducing medications, such as angiotensin-converting enzyme inhibitors and angiotensin receptor blockers, and beta-blockers tend to be poorly tolerated. Indeed, some patients with significant postural hypotension may benefit from vasoconstricting medications, such as midodrine.

Atrial arrhythmias, such as atrial fibrillation and atrial flutter, are common in amyloid cardiomyopathy. The loss of atrioventricular synchrony can dramatically worsen heart failure in these patients. Thus, effort should be made to restore sinus rhythm. Direct current cardioversion has a high success rate.[23] Importantly, cardiac amyloid patients with atrial fibrillation or flutter are at increased risk for intracardiac thrombus formation and should receive systemic anticoagulation with warfarin or a direct oral anticoagulant, regardless of the presence of other risk factors for cardioembolism (ie, CHADS2VASC score).[24] Because of the relatively high rates of persistent left atrial thrombus despite therapeutic anticoagulation, some centers recommend transesophageal echocardiography before cardioversion in all patients with amyloidosis, regardless of the duration of preceding therapeutic anticoagulation. Antiarrhythmic options are limited due to the presence of heart failure and beta-blocker intolerance. Amiodarone is a reasonable first-line choice and is usually well tolerated. Digoxin toxicity, owing to abnormal drug binding to amyloid fibrils, has been described.[25] However, digoxin use is generally safe with close monitoring of drug levels and for signs of toxicity. Because atrial amyloid infiltration is diffuse, catheter ablation procedures are associated with a high rate of recurrent atrial arrhythmias.[26,27]

Amyloid cardiomyopathy is associated with conduction system disease, including sinus bradycardia and atrioventricular nodal block. Indications for permanent pacemaker implantation follow the society guidelines and are generally based on the severity of conduction disease and presence of symptoms.[28] Sudden cardiac death is another complication encountered in amyloid cardiomyopathy. Causes include pulseless electrical activity, bradycardia, and ventricular arrhythmias. Pulseless electrical activity is caused by electromechanical dissociation, which is not amenable to implantable cardioverter-defibrillator (ICD) therapy.[29] A small retrospective study of ICD implantation in amyloid cardiomyopathy showed that despite a high rate of appropriate ICD shocks, there was no difference in survival compared with controls.[30] Thus, the role of an implantable cardioverter-defibrillation for primary prevention of sudden death in the cardiac amyloidosis population is uncertain. Secondary prevention ICD implantation may be beneficial in select, high-risk patients (eg, prior ventricular tachycardia, nonpostural syncope), but further studies are needed.[31]

AL amyloidosis patients with significant cardiac involvement may develop severe heart failure that is refractory to the abovementioned therapies. Heart transplantation may be considered for patients in whom the burden of extracardiac amyloid deposition is limited, and optimal control of the circulating amyloidogenic free light chain has been achieved. A single-center study demonstrated that in these carefully selected patients, short- to intermediate-term heart transplantation outcomes are comparable to those transplanted for other causes of heart failure.[32] Moreover, a study of the United Network for Organ Sharing registry showed that contemporary heart transplant outcomes in cardiac amyloidosis patients are improving and are similar to outcomes for nonamyloid patients.[33] Left ventricular assist devices are rarely used in cardiac amyloidosis patients but are technically feasible in certain cases.[34] Small left ventricular cavity size, right ventricular failure, and multiorgan dysfunction limit wider use of this therapy.

Anti-Plasma Cell Therapies for Immunoglobulin Light Chains Cardiomyopathy

The primary goal of therapy in AL amyloidosis is to eliminate the amyloidogenic plasma cell clone and prevent further end-organ damage. Complete hematologic remission is characterized by normalization of circulating free light chains and the absence of monoclonal protein by serum and urine immunofixation.[35] AL amyloidosis was first successfully treated with a regimen of melphalan, an alkylating agent, and prednisone.[36] Notably, patients with predominant cardiac involvement had minimal response to treatment. Subsequently, protocols were developed using high-dose melphalan followed by rescue with autologous stem cell transplantation.[37] This more intensive therapy appeared to lead to longer remission and improved survival, although interpretation was limited by the lack of randomized studies and the potential for significant differences in the populations who received each therapy. Autologous stem cell transplantation may be poorly tolerated in many patients, particularly those with significant cardiac disease, multiorgan dysfunction, and advanced age. In the only randomized controlled trial of high-dose melphalan and stem cell transplantation compared with melphalan and dexamethasone, median survival was actually longer in the melphalan and dexamethasone group (56.9 months vs 22.2 months in the high-dose melphalan plus stem cell transplantation group; $P = .04$).[38] The survival advantage of melphalan and dexamethasone persisted even with a 6-month landmark analysis, only considering patients who received the intended therapy and lived at least 6 months, presumably largely discounting the effects of acute treatment-related mortality from the stem cell transplantation. Importantly, the non–stem cell transplant regimen (melphalan and dexamethasone) used in that trial, published in 2007, is far inferior to the options today, further raising the potential that stem cell transplantation should not be the preferred therapy for most patients with the disease. Indeed, over the past decade, significant advancements have been made for identifying more targeted anti-plasma cell therapies that are also better tolerated with AL amyloid patients with severe cardiac involvement[39,40] (summarized in **Table 2**).

Proteasome inhibitors

Proteasomes are responsible for maintaining proteostasis by degrading damaged or excess proteins. In AL amyloidosis, the aberrant plasma cell clone overproduces a misfolded and cytotoxic light chain. Proteasomes are important for protecting these plasma cells from light chain–mediated damage and subsequent cell death. Therefore, proteasome inhibition is an attractive target for selectively eliminating plasma cells producing amyloidogenic light chain.[41] Indeed, amyloidogenic light chains increase plasma cell susceptibility to proteasome inhibitor toxicity.[42] Currently, 3 proteasome inhibitors have been studied for AL amyloidosis.

Bortezomib An early retrospective study investigated bortezomib with dexamethasone in 20 patients with relapsed AL amyloidosis; 15% achieved complete hematologic remission.[43] In a larger study of bortezomib with or without dexamethasone in AL patients as either initial or subsequent therapy (n = 94), there was a similarly favorable rate of complete hematologic remission (25%).[44] Subsequent studies evaluated a regimen of bortezomib, dexamethasone, and cyclophosphamide, an alkylating agent, and demonstrated high rates of complete hematologic remission (71% and 65%, respectively).[45,46] These studies revealed high rates of peripheral neuropathy; however, this complication may be attenuated by using subcutaneous rather than intravenous bortezomib.[47]

Table 2
Chemotherapy drugs for immunoglobulin light chains amyloidosis

Drug Name	Drug Class	Administration Route	Adverse Effects
Bortezomib	Proteasome inhibitor	Intravenous or subcutaneous	Peripheral neuropathy
Carfilzomib	Proteasome inhibitor	Intravenous	Heart failure, arrhythmia, hypertension, thrombosis
Ixazomib	Proteasome inhibitor	Oral	Skin reactions, diarrhea
Daratumumab	Human anti-CD38 monoclonal antibody	Intravenous	Mild infusion-related reaction
Lenalidomide	Immunomodulator	Oral	Thromboembolism, cytopenias, fluid retention
Pomalidomide	Immunomodulator	Oral	Thromboembolism, cytopenias, fluid retention

Bortezomib appears to be effective even in patients with advanced cardiac disease. A large retrospective study (n = 230) of bortezomib, dexamethasone, and cyclophosphamide included 43 patients with advanced cardiac disease (Mayo stage III with NT-proBNP >8500). In this high-risk subgroup, patients who achieved at least a partial hematologic response had a 2-year survival of 67%.[48] In a single-center retrospective study of patients with symptomatic AL amyloid cardiomyopathy, a bortezomib-based regimen was associated with improved survival (n = 106, hazard ratio 0.209, P = .006).[49] Based on the above retrospective studies, bortezomib-based regimens have already been adopted as first-line therapy for AL amyloidosis. The only randomized controlled trial to date for bortezomib in AL amyloidosis (melphalan/dexamethasone with or without bortezomib) has completed enrollment of 110 patients, but detailed results are not yet available.[50]

Carfilzomib Carfilzomib is a second-generation proteasome inhibitor used in multiple myeloma. In a phase 1/2 trial of patients with refractory or relapsed AL amyloidosis, 63% had some degree of hematologic response.[51] Notably, there were several severe adverse events (eg, heart failure, ventricular tachycardia, hypertension, hypoxia). In the authors' experience, carefully selected patients can still benefit from carfilzomib if they are refractory to bortezomib, even if there is cardiac involvement present.

Ixazomib Ixazomib is an oral second-generation proteasome inhibitor. A phase 1/2 study assessed the safety and efficacy of ixazomib in 27 patients with AL amyloidosis refractory to one or more lines of treatment.[52] The progression-free and overall survival rates at 1 year were 60% and 85%, respectively. The most frequent adverse events were cutaneous and gastrointestinal symptoms. There was no evidence of severe peripheral neuropathy. A phase 3 study is actively enrolling with patients with refractory or relapsed AL amyloidosis and randomizing to ixazomib and dexamethasone or physician's choice (dexamethasone plus melphalan, cyclophosphamide, thalidomide, or lenalidomide).[53]

Daratumumab

Daratumumab is a humanized monoclonal antibody against CD38, a protein that is highly expressed on aberrant plasma cells. Early studies of daratumumab in AL amyloidosis patients have shown high response rates. In a retrospective of study of 25 AL amyloidosis patients who were heavily pretreated, 76% achieved a hematologic response (36% with complete remission).[54] The drug was well tolerated with only minor infusion-related reactions reported. Two phase 2 studies showed similar safety and efficacy.[55,56] Given these results, there may be a role for daratumumab in a first-line treatment regimen. Currently, a phase 3 randomized controlled is enrolling newly diagnosed AL amyloidosis patients to first-line therapy (bortezomib, dexamethasone, and cyclophosphamide) with or without daratumumab.[57]

Immunomodulators

Immunomodulators function through a variety of mechanisms to costimulate T cells and natural killer cells, inhibit cell proliferation, and modulate protein degradation.[58] Thalidomide, a first-generation immunomodulator, has long been used to treat multiple myeloma.[59] Second-generation immunomodulators, lenalidomide and pomalidomide, have been studied for treating AL amyloidosis.

Early studies of lenalidomide and dexamethasone in patients with relapsed or refractory AL amyloidosis revealed modest rates of hematologic response, but with rates of severe adverse events, including neutropenia, thrombocytopenia, and venous thromboembolism.[60–62] A recent single-center prospective study evaluated a regimen of lenalidomide, melphalan, and dexamethasone in 50 previously untreated patients with AL amyloidosis; 36% of the patients had advanced cardiac disease (Mayo stage 3).[63] The overall hematologic remission rate was 68% (18% with complete remission). The median overall survival was 67.5 months. In addition to cytopenias, cardiac adverse events were noted with this regimen (eg, worsening heart failure, hypotension, atrial fibrillation).

Pomalidomide with dexamethasone has been investigated for previously treated AL amyloidosis and showed hematologic response rates of 48% to 68%.[64–66] The most common adverse events were fluid retention, cytopenias, arrhythmia, and infection.

SUMMARY

AL cardiac amyloidosis remains a deadly, underdiagnosed disease. Over the past decade, crucial advances in plasma cell-directed therapies have dramatically improved the rates of hematologic remission and overall survival. Early diagnosis is crucial to achieve the maximum benefit of these therapies and avoid irreversible complications or end-organ damage.

REFERENCES

1. Alexander KM, Orav J, Singh A, et al. Geographic disparities in reported US amyloidosis mortality

from 1979 to 2015: potential underdetection of cardiac amyloidosis. JAMA Cardiol 2018;3(9): 865–70.

2. Gonzalez-Lopez E, Gallego-Delgado M, Guzzo-Merello G, et al. Wild-type transthyretin amyloidosis as a cause of heart failure with preserved ejection fraction. Eur Heart J 2015;36(38):2585–94.

3. Kyle RA, Linos A, Beard CM, et al. Incidence and natural history of primary systemic amyloidosis in Olmsted County, Minnesota, 1950 through 1989. Blood 1992;79(7):1817–22.

4. Falk RH, Alexander KM, Liao R, et al. AL (light-chain) cardiac amyloidosis: a review of diagnosis and therapy. J Am Coll Cardiol 2016;68(12):1323–41.

5. Mussinelli R, Salinaro F, Alogna A, et al. Diagnostic and prognostic value of low QRS voltages in cardiac AL amyloidosis. Ann Noninvasive Electrocardiol 2013;18(3):271–80.

6. Boldrini M, Salinaro F, Mussinelli R, et al. Prevalence and prognostic value of conduction disturbances at the time of diagnosis of cardiac AL amyloidosis. Ann Noninvasive Electrocardiol 2013;18(4):327–35.

7. Phelan D, Collier P, Thavendiranathan P, et al. Relative apical sparing of longitudinal strain using two-dimensional speckle-tracking echocardiography is both sensitive and specific for the diagnosis of cardiac amyloidosis. Heart 2012;98(19): 1442–8.

8. Quarta CC, Falk RH. Longitudinal strain imaging in light-chain cardiac amyloidosis: can it help to refine the approach to treatment? J Am Coll Cardiol 2012; 60(12):1077–8.

9. Fontana M, Chung R, Hawkins PN, et al. Cardiovascular magnetic resonance for amyloidosis. Heart Fail Rev 2015;20(2):133–44.

10. Fontana M, Pica S, Reant P, et al. Prognostic value of late gadolinium enhancement cardiovascular magnetic resonance in cardiac amyloidosis. Circulation 2015;132(16):1570–9.

11. Banypersad SM, Fontana M, Maestrini V, et al. T1 mapping and survival in systemic light-chain amyloidosis. Eur Heart J 2015;36(4):244–51.

12. Ehman EC, El-Sady MS, Kijewski MF, et al. Early detection of multiorgan light chain (AL) amyloidosis by whole body (18)F-florbetapir PET/CT. J Nucl Med 2019. [Epub ahead of print].

13. Pilebro B, Arvidsson S, Lindqvist P, et al. Positron emission tomography (PET) utilizing Pittsburgh compound B (PIB) for detection of amyloid heart deposits in hereditary transthyretin amyloidosis (ATTR). J Nucl Cardiol 2018;25(1):240–8.

14. Law WP, Wang WY, Moore PT, et al. Cardiac amyloid imaging with 18F-florbetaben PET: a pilot study. J Nucl Med 2016;57(11):1733–9.

15. Baratto L, Park SY, Hatami N, et al. 18)F-florbetaben whole-body PET/MRI for evaluation of systemic amyloid deposition. EJNMMI Res 2018;8(1):66.

16. Molecular imaging of primary amyloid cardiomyopathy. Available at: https://ClinicalTrials.gov/show/NCT02641145. Accessed July 9, 2019.

17. Deckers JW, Hare JM, Baughman KL. Complications of transvenous right ventricular endomyocardial biopsy in adult patients with cardiomyopathy: a seven-year survey of 546 consecutive diagnostic procedures in a tertiary referral center. J Am Coll Cardiol 1992;19(1):43–7.

18. Holzmann M, Nicko A, Kuhl U, et al. Complication rate of right ventricular endomyocardial biopsy via the femoral approach: a retrospective and prospective study analyzing 3048 diagnostic procedures over an 11-year period. Circulation 2008;118(17): 1722–8.

19. Gertz MA, Li CY, Shirahama T, et al. Utility of subcutaneous fat aspiration for the diagnosis of systemic amyloidosis (immunoglobulin light chain). Arch Intern Med 1988;148(7):929–33.

20. Pinney JH, Whelan CJ, Petrie A, et al. Senile systemic amyloidosis: clinical features at presentation and outcome. J Am Heart Assoc 2013;2(2):e000098.

21. Geller HI, Singh A, Mirto TM, et al. Prevalence of monoclonal gammopathy in wild-type transthyretin amyloidosis. Mayo Clin Proc 2017;92(12):1800–5.

22. Sethi S, Vrana JA, Theis JD, et al. Laser microdissection and mass spectrometry-based proteomics aids the diagnosis and typing of renal amyloidosis. Kidney Int 2012;82(2):226–34.

23. El-Am EA, Dispenzieri A, Melduni RM, et al. Direct current cardioversion of atrial arrhythmias in adults with cardiac amyloidosis. J Am Coll Cardiol 2019; 73(5):589–97.

24. Feng D, Syed IS, Martinez M, et al. Intracardiac thrombosis and anticoagulation therapy in cardiac amyloidosis. Circulation 2009;119(18):2490–7.

25. Rubinow A, Skinner M, Cohen AS. Digoxin sensitivity in amyloid cardiomyopathy. Circulation 1981;63(6): 1285–8.

26. Barbhaiya CR, Kumar S, Baldinger SH, et al. Electrophysiologic assessment of conduction abnormalities and atrial arrhythmias associated with amyloid cardiomyopathy. Heart Rhythm 2016;13(2):383–90.

27. Tan NY, Mohsin Y, Hodge DO, et al. Catheter ablation for atrial arrhythmias in patients with cardiac amyloidosis. J Cardiovasc Electrophysiol 2016; 27(10):1167–73.

28. Kusumoto FM, Schoenfeld MH, Barrett C, et al. 2018 ACC/AHA/HRS guideline on the evaluation and management of patients with bradycardia and cardiac conduction delay: a report of the American College of Cardiology/American Heart Association Task Force on Clinical Practice Guidelines and the Heart Rhythm Society. J Am Coll Cardiol 2019;74(7): 932–87.

29. Kristen AV, Dengler TJ, Hegenbart U, et al. Prophylactic implantation of cardioverter-defibrillator in

patients with severe cardiac amyloidosis and high risk for sudden cardiac death. Heart Rhythm 2008; 5(2):235–40.

30. Lin G, Dispenzieri A, Kyle R, et al. Implantable cardioverter defibrillators in patients with cardiac amyloidosis. J Cardiovasc Electrophysiol 2013; 24(7):793–8.

31. Varr BC, Zarafshar S, Coakley T, et al. Implantable cardioverter-defibrillator placement in patients with cardiac amyloidosis. Heart Rhythm 2014;11(1): 158–62.

32. Davis MK, Kale P, Liedtke M, et al. Outcomes after heart transplantation for amyloid cardiomyopathy in the modern era. Am J Transplant 2015;15(3):650–8.

33. Davis MK, Lee PH, Witteles RM. Changing outcomes after heart transplantation in patients with amyloid cardiomyopathy. J Heart Lung Transplant 2015;34(5):658–66.

34. Swiecicki PL, Edwards BS, Kushwaha SS, et al. Left ventricular device implantation for advanced cardiac amyloidosis. J Heart Lung Transplant 2013; 32(5):563–8.

35. Comenzo RL, Reece D, Palladini G, et al. Consensus guidelines for the conduct and reporting of clinical trials in systemic light-chain amyloidosis. Leukemia 2012;26(11):2317–25.

36. Kyle RA, Gertz MA, Greipp PR, et al. A trial of three regimens for primary amyloidosis: colchicine alone, melphalan and prednisone, and melphalan, prednisone, and colchicine. N Engl J Med 1997;336(17): 1202–7.

37. Comenzo RL, Vosburgh E, Falk RH, et al. Dose-intensive melphalan with blood stem-cell support for the treatment of AL (amyloid light-chain) amyloidosis: survival and responses in 25 patients. Blood 1998;91(10):3662–70.

38. Jaccard A, Moreau P, Leblond V, et al. High-dose melphalan versus melphalan plus dexamethasone for AL amyloidosis. N Engl J Med 2007;357(11): 1083–93.

39. Kastritis E, Dimopoulos MA. Recent advances in the management of AL amyloidosis. Br J Haematol 2016;172(2):170–86.

40. Alexander KM, Singh A, Falk RH. Novel pharmacotherapies for cardiac amyloidosis. Pharmacol Ther 2017;180:129–38.

41. Sitia R, Palladini G, Merlini G. Bortezomib in the treatment of AL amyloidosis: targeted therapy? Haematologica 2007;92(10):1302–7.

42. Oliva L, Orfanelli U, Resnati M, et al. The amyloidogenic light chain is a stressor that sensitizes plasma cells to proteasome inhibitor toxicity. Blood 2017; 129(15):2132–42.

43. Wechalekar AD, Lachmann HJ, Offer M, et al. Efficacy of bortezomib in systemic AL amyloidosis with relapsed/refractory clonal disease. Haematologica 2008;93(2):295–8.

44. Kastritis E, Wechalekar AD, Dimopoulos MA, et al. Bortezomib with or without dexamethasone in primary systemic (light chain) amyloidosis. J Clin Oncol 2010;28(6):1031–7.

45. Mikhael JR, Schuster SR, Jimenez-Zepeda VH, et al. Cyclophosphamide-bortezomib-dexamethasone (CyBorD) produces rapid and complete hematologic response in patients with AL amyloidosis. Blood 2012;119(19):4391–4.

46. Venner CP, Lane T, Foard D, et al. Cyclophosphamide, bortezomib, and dexamethasone therapy in AL amyloidosis is associated with high clonal response rates and prolonged progression-free survival. Blood 2012;119(19):4387–90.

47. Shah G, Kaul E, Fallo S, et al. Bortezomib subcutaneous injection in combination regimens for myeloma or systemic light-chain amyloidosis: a retrospective chart review of response rates and toxicity in newly diagnosed patients. Clin Ther 2013;35(10):1614–20.

48. Palladini G, Sachchithanantham S, Milani P, et al. A European Collaborative Study of cyclophosphamide, bortezomib, and dexamethasone in upfront treatment of systemic AL amyloidosis. Blood 2015; 126(5):612–5.

49. Sperry BW, Ikram A, Hachamovitch R, et al. Efficacy of chemotherapy for light-chain amyloidosis in patients presenting with symptomatic heart failure. J Am Coll Cardiol 2016;67(25): 2941–8.

50. A trial for systemic light-chain (AL) amyloidosis. Available at: https://ClinicalTrials.gov/show/NCT01277016. Accessed July 9, 2019.

51. A safety study of carfilzomib in patients with previously-treated systemic light chain amyloidosis. Available at: https://ClinicalTrials.gov/show/NCT01789242. Accessed July 9, 2019.

52. Sanchorawala V, Palladini G, Kukreti V, et al. A phase 1/2 study of the oral proteasome inhibitor ixazomib in relapsed or refractory AL amyloidosis. Blood 2017;130(5):597–605.

53. Study of dexamethasone plus IXAZOMIB (MLN9708) or physicians choice of treatment in relapsed or refractory systemic light chain (AL) amyloidosis. Available at: https://ClinicalTrials.gov/show/NCT01659658. Accessed July 9, 2019.

54. Kaufman GP, Schrier SL, Lafayette RA, et al. Daratumumab yields rapid and deep hematologic responses in patients with heavily pretreated AL amyloidosis. Blood 2017;130(7):900–2.

55. Daratumumab for the treatment of patients with AL amyloidosis. Available at: https://ClinicalTrials.gov/show/NCT02841033. Accessed July 9, 2019.

56. Daratumumab therapy for patients with refractory or relapsed AL amyloidosis. Available at: https://ClinicalTrials.gov/show/NCT02816476. Accessed July 9, 2019.

57. A study to evaluate the efficacy and safety of dar-atumumab in combination with cyclophosphamide, bortezomib and dexamethasone (CyBorD) compared to CyBorD alone in newly diagnosed systemic amy-loid light-chain (AL) amyloidosis. Available at: https://ClinicalTrials.gov/show/NCT03201965. Accessed July 9, 2019.

58. Quach H, Ritchie D, Stewart AK, et al. Mechanism of action of immunomodulatory drugs (IMiDS) in multi-ple myeloma. Leukemia 2010;24(1):22–32.

59. Singhal S, Mehta J, Desikan R, et al. Antitumor activ-ity of thalidomide in refractory multiple myeloma. N Engl J Med 1999;341(21):1565–71.

60. Dispenzieri A, Lacy MQ, Zeldenrust SR, et al. The activity of lenalidomide with or without dexametha-sone in patients with primary systemic amyloidosis. Blood 2007;109(2):465–70.

61. Sanchorawala V, Wright DG, Rosenzweig M, et al. Lenalidomide and dexamethasone in the treatment of AL amyloidosis: results of a phase 2 trial. Blood 2007;109(2):492–6.

62. Mahmood S, Venner CP, Sachchithanantham S, et al. Lenalidomide and dexamethasone for sys-temic AL amyloidosis following prior treatment with thalidomide or bortezomib regimens. Br J Haematol 2014;166(6):842–8.

63. Hegenbart U, Bochtler T, Benner A, et al. Lenalido-mide/melphalan/dexamethasone in newly diag-nosed patients with immunoglobulin light chain amyloidosis: results of a prospective phase 2 study with long-term follow up. Haematologica 2017; 102(8):1424–31.

64. Dispenzieri A, Buadi F, Laumann K, et al. Activity of pomalidomide in patients with immunoglobulin light-chain amyloidosis. Blood 2012;119(23):5397–404.

65. Sanchorawala V, Shelton AC, Lo S, et al. Pomalido-mide and dexamethasone in the treatment of AL amyloidosis: results of a phase 1 and 2 trial. Blood 2016;128(8):1059–62.

66. Palladini G, Milani P, Foli A, et al. A phase 2 trial of pomalidomide and dexamethasone rescue treat-ment in patients with AL amyloidosis. Blood 2017; 129(15):2120–3.

Carcinoid Heart Disease
A Guide for Clinicians

Daniel Perry, MD, Salim S. Hayek, MD*

KEYWORDS

- Carcinoid syndrome • HIAA • Tricuspid valve • Pulmonic valve • Regurgitation • Right heart failure

KEY POINTS

- Carcinoid heart disease is the collective term for all cardiac manifestations that develop in patients with carcinoid malignancies, including valvular disease, heart failure, and metastatic tumor involvement.
- The cardiac manifestations of carcinoid tumors are attributed to the paraneoplastic effects of vasoactive substances released by the malignant cells, including 5-hydroxytryptamine (serotonin), histamine, tachykinins, transforming growth factor β, and prostaglandins.
- The clinical manifestations of carcinoid heart disease include valvular destruction, leading to valvular regurgitation and stenosis, right-sided heart failure, and metastatic carcinoid disease.
- A combination of biomarkers and cardiac imaging is used in the screening and diagnosis of carcinoid heart disease in patients with carcinoid syndrome, most importantly echocardiography and measurement of N-terminal pro–B-type natriuretic peptide.
- The management of carcinoid heart disease involves both medical and surgical treatment and requires a multidisciplinary approach for optimized care.

 Video content accompanies this article at http://www.cardiology.theclinics.com.

DEFINITION AND EPIDEMIOLOGY

Carcinoid tumors are a rare subset of neuroendocrine tumors that originate from the gastrointestinal tract (55%) and bronchopulmonary system (30%).[1] The incidence is 38.4 per 1 million individuals and is higher in black men compared with whites, with an average age of diagnosis between ages 55 and 60 years.[2] Carcinoid tumors have profound cardiovascular and noncardiovascular effects caused by the release of various vasoactive substances, including serotonin, 5-hydroxytryptopan, histamine, bradykinin, tachykinins, and prostaglandins. The constellation of symptoms attributed to these effects is called the carcinoid syndrome, which consists of flushing, hypermotility of the gastrointestinal tract, hypotension, and bronchospasm. Carcinoid heart disease is the collective term for all cardiac manifestations that develop in patients with carcinoid malignancies, including valvular disease, heart failure, and metastatic tumor involvement.

Cardiac involvement eventually occurs in 50% of patients with carcinoid syndrome and is the presenting symptom of carcinoid disease 20% of the time.[3,4] Most patients with carcinoid heart disease present in the fifth to seventh decades of life.[5] The right side of the heart is the most often affected, specifically the tricuspid and pulmonary valves. Progressive valvular disease leads to the development of edema, ascites, and right-sided heart failure. Carcinoid heart disease is a major cause of

Disclosure Statement: The authors have nothing to disclose.
Division of Cardiology, Department of Medicine, University of Michigan, 1500 East Medical Center Drive, Ann Arbor, MI 48109, USA
* Corresponding author. University of Michigan Frankel Cardiovascular Center, 1500 East Medical Center Drive, CVC #2709, Ann Arbor, MI 48109.
E-mail address: shayek@med.umich.edu

Cardiol Clin 37 (2019) 497–503
https://doi.org/10.1016/j.ccl.2019.07.014

morbidity and mortality in patients with carcinoid syndrome. Untreated, the 3-year survival of carcinoid heart disease is 31%, approximately half the survival rate of carcinoid patients without cardiac involvement.[3] Diagnosis and management of carcinoid heart disease are challenging, because the initial presentation can be subtle, and the disease can progress quickly leading to high morbidity. This article discusses various aspects of carcinoid heart disease and highlights the challenges faced by clinicians when managing the cardiovascular manifestations of carcinoid malignancies.

PATHOPHYSIOLOGY OF CARCINOID HEART DISEASE

The cardiac manifestations of carcinoid tumors are attributed to the paraneoplastic effects of vasoactive substances released by the malignant cells, including 5-hydroxytryptamine (serotonin), histamine, tachykinins, transforming growth factor β (TGF-β), and prostaglandins.[5] Normally these substances are metabolized and inactivated by the liver and lung; however, metastatic disease involving the liver exposes the right-sided cardiac structures to large quantities of hormones. The exact mechanism of valvular disease in carcinoid syndrome is unknown. Some of these substances, including serotonin and TGF-β, are thought to induce proliferation of fibroblasts, leading to the deposition of plaques on endocardial surfaces, including valve leaflets, subvalvular apparatus, and cardiac chambers.[6] These plaques are made of smooth muscle cells, myofibroblasts, extracellular matrix, and an overlying endothelial layer. Plaque formation causes annular constriction, thickening of valve leaflets, and fusion of the subvalvular apparatus,[7] eventually leading to noncoaptation of the valve leaflets and valvular regurgitation.[8]

Patients with carcinoid heart disease have significantly higher levels of serotonin, platelet serotonin, and urinary 5-hydroxyindoleacetic acid (5-HIAA) levels than carcinoid patients without cardiac involvement.[9,10] Additionally, serotonergic drugs and other structurally similar medications that activate serotonin receptors have been associated with similar valve lesions as those seen in carcinoid heart disease, supporting the involvement of serotonin in the pathogenesis of carcinoid-related valvular disease.[11]

CLINICAL MANIFESTATIONS

The clinical manifestations of carcinoid heart disease are due to progressive valvular destruction,

leading to valvular regurgitation and stenosis, right-sided heart failure, and metastatic carcinoid disease. Early valvular disease is often asymptomatic and is typically diagnosed a year and a half after the diagnosis of carcinoid syndrome.[12] Valvular involvement ranges from mild disease causing stiff thickened leaflets with trivial or mild regurgitation to severe disease with fixed, retracted leaflets with severe regurgitation with or without accompanying stenosis.[13] As tricuspid and pulmonic valvular disease worsens, progressively elevated right ventricular pressure leads to dilatation of the ventricle and right-sided heart failure causing peripheral edema and ascites.[14] Hormone levels are a determinant of severity of disease, because elevated 5-HIAA levels have been correlated with progression of carcinoid heart disease.[15] On pathology, the affected valves typically appear white with thickened leaflets and subvalvular apparatus. In advanced disease, carcinoid plaques can be seen in the endocardial lining of the chambers of the heart. Left-sided cardiac disease is rare, occurring in less than 10% of patients with carcinoid heart disease because vasoactive hormones are inactivated in the pulmonary vasculature and do not reach left-sided cardiac structures.[3] Left-sided heart disease, however, is more likely to develop in patients with right-to-left shunts (patent foramen ovale and atrial septal defects), poorly controlled disease with high levels of circulating hormones, or bronchopulmonary carcinoid disease, owing to higher levels of vasoactive hormones reaching the left side of the heart. Metastatic disease to the heart is rare, occurring in 4% of patients with carcinoid syndrome.[13]

THE PHYSICAL EXAMINATION

Physical examination may be normal at the time of diagnosis of carcinoid heart disease. Early physical examination findings include murmurs of tricuspid and pulmonic valve regurgitation and less frequently stenosis as well as elevated jugular venous pressure.[16] A palpable right ventricular impulse also may be present. With more advanced disease, additional findings of right-sided heart failure develop, including lower extremity edema, ascites, and hepatomegaly. The sensitivity of the physical examination is poor, with 1 study showing that at least 37% of patients with carcinoid heart disease diagnosed via screening echocardiography had no clinical signs of cardiac abnormalities by physical examination.[17]

Screening, Diagnosis and Monitoring

Early diagnosis of carcinoid heart disease is critical given its impact on morbidity and mortality. The American College of Cardiology issued guidelines in 2017 for the diagnosis and management of carcinoid heart disease as well as its surveillance.[18] Patients diagnosed with a serotonin-producing metastatic neuroendocrine tumor should have a cardiovascular evaluation with cardiac imaging performed at diagnosis and biomarker assessment every 6 months, with repeat imaging should biomarker levels rise or physical examination findings of carcinoid heart disease develop (**Fig. 1**).

Imaging

Transthoracic echocardiography (TTE) is the primary imaging modality used to assess carcinoid heart disease and should be performed at the time of diagnosis of a neuroendocrine tumor. Repeat TTE should be performed in patients with carcinoid who present with signs or symptoms suggestive of cardiac involvement, or if biomarkers are elevated.[18] If there is evidence for carcinoid heart disease or other concerning pathology seen on TTE, patients should be referred to a cardiologist with experience managing carcinoid heart disease. For patients with known carcinoid heart disease, TTE should be performed every 3 months to 6 months to monitor for progression of disease, or earlier if there is a change in clinical status. An agitated saline "bubble study" should be done to evaluate for right-to-left shunts, which if present significantly increase the risk of developing left-sided valvular disease. Transesophageal echocardiography is used only if valves are not adequately visualized or in preparation for valvular surgery.

Echocardiographic findings of carcinoid heart disease range from mild, isolated thickening of a single-valve leaflet with no significant reduction in leaflet mobility, to advanced thickening, retraction, and immobility of multiple valves with associated severe valve dysfunction.[13] Abnormalities of the tricuspid valve were visualized by TTE in 90% of patients with carcinoid heart disease. Mild changes consist of thickening of the valve leaflets and subvalvular apparatus with disruption of the normal curvature of the leaflets, causing them to appear straightened (**Fig. 2**A). The diseased leaflets move in a stiff board-like fashion as opposed to the normal undulating motion. In severe cases, leaflets were fixed and retracted and failed to coapt, causing severe tricuspid regurgitation and a dagger-shape on Doppler assessment (Videos 1 and 2). The right ventricle is dilated in 93% of patients with severe tricuspid regurgitation. Pulmonary valve abnormalities are seen in 69% of patients with carcinoid heart disease, with morphologic changes similar to that in tricuspid valve disease (**Fig. 2**B, Video 3). A third of patients with carcinoid heart disease have evidence of left-sided valvular involvement, and among those 87% were associated with a patent foramen ovale, and the remaining had bronchial carcinoid metastases. Patients with left-sided disease similarly have diffuse thickening of aortic and mitral valve leaflets. TTE also can be used to assess right-sided heart function and chamber size in advanced disease. Cardiac magnetic resonance imaging (MRI) and computed tomography can be used as alternatives if echo windows are poor but are not routinely used. MRI has the added benefit of detecting myocardial metastases and extension of disease into extracardiac structures.

Biomarkers

N-terminal pro–B-type natriuretic peptide N-terminal pro–B-type natriuretic peptide (NT-proBNP) is the most useful biomarker in screening for cardiac involvement, with a sensitivity for the detection of carcinoid heart disease of 92% and specificity of 91%.[19] Pro-BNP is released by the atria and ventricles in response to wall stress from volume and pressure overload and is cleaved into physiologically active BNP and inactive degradation product NT-proBNP.[20] Median NT-proBNP levels are significantly higher in patients with carcinoid heart disease than in patients without cardiac involvement.[21] Serum NT-proBNP level should be measured every 6 months in all patients with carcinoid syndrome without known carcinoid heart disease. At a cutoff level of 260 pg/mL, NT-proBNP is used as a screening biomarker, with follow-up echocardiogram if levels are above this threshold.[21] Data for use of BNP levels as

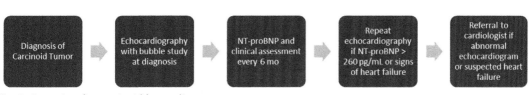

Fig. 1. Screening for carcinoid heart disease.

A   **B**

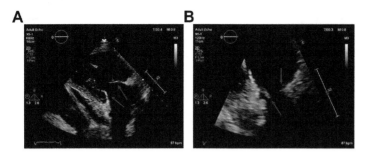

Fig. 2. Echocardiographic images of tricuspid and pulmonic valves in carcinoid heart disease. (*A*) Right ventricular inflow view of the tricuspid valve in systole. (*B*) Short axis, basal view of the pulmonic valve. Note the thickened valves (*red arrows*) with loss of curvature and lack of coaptation.

opposed to NT-proBNP levels are limited; thus, BNP is not currently recommended for screening.

Chromogranin A Chromogranin A is a glycoprotein that is released by neuroendocrine tumor cells. Levels of chromogranin A are elevated in more than 80% of patients with advanced carcinoid tumors[22]; however, its specificity for the detection of severe carcinoid heart disease is only 30%. Due to its low specificity, chromogranin A levels are not recommended as a screening test for carcinoid heart disease and are not used routinely in clinical practice. Chromogranin A, however, may be useful for assessing neuroendocrine tumor recurrence or tumor progression[23] and can provide prognostic information for overall survival when used together with NT-proBNP. In patients with normal chromogranin A levels, 81% had survived after 5 years. In patients with elevated chromogranin A and normal NT-proBNP survival dropped to 44% and with elevated levels of both chromogranin A and NT-proBNP levels survival was only 16%.[19]

5-Hydroxyindoleacetic acid 5-HIAA is produced by the metabolism of serotonin released by carcinoid tumors. Plasma and urinary levels of 5-HIAA are significantly higher in patients with carcinoid heart disease than without cardiac involvement.[10,24] Elevated 24-hour urine 5-HIAA or plasma 5-HIAA levels are needed for diagnosis of carcinoid syndrome and also are useful in identifying patients with carcinoid syndrome who are at a higher risk of developing carcinoid heart disease. Urinary 5-HIAA levels greater than 300 mmol/24 hours confers a 2-fold to 3-fold increase in the risk of developing or progression of carcinoid heart disease in patients with carcinoid syndrome; however, guidelines for the use of urinary 5-HIAA levels clinically for carcinoid heart disease are absent.[25]

No biomarker has been proved useful in predicting the development of left-sided heart disease.

TREATMENT OF CARCINOID HEART DISEASE

The management of carcinoid heart disease involves both medical and surgical interventions and requires a multidisciplinary approach for optimized care. Therapy is aimed at managing heart failure symptoms, lowering circulating vasoactive hormone levels, and surgical valve replacement in advanced disease.

Medical Management

Medical management has 2 aims: (1) preventing progression to right-sided heart failure and (2) management of symptoms and hypervolemia. For patients with symptomatic carcinoid, medical therapy with somatostatin analogues, such as octreotide and lanreotide, is the primary treatment. These medications produce both symptomatic improvement and reduction in 5-HIAA urinary secretion and serum serotonin concentrations. Although these medications have not been shown to reverse valvular heart disease that is already present,[10] they increasingly are used in asymptomatic patients who have elevated levels of 5-HIAA to lower the levels of circulating hormone and reduce the risk of developing carcinoid heart disease. Telotristat etiprate is an inhibitor of tryptophan hydroxylase, an enzyme involved in the conversion of tryptophan to serotonin, which has been approved in combination with somatostatin analog therapy for the treatment of adults with carcinoid syndrome diarrhea uncontrolled by somatostatin analog therapy. Whether telotristat etiprate reduces the development or progression of carcinoid heart disease is unclear; however, several studies have shown a reduction in 5-HIAA levels in patients treated with telotristat etiprate, suggesting it may be useful in preventing carcinoid heart disease in patients with high levels of serotonin.[26–28]

Progressive tricuspid and pulmonary valve disease eventually leads to right-sided heart failure, for which medical therapy is limited. Diuretics are used to control symptoms by lowering cardiac preload and reducing edema and ascites; however, they must be dosed carefully because volume depletion can cause a reduction in cardiac output due to right-sided heart failure being a preload-dependent state, leading to hypotension and acute kidney injury.[29] Similarly, conservative measures, such as dietary and fluid restriction and compressive stockings, are adjunctive and can help minimize diuretic requirements.

Surgical Management

Valvular surgery should be considered in patients with well-controlled metastatic disease but severe valvular involvement who are symptomatic despite medical therapy or have evidence of right ventricular dysfunction.[30] Valve replacement is effective in both relieving symptoms and improving outcomes. In patients with severe symptomatic carcinoid heart disease, survival was 40% at 2 years in patients treated surgically compared with 8% in patients treated without surgery.[31] Given the complexity of the procedures, valvular surgery should be performed at experienced medical centers with a team-based approach among surgeons, cardiologists, and anesthesiologists who are experienced in treating patients with carcinoid syndrome. The optimal timing of valve surgery is unknown. Patients with carcinoid heart disease should be referred for surgical evaluation as soon as they develop symptoms (fatigue, dyspnea, and edema) or asymptomatic evidence of right ventricular dysfunction observed by echocardiography.[18] Tricuspid valve replacement is the most common procedure performed, but multiple valves can be replaced. Both bioprosthetic and mechanical valves have been used, and the choice on type of valve used should be made on a case-by-case basis after considering patient factors, such as bleeding risk and life expectancy.[6] If a patent foramen is present, this should be closed at the time of surgery to reduce the likelihood of developing left-sided carcinoid heart disease. Carcinoid syndrome complicates surgery, because anesthesia can lead to carcinoid crisis by triggering the release of large quantities of vasoactive hormones, inducing life-threatening hypotension, bronchoconstriction, and arrhythmias.[32] As a preventive measure, octreotide typically is administered prior to anesthesia and continued throughout the procedure and postoperatively until the patient is stable.[33,34]

Percutaneous catheter-based valvular procedures are being explored as a treatment option in patients with severe disease who are not candidates for surgery. Data are limited for this novel technique; however, case reports describe the successful use of percutaneous valves on native pulmonary valves affected by carcinoid heart disease[35] as well as in patients with carcinoid heart disease who have dysfunctional bioprosthetic pulmonary and tricuspid valves (valve-in-valve approach).[36–38]

SUMMARY

Carcinoid heart disease refers to collection of cardiac manifestations that present in patients with carcinoid tumors, including valvular disease, right-sided heart failure, and metastatic tumor involvement. It is a cause of significant morbidity and mortality among patients with carcinoid tumors. Diagnosing carcinoid heart disease requires adequate screening protocols and a high index of suspicion, because the initial symptoms often are absent or mild. A combination of biomarkers and cardiac imaging is used in the screening and diagnosis of carcinoid heart disease in patients with carcinoid syndrome, most importantly echocardiography and measurement of NT-proBNP. Treatment is centered around controlling heart failure symptoms, reducing systemic levels of vasoactive tumor hormone, and valve replacement surgery in severe disease. Transcatheter approaches are emerging and may lead to a paradigm shift in the approach to treating severe carcinoid heart disease. A multidisciplinary approach should be used at an experienced medical center for optimal management of this complex and challenging disease.

SUPPLEMENTARY DATA

Supplementary data related to this article can be found online at https://doi.org/10.1016/j.ccl.2019.07.014.

REFERENCES

1. Maggard MA, O'Connell JB, Ko CY. Updated population-based review of carcinoid tumors. Ann Surg 2004;240(1):117–22.
2. Yao JC, Hassan M, Phan A, et al. One hundred years after "carcinoid": epidemiology of and prognostic factors for neuroendocrine tumors in 35,825 cases in the United States. J Clin Oncol 2008;26(18):3063–72.
3. Pellikka PA, Tajik AJ, Khandheria BK, et al. Carcinoid heart disease. Clinical and echocardiographic spectrum in 74 patients. Circulation 1993;87(4):1188–96.
4. Lundin L, Norheim I, Landelius J, et al. Carcinoid heart disease: relationship of circulating vasoactive

substances to ultrasound-detectable cardiac abnormalities. Circulation 1988;77(2):264–9.

5. Fox DJ, Khattar RS. Carcinoid heart disease: presentation, diagnosis, and management. Heart 2004;90(10):1224–8.

6. Grozinsky-Glasberg S, Grossman AB, Gross DJ. Carcinoid heart disease: from pathophysiology to treatment–'something in the way it moves'. Neuroendocrinology 2015;101(4):263–73.

7. Yuan SM. Valvular disorders in carcinoid heart disease. Braz J Cardiovasc Surg 2016;31(5):400–5.

8. Warner RRP, Castillo JG. Carcinoid heart disease: the challenge of the unknown known. J Am Coll Cardiol 2015;66(20):2197–200.

9. Robiolio PA, Rigolin VH, Wilson JS, et al. Carcinoid heart disease. Correlation of high serotonin levels with valvular abnormalities detected by cardiac catheterization and echocardiography. Circulation 1995;92(4):790–5.

10. Denney WD, Kemp WE Jr, Anthony LB, et al. Echocardiographic and biochemical evaluation of the development and progression of carcinoid heart disease. J Am Coll Cardiol 1998;32(4):1017–22.

11. Rothman RB, Baumann MH, Savage JE, et al. Evidence for possible involvement of 5-HT(2B) receptors in the cardiac valvulopathy associated with fenfluramine and other serotonergic medications. Circulation 2000;102(23):2836–41.

12. Moller JE, Pellikka PA, Bernheim AM, et al. Prognosis of carcinoid heart disease: analysis of 200 cases over two decades. Circulation 2005;112(21):3320–7.

13. Bhattacharyya S, Toumpanakis C, Burke M, et al. Features of carcinoid heart disease identified by 2- and 3-dimensional echocardiography and cardiac MRI. Circ Cardiovasc Imaging 2010;3(1):103–11.

14. Bruce CJ, Connolly HM. Right-sided valve disease deserves a little more respect. Circulation 2009;119(20):2726–34.

15. Moller JE, Connolly HM, Rubin J, et al. Factors associated with progression of carcinoid heart disease. N Engl J Med 2003;348(11):1005–15.

16. Ross EM, Roberts WC. The carcinoid syndrome: comparison of 21 necropsy subjects with carcinoid heart disease to 15 necropsy subjects without carcinoid heart disease. Am J Med 1985;79(3):339–54.

17. Bhattacharyya S, Toumpanakis C, Caplin ME, et al. Analysis of 150 patients with carcinoid syndrome seen in a single year at one institution in the first decade of the twenty-first century. Am J Cardiol 2008;101(3):378–81.

18. Davar J, Connolly HM, Caplin ME, et al. Diagnosing and managing carcinoid heart disease in patients with neuroendocrine tumors: an expert statement. J Am Coll Cardiol 2017;69(10):1288–304.

19. Korse CM, Taal BG, de Groot CA, et al. Chromogranin-A and N-terminal pro-brain natriuretic peptide:

an excellent pair of biomarkers for diagnostics in patients with neuroendocrine tumor. J Clin Oncol 2009;27(26):4293–9.

20. Valli N, Gobinet A, Bordenave L. Review of 10 years of the clinical use of brain natriuretic peptide in cardiology. J Lab Clin Med 1999;134(5):437–44.

21. Bhattacharyya S, Toumpanakis C, Caplin ME, et al. Usefulness of N-terminal pro-brain natriuretic peptide as a biomarker of the presence of carcinoid heart disease. Am J Cardiol 2008;102(7):938–42.

22. Bhattacharyya S, Gujral DM, Toumpanakis C, et al. A stepwise approach to the management of metastatic midgut carcinoid tumor. Nat Rev Clin Oncol 2009;6(7):429–33.

23. Askew JW, Connolly HM. Carcinoid valve disease. Curr Treat Options Cardiovasc Med 2013;15(5):544–55.

24. Zuetenhorst JM, Bonfrer JM, Korse CM, et al. Carcinoid heart disease: the role of urinary 5-hydroxyindoleacetic acid excretion and plasma levels of atrial natriuretic peptide, transforming growth factor-beta and fibroblast growth factor. Cancer 2003;97(7):1609–15.

25. Bhattacharyya S, Toumpanakis C, Chilkunda D, et al. Risk factors for the development and progression of carcinoid heart disease. Am J Cardiol 2011;107(8):1221–6.

26. Kulke MH, O'Dorisio T, Phan A, et al. Telotristat etiprate, a novel serotonin synthesis inhibitor, in patients with carcinoid syndrome and diarrhea not adequately controlled by octreotide. Endocr Relat Cancer 2014;21(5):705–14.

27. Pavel M, Horsch D, Caplin M, et al. Telotristat etiprate for carcinoid syndrome: a single-arm, multicenter trial. J Clin Endocrinol Metab 2015;100(4):1511–9.

28. Kulke MH, Horsch D, Caplin ME, et al. Telotristat ethyl, a tryptophan hydroxylase inhibitor for the treatment of carcinoid syndrome. J Clin Oncol 2017;35(1):14–23.

29. Bernheim AM, Connolly HM, Hobday TJ, et al. Carcinoid heart disease. Prog Cardiovasc Dis 2007;49(6):439–51.

30. Connolly HM, Schaff HV, Abel MD, et al. Early and late outcomes of surgical treatment in carcinoid heart disease. J Am Coll Cardiol 2015;66(20):2189–96.

31. Connolly HM, Nishimura RA, Smith HC, et al. Outcome of cardiac surgery for carcinoid heart disease. J Am Coll Cardiol 1995;25(2):410–6.

32. Mason RA, Steane PA. Carcinoid syndrome: its relevance to the anaesthetist. Anaesthesia 1976;31(2):228–42.

33. Vaughan DJ, Brunner MD. Anesthesia for patients with carcinoid syndrome. Int Anesthesiol Clin 1997;35(4):129–42.

34. Weingarten TN, Abel MD, Connolly HM, et al. Intraoperative management of patients with carcinoid heart disease having valvular surgery: a review of one hundred consecutive cases. Anesth Analg 2007;105(5):1192–9. table of contents.

35. Heidecker B, Moore P, Bergsland EK, et al. Transcatheter pulmonic valve replacement in carcinoid heart disease. Eur Heart J Cardiovasc Imaging 2015;16(9):1046.

36. Hon JK, Cheung A, Ye J, et al. Transatrial transcatheter tricuspid valve-in-valve implantation of balloon expandable bioprosthesis. Ann Thorac Surg 2010; 90(5):1696–7.

37. Khan JN, Doshi SN, Rooney SJ, et al. Transcatheter pulmonary and tricuspid valve-in-valve replacement for bioprosthesis degeneration in carcinoid heart disease. Eur Heart J Cardiovasc Imaging 2016; 17(1):114.

38. Conradi L, Schaefer A, Mueller GC, et al. Carcinoid heart valve disease: transcatheter pulmonary valve-in-valve implantation in failing biological xenografts. J Heart Valve Dis 2015;24(1):110–4.

Role of Cardiovascular Biomarkers in the Risk Stratification, Monitoring, and Management of Patients with Cancer

Christopher W. Hoeger, MD[a], Salim S. Hayek, MD[b],*

KEYWORDS

- Biomarkers • Troponin • Brain natriuretic peptide • Cardiotoxicity • Cancer • Chemotherapy
- Anthracycline • Trastuzumab

KEY POINTS

- Cardiovascular biomarkers are being explored in the prediction, diagnosis, and management of the cardiotoxic effects of cancer therapies.
- Troponin and B-type natriuretic peptides are most studied and most commonly used biomarkers clinically.
- Biomarkers can be incorporated into a multimodal strategy that includes cardiovascular imaging to predict and monitor for cardiotoxicity. Abnormal biomarker testing during or after cardiotoxic cancer therapy should prompt further investigation for cardiac dysfunction.
- Overall, most studies are small in sample size and are inconclusive. Larger, well-powered studies are needed to delineate care strategies using biomarkers in the prediction and management of the cardiovascular effects of cancer therapy.

INTRODUCTION

The explosive growth of novel cancer therapies in the last decade has led to dramatic improvements in the survival of patients with cancer.[1] The occurrence of poorly understood cardiovascular toxicities attributed to cancer therapy threatens to offset the benefits of potent new treatments.[2,3] Cancer therapies have been associated with a wide range of cardiovascular manifestations including heart failure, myocardial ischemia, myocarditis, hypertension, pulmonary hypertension, pericardial diseases, thromboembolism, arrhythmias, and radiation-induced cardiovascular disease.[4]

The prevention, diagnosis and management of cardiovascular toxicity in cancer therapy present a major clinical challenge. Although such toxicity is often a defined risk of therapy, it can present idiopathically. For example, the current diagnostic standard for drug-induced cardiomyopathy is echocardiography, which is an insensitive modality that reflects cardiac damage that has already occurred. Blood-based biomarkers can be cost-effective alternatives to imaging for screening or monitoring patients at risk of cardiotoxicity and can detect subclinical disease (**Table 1**).[5,6]

In this review, we delineate the current state of biomarker research and clinical applications in

Disclosure: The authors have nothing to disclose.
[a] Department of Medicine, University of Michigan, 1500 East Medical Center Drive, Ann Arbor, MI 48109, USA;
[b] Division of Cardiology, Department of Medicine, University of Michigan, University of Michigan Frankel Cardiovascular Center, 1500 East Medical Center Drive, CVC #2709, Ann Arbor, MI 48109, USA
* Corresponding author.
E-mail address: shayek@med.umich.edu

Cardiol Clin 37 (2019) 505–523
https://doi.org/10.1016/j.ccl.2019.07.015
0733-8651/19/© 2019 Elsevier Inc. All rights reserved.

cardiology.theclinics.com

Table 1
Biomarkers of cardiovascular disease, their physiologic roles and clinical implications

Biomarker	Biologic Role	Clinical Implications
Troponin I/T	Calcium-mediated interaction of actin and myosin in cardiac myocytes	Diagnosis of myocardial injury, including STEMI, drug-induced cardiac injury
Brain natriuretic peptides – BNP/NT-proBNP	Released by ventricles in volume overload or wall stress, induces natriuresis to maintain euvolemia	Diagnosis and prognostication in heart failure, prognostication in acute coronary syndrome, coronary artery disease, and valvular heart disease
C-Reactive protein	Classical acute phase protein that is a sensitive systemic marker and mediator of inflammation and tissue damage	Assessment of disease activity in inflammatory conditions, diagnosis and management of infection, classification of inflammatory disease; cardiovascular disease risk stratification; risk stratification for anti-inflammatory use after acute coronary syndromes
Myeloperoxidase	Enzyme secreted by neutrophils involved in reactive oxygen species generation, lipid peroxidation, nitric oxide synthase inhibition, and scavenging of nitric oxide	Associated with adverse prognosis in heart failure
miRNAs	Small, noncoding nucleic acids that bind to and inhibit transcription of mRNA	Monitoring response to heart failure therapies, potential therapeutic target
GDF-15	Member of the transforming growth factor β cytokine superfamily, produced in response to injury, inflammation, and oxidative stress	Possible marker of outcomes in acute coronary syndromes and heart failure
Galactin-3	Soluble β-galactoside-binding lectin associated with myocardial fibrosis, thought to be a mediator of aldosterone-induced fibrosis and vascular inflammation	Associated with outcomes in heart failure, risk of incident heart failure and mortality in the community
ST2	Interleukin-1 (IL-1) receptor family that is a decoy receptor for IL-33 in the systemic circulation, which stimulates cellular inflammatory response	Predictor of mortality or transplant in patients with severe chronic heart failure and mortality in acute heart failure
Peripheral blood mononuclear cell gene expression	Thought to reflect transcription of genes in target organs (ie, heart)	Associated with disease activity in rheumatologic disease, cancer, and asthma
Arginine-nitric oxide metabolites	Mediator of endothelial dysfunction and oxidative stress	Associated with mortality in acute coronary syndromes, myocardial infarction, and congestive heart failure
Soluble urokinase plasminogen receptor activator	Receptor expressed on a variety of immune cells that is involved in cellular migration, adhesion, angiogenesis, fibrinolysis, and cell proliferation, released from cells during inflammatory stimulation	Associated with incidence of chronic kidney disease, cancer, cardiovascular disease, diabetes, and mortality
Immunoglobulin E	Defense against parasitic disease and involved in pathogenesis of allergic diseases	Not studied as a biomarker in other disease states

cardio-oncology including pretreatment risk stratification, monitoring for cardiovascular toxicity during and after therapy, and, lastly, biomarker-guided prevention of toxicity.

PRETREATMENT RISK STRATIFICATION
Overview

Biomarkers have been mostly studied in the diagnosis of heart failure secondary to anthracyclines, trastuzumab, tyrosine kinase inhibitors (TKIs), and radiation therapy (**Table 2**).[7] Clinical trial data to guide the use of biomarkers in the risk stratification of patients before cancer therapy is lacking, and recommendations for their use are largely based on expert opinion.

Current Guidelines

The European Society of Cardiology (ESC), American Society of Clinical Oncology (ASMO), European Society of Medical Oncology (ESMO), and Canadian Cardiovascular Society have published recommendations on the use of biomarkers in patients with cancer receiving cardiotoxic treatment.[5,8–10] The ESC recommends consideration of baseline biomarker measurement (either troponin or brain natriuretic peptide [BNP]) with serial measurements to determine cardiac response to treatment,[5] whereas the ESMO guidelines note a "strong case to incorporate their use in the clinical trial setting" but fall short of making a recommendation on their clinical implementation.[9]

Evidence

Troponin in the prediction of cardiotoxicity attributed to trastuzumab
The largest study published to date is an analysis of a subset of the Herceptin Adjuvant study, in which 533 patients with breast cancer undergoing trastuzumab therapy had serial measurements of high-sensitivity troponins I (hs-TnI) and T (hs-TnT reported as abnormal, which is defined as >40 ng/L and >14 ng/L for hs-TnI and hs-TnT, respectively). Whereas a small number of events were noted (7.8%), an increased baseline troponin was associated with a 4-fold risk in developing cardiotoxicity.[11] These findings were confirmed in another study of 251 patients with breast cancer undergoing treatment, which found that 17% of the patients who later developed trastuzumab-induced cardiomyopathy had a positive conventional troponin I at baseline (>0.08 ng/mL), compared with none of the patients in the subgroup who did not develop cardiomyopathy.[12] Both studies, however, had a high prevalence of previous anthracyclines exposure (90% and

78%, respectively); thus, whether pretreatment troponin levels are predictive of cardiac dysfunction after trastuzumab therapy alone remains unclear.

Troponins in the prediction of anthracycline toxicity
There is less evidence available supporting the use of troponin for risk stratification before anthracycline treatment. In several studies, pretreatment conventional TnI[13–16] and hs-TnI[17] were normal in all subjects and thus not predictive of cardiovascular outcomes. Several other studies have found no association between conventional TnI,[18] hs-TnI,[19] or hs-TnT[20,21] and cardiovascular outcomes after anthracycline therapy. The absence of an association is likely due to the overall low prevalence of patients with previous cardiovascular disease or risk factors in these studies.

B-Natriuretic peptide in the prediction of anthracycline toxicity
In a study of 53 patients with breast cancer undergoing anthracycline treatment, patients with a decreased left ventricular ejection fraction (LVEF) by $\geq$10% at follow-up had pretreatment levels of BNP of 55.5 $\pm$ 72.3 pg/mL, whereas those who did not develop cardiac dysfunction had a baseline of 26.1 $\pm$ 21.4 pg/mL.[19] A similar study from Lenihan and colleagues,[18] found that patients who experienced a cardiac event had a trend toward higher baseline levels of BNP. However, several other studies found no association between pretreatment BNP or the N-terminal prohormone of BNP (NT-proBNP) and cardiovascular outcomes.[11,20,22–25] Potential explanations for these divergent findings include small sample sizes, variable follow-up time, and differing definitions of cardiovascular toxicity.

Immunoglobulin E
One intriguing case-control study of patients with and without with a diagnosis of cardiac dysfunction because cancer therapy identified immunoglobulin E (IgE) levels as a main differentiator between cases and controls among thousands of proteins analyzed. This difference was seen across all time points of samples and was validated in a study of 35 subjects that found a significantly lower risk of cardiac dysfunction with higher baseline IgE levels ($P = .018$).[26] The authors of this study postulated that decreased IgE levels represent dysregulation of the cytokine response ratio of Th1 to Th2 that could adversely affect myocardial inflammation, and thus higher IgE levels would be associated with more favorable cardiac outcomes.

Table 2
Observational studies of biomarkers in cardio-oncology

Cancer Therapy	Malignancy Type	Biomarkers	Sample Size	Age, y	% Male	Other Characteristics	Primary Outcome	Findings	Reference
Anthracyclines	Breast	miRNA	56	50	0	Ancillary study from "Carvedilol Effect on Chemotherapy-induced Cardiotoxicity" (CECCY) trial	Reduction in LVEF ≥10% or LVEF <50% during or after treatment	17.9% experienced primary outcome, miR-1 showed greater AUC than TnI to predict cardiotoxicity (AUC = 0.851 and 0.544, $P = .0016$), miR-208a undetectable after treatment	Rigaud et al,[27] 2016
Anthracyclines	Breast	miRNA	59		0		Reduction in LVEF at 12 wk	11% experienced primary outcome. TnI increased 8.3 (±1.9) to 123.4 pg/mL (±10.0) in patients who experienced primary outcome. miR-208a not detected in any patients	Oliveira-Carvalho et al,[41] 2015
Anthracyclines	Breast	Peripheral blood cell transcriptome	33		0		Decline in LVEF by >10% or <50% by multigated acquisition scan after treatment	67 differentially expressed genes ($P<.05$) after treatment in those who experienced primary outcome	Todorova et al,[46] 2016
Anthracyclines	Breast	TnI	211	46	0		Change in LVEF by echocardiography at 14 mo	70 patients had TnI increased >0.5 ng/mL, TnI level correlated with LVEF decrease ($r = -0.92$, $P<.0001$)	Cardinale et al,[14] 2002
Anthracyclines	Breast	TnI	50	58	2		LVEF < 50% or clinical heart failure at 3 y	Change in troponin at 5 mo was associated with primary outcome by AUC analysis (AUC = 0.69)	Garrone et al,[17] 2011
Anthracyclines	Breast	TnI and BNP	53	55	2		Decline in LVEF by ≥10% or overt heart failure at 1 y	Pretreatment BNP nearly correlated with LVEF at 1 y ($P = .07$, hazard ratio [HR] =0.96-1)	Feola et al,[19] 2011

Anthracyclines	Breast	TnI, NT-proBNP, Gal-3ST2, sFlt-1, Interleukin-6 (IL-6), and tumor necrosis factor alpha (TNF-α)	55	53	0		LVEF and biomarker levels 1 y after treatment	NT-proBNP increased in 18.2% of patients (age adjusted cutoffs). TnI, TNF-α, Gal-3, IL-6, ST2, and sFlt-1 normal in all patients. NT-proBNP and LVEF were correlated (r = −0.564, P≤.01)	van Boxtel et al,[59] 2015
Anthracyclines	Breast, leukemia, lymphoma, and others	TnT and NT-proBNP	100	46	48		Change in LVEF, measures of diastolic function, or Tei index at 12 mo	No patients had abnormal TnT levels (>0.1 ng/mL). No significant change in NT-proBNP during therapy	Dodos et al,[22] 2008
Anthracyclines	Breast, lymphoma, and others	TnI	179	46	23	Not all patients received anthracyclines	LVEF at 1–12 mo after treatment	TnI ≥ 0.08 μg/mL associated with average decrease of 18% in LVEF vs 2.5% decrease in patients with TnI < 0.08 μg/mL	Sandri et al,[16] 2003
Anthracyclines	Breast, lymphoma, lung, and ovarian	TnI	204	45	19	Not all patients received anthracyclines	LVEF at 7 mo after treatment	Increases in TnI after treatment associated with primary outcome (r = −0.87, P<.0001)	Cardinale et al,[13] 2000
Anthracyclines	Breast, lymphoma, myeloma, ovarian, lung, germ cell, and sarcoma	TnI	703	47	31	33% of patients received chest radiotherapy	Cardiac death, pulmonary edema/heart failure, LVEF reduction by >25%, life-threatening arrhythmia at 3 y	Increased rate of cardiac events in persistently increased vs only acute increased TnI (84% vs 37%, P<.001). TnI group had 1% event rate	Cardinale et al,[31] 2004
Anthracyclines	Breast, sarcoma, and lymphoma	TnI and BNP	109	56	48		Reduction in LVEF by >15 or >10 points to <50%, symptomatic heart failure, symptomatic arrhythmia, sudden cardiac death, acute coronary syndromes at 1 y	10.1% incidence of primary outcome, all of these patients had at least 1 BNP >100 pg/mL	Lenihan et al,[18] 2016
Anthracyclines	Leukemia	BNP and atrial natriuretic peptide (ANP)	13	52	23		New heart failure, LVEF <50%, decrease in LVEV by >10, or cardiomegaly during or after treatment	BNP increased to >40 pg/mL in all patients who experienced the primary outcome (61.5%) and none who did not	Okumura et al,[36] 2000

(continued on next page)

Table 2
(continued)

Cancer Therapy	Malignancy Type	Biomarkers	Sample Size	Age, y	% Male	Other Characteristics	Primary Outcome	Findings	Reference
Anthracyclines	Leukemia	TnT and NT-proBNP	19	6	63		Clinical heart failure	No significant increases of TnT or NT-proBNP	Ruggiero et al,[20] 2013
Anthracyclines	Leukemia	TnT and NT-proBNP	50	12	60	Asymptomatic childhood cancer survivors	Tissue Doppler imaging (TDI) 4 y after treatment	26% had abnormal TDI, abnormal TDI associated with higher NT-proBNP (1127.7 ± 689.91 vs 159.24 ± 59.33, $P = .000$)	Sherief et al,[56] 2012
Anthracyclines	Leukemia	TnT, NT-proBNP, and hsCRP	156	8	47		Echocardiographic parameters of left ventricular (LV) remodeling 4 y after treatment	Increase in TnT within 90 d associated with abnormally reduced LV mass and LV end-diastolic posterior wall thickness at 4 y ($P<.01$), increase in NT-proBNP associated with abnormal LV thickness-to-dimension ratio ($P = .01$), no association with hsCRP and outcomes	Lipshultz et al,[21] 2012
Anthracyclines	Leukemia and lymphoma	TnT	79	59	54		LVEF change 3 mo after treatment	Greater decrease in LVEF seen in patients with TnT increase ≥0.03 ng/mL (10% vs 2%, $P = .017$)	Auner et al,[32] 2003
Anthracyclines	Leukemia and lymphoma	TnT, BNP, NT-proBNP, Gal-3, and ST2	150	25	57	Childhood cancer survivors with LVEF >50%	Echocardiographic parameters of LV remodeling 13 y after treatment	No association between biomarkers and primary outcome	Armenian et al,[58] 2014
Anthracyclines	Leukemia and solid tumors	TnT and NT-proBNP	122	21	62	Asymptomatic childhood cancer survivors	Echocardiographic parameters of LV remodeling and biomarker levels 13.8 y after treatment	Sex-adjusted NT-proBNP increased in 13% of population. No association with TnT and outcomes	Mavinkurve-Groothuis et al,[61] 2009
Anthracyclines	Lymphoma	BNP, ANP, and NT-proANP	28	53	61		Change in LVEF and new heart failure within 4 wk of treatment	Change in ANP and LVEF correlated ($r = -0.447$, $P = 0.029$), with nonsignificant trend between change in NT-proANP and LVEF ($r = -0.390$, $P = .059$)	Nousiainen et al,[25] 1999

Drug	Cancer Type	Biomarker	n			Endpoint	Results	Reference
Anthracyclines	Lymphoma and solid tumors	TnI and GDF-15	38	7	55	Biomarker levels 1.9 y after treatment	GDF-15 increased after treatment (631.12 ± 230.2 vs 530 ± 132.14, P = .027), and TnI was not (0.12 ± 0.03 vs 0.12 ± 0.03)	Arslan et al,[57] 2013
Anthracyclines	Lymphoma and solid tumors	NT-proBNP	80	6	50	Biomarker levels and TDI 3.9 y after treatment	85.7% of patients with abnormal TDI had increased NT-proBNP vs 0% with normal TDI	Zidan et al,[60] 2015
Anthracyclines	Unspecified	BNP and ANP	34	12	53	LVEF after chemotherapy	BNP and ANP levels correlated inversely with LVEF (r = −0.43, P<.01; and r = −0.32, P<.05, respectively)	Hayakawa et al,[37] 2001
Anthracyclines	Unspecified	miRNA	24	10	71	Biomarkers before and 24 h after chemotherapy	miRNA increased after chemotherapy (24-h MANOVA, P = .024). miR-29b and miR-499 levels were most increased in subjects with increased hs-TnT	Leger et al,[39] 2017
Anthracyclines and trastuzumab	Breast	Arginine-NO	170	48	0	Reduction in ejection fraction (EF) by ≥10 to an absolute value of <50% at up to 5 y after treatment	Levels of asymmetric dimethylarginine (ADMA) and N-monomethylarginine (MMA) at 2 mo (HR = 3.33, 95% CI 1.12–9.96 for ADMA and HR = 2.70, 95% CI 1.35–5.41 for MMA) and arginine at 1 mo (HR = 0.78, 95% CI 0.64-0.97)	Finkelman et al,[28] 2017
Anthracyclines and trastuzumab	Breast	Hs-TnI, NT-proBNP, and ST2	81	50	0	Cardiomyopathy with decreased LVEF, symptomatic reduction of LVEF by ≥5 points to <55%, or asymptomatic reduction of LVEF by ≥ 10 points to < 55% at 15 mo	Elevated usTnI (≥30 μg/mL) at end of treatment predictive of primary outcome (P = .04), NT-proBNP and ST2 were not (P = .39 and P = .78, respectively)	Sawaya et al,[66] 2012

(continued on next page)

Table 2
(continued)

Cancer Therapy	Malignancy Type	Biomarkers	Sample Size	Age, y	% Male	Other Characteristics	Primary Outcome	Findings	Reference
Anthracyclines and trastuzumab	Breast	Hs-TnT	19	53	0		LVEF decrease of ≥5 at 6 mo after treatment	hs-TnT increased in group who experienced primary outcome vs those who did not (11.0 ± 7.8 pg/mL vs 4.0 ± 1.4 pg/mL, $P<.01$). hs-TnT >5.5 pg/mL at 6 mo had 78% sensitivity and 80% specificity for predicting a reduction of LVEF at 15 mo	Katsurada et al,[33] 2014
Anthracyclines and trastuzumab	Breast	TnI, CRP, GDF-15, MPO, PIGF, sFlt-1, and Gal-3	78	50	0		Symptomatic reduction in LVEF by ≥5 points to <55% or an asymptomatic reduction by ≥10 points to <55% up to 15 mo after treatment	TnI, CRP, GDF-15, MPO, PIGF, and sFlt-1 levels increased from before treatment to 3 mo after ($P<.05$). TnI (HR = 1.38 per SD, 95% CI 1.05–1.81, $P = .02$) and MPO (HR = 1.34 per SD, 95% CI 1.00–1.80; $P = .048$) associated with primary outcome individually and in models combining both markers ($P = .007$ and $P = .03$, respectively). The risk of cardiotoxicity was 46.5% in patients with the largest changes in both markers (ΔTnI > 121.8 μg/L; ΔMPO > 422.6 pmol/L)	Ky et al,[29] 2014
Anthracyclines and trastuzumab	Breast	TnI, TnT, and NT-proBNP	100	66	0		Mortality at 12 mo	NT-proBNP increased after treatment (max 327 pg/mL in HER2+ group and 150 in HER2− group), levels at 3–12 mo associated with mortality by AUC analysis. No association between TnI or pretreatment NT-proBNP and mortality	De Iuliis et al,[24] 2016

Treatment	Cancer	Biomarker(s)				Comparison	Timing	Findings	Study
Anthracyclines and trastuzumab	Breast	TnT, NT-proBNP, miRNAs, and sST2	45	49	0		Change in biomarker levels 3 mo after treatment	Significant increases in all biomarkers, along with miRNAs miR-126-3p, miR-199a-3p, miR-423-5p, miR-34a-5p after treatment	Frères et al,[40] 2018
Anthracyclines and trastuzumab	Breast	Hs-TnI and NT-proBNP	43	49	0		Symptomatic reduction in LVEF by ≥5 points to <55% or an asymptomatic reduction by ≥10 points to <55% at 6 mo after treatment	TnI > 0.015 pg/mL at 3 mo associated with primary outcome (odds ratio = 9, 95% CI 1.8–50, $P = .006$)	Sawaya et al,[23] 2011
Anthracyclines and trastuzumab	Breast	TnI, CRP, GDF-15, MPO, PlGF, sFlt-1, and Gal-3	78	49	0		Symptomatic reduction in LVEF by ≥ 5 points to < 55% or an asymptomatic reduction by ≥ 10 points to < 55% up to 15 mo after treatment	Increases in MPO, PlGF, and GDF-15 were associated with the primary outcome (MPO HR = 1.38, 95% CI 1.10–1.71, $P = .02$; PlGF HR = 3.78 95%, CI 1.30–11.0, $P = .047$; GDF-15 HR = 1.71 95% CI 1.15–2.55, $P = .01$)	Putt et al,[34] 2015
Radiation	Breast	BNP	59	58	0	Some patients received anthracyclines	Posttreatment changes in BNP at 12 mo	BNP increased to 38 ± 23 to 43 ± 28 pg/mL, $P = .002$. BNP increase correlated with cardiac radiation dose ($P = .03$)	D'Errico et al,[53] 2015
Radiation	Breast	TnI	75	53	0	Left- and right-sided chest radiation groups were compared	TnI levels after treatment	TnI in left-sided radiation was increased after treatment (0.021 ± 0.01 to 0.027 ± 0.02 ng/mL, $P = .38$) but not in right-sided radiation (0.020 ± 0.02 to 0.021 ± 0.01 ng/mL, $P = .8$)	Erven et al,[50] 2013
Radiation	Breast	TnI and NT-proBNP	60	55	0	Left-sided radiation patients compared with nontreated controls	Biomarker levels after treatment	NT-proBNP levels were significantly higher ($P = .03$) in the treatment group (median 90.0 pg/mL; range, 16.7–333.1 pg/mL vs median 63.2 pg/mL; range, 11.0–172.5 pg/mL). TnI remained <0.07 ng/mL in both groups	D'Errico et al,[52] 2012

(continued on next page)

Table 2 (continued)

Cancer Therapy	Malignancy Type	Biomarkers	Sample Size	Age, y	% Male	Other Characteristics	Primary Outcome	Findings	Reference
Radiation	Breast and lung	TnI and BNP	23	62	61		Biomarker levels before and after treatment	TnI and BNP increased after treatment (0.007 ± 0.008 to 0.014 ± 0.01 ng/mL, 123 ± 147 to 159 ± 184 pg/mL, respectively)	Nellessen et al,[51] 2010
Radiation	Breast, lung, lymphoma	Hs-TnT, NT-proBNP, PlGF, and GDF-15	87	53	15	Treated with proton RT	Posttreatment changes in biomarker levels, LVEF, and strain	In lung cancer/lymphoma, PlGF increased from a median interquartile range of 20 ng/L (16–26) to 22 ng/L (16–30) (P = .005), and GDF-15 increased from 1171 ng/L (755–2493) to 1887 ng/L (903–3763) (P = .006) at median 20 d after treatment. hs-TnT and NT-proBNP did not increase after treatment. No significant increases in biomarker levels after breast cancer therapy. No association between biomarker levels and echocardiographic measurements	Demissei et al,[54] 2019
Trastuzumab	Breast	TnI	251	50	0		Decrease in LVEF by >10 points to <50% after treatment with average follow-up 2.8 y	TnI increase >0.08 ng/mL independently predicted the primary outcome in a multivariate analysis (HR = 22.9, 95% CI 11.6–45.5, P<.001) and of lack of LVEF recovery to >50% (HR =2.88, 95% CI 1.78–4.65, P < .001)	Cardinale et al,[12] 2010

Drug	Cancer	Biomarker	N			Definition	Findings	Reference
Trastuzumab	Breast	TnI, BNP, and hsCRP	54	55	0	Decrease in LVEF by ≥15 points or to a value <50% at average follow-up 3.3 y	Abnormal hsCRP (≥3 mg/L) predicted the primary outcome with a sensitivity of 92.9% (95% CI 66.1–99.8) and specificity of 45.7% (95% CI 28.8–63.4), normal hsCRP had a negative predictive value of 94.1% (95% CI 70.3–99.9)	Onitilo et al,[38] 2012
Trastuzumab	Breast	TnI, TnT, and NT-proBNP	533	50	0	Decrease in LVEF by ≥10 points to <50%, symptomatic NYHA class III or IV heart failure, or cardiac death	Elevated pretreatment TnI (>40 ng/L) and TnT (>14 ng/L) were associated with an increased risk of significant decrease in LVEF (HR = 4.52, $P<.001$ and HR = 3.57, $P<.001$, respectively)	Zardavas et al,[11] 2017
Tyrosine kinase inhibitors (TKIs)	Renal cell carcinoma	Hs-TnI and BNP	90	63	66	Decrease in LVEF by ≥10 points to <50% at up to 33 wk after treatment	Modest association with BNP increase and LVEF change at 7 mo (0.4% decrease in LVEF per 100-unit increase in BNP, $P = .007$), no association with hs-TnI (0.1% decrease in LVEF per 10 unit increase in hs-TnT, $P = .407$)	Narayan et al,[49] 2017
TKIs	Renal cell carcinoma	TnT	89	66	63	Increased cardiac enzymes, symptomatic arrhythmia requiring treatment, new LV dysfunction, or acute coronary syndromes during treatment	10% of patients had increased TnT during treatment with unclear relationship to outcomes	Schmidinger et al,[48] 2008
TKIs and vascular endothelial growth factor (VEGF) inhibitors	Renal cell carcinoma	TnI and NT-proBNP	159	61	77	Symptomatic heart failure, EF <50% or >10-point drop from baseline, increased biomarkers, or new hypertension during treatment	24% developed increased NT-proBNP with 31% of this group also developing a decreased LVEF, 3% developed increased TnI	Hall et al,[3] 2013

Other biomarkers

Studies of other biomarkers, including microRNAs (miRNAs), arginine-nitric oxide (NO) metabolites, C-reactive protein (CRP), growth differentiation factor-15 (GDF-15), myeloperoxidase (MPO), placental growth factor (PIGF), fms-like tyrosine kinase 1 (sFLT-1), and galectin-3 (Gal-3) have not demonstrated an association between pretreatment biomarker levels and cardiovascular outcomes.[27–29]

SUMMARY

Definite conclusions are impossible to derive given the limited sample sizes in most of the studies. However, the association between pretreatment biomarkers and incident cardiotoxicity was more evident in patients already at risk, such as those who have received anthracyclines or who have known cardiovascular risk factors and disease. Thus, there is no sufficient evidence to recommend routine pretherapy biomarker measurements. Elevated biomarkers, if obtained for other clinical indications, should prompt obtaining an echocardiogram if not already done.

MONITORING FOR CARDIOVASCULAR TOXICITY DURING THERAPY
Current Guidelines

The American Society of Echocardiography and European Society of Cardiovascular Imaging have established joint guidelines for the monitoring of cardiac toxicity of cancer therapy, and suggest routine troponin measurement along with traditional echocardiography and strain imaging at baseline as well as after every cycle of cardiotoxic therapy (specifically anthracyclines, mitoxantrone, and trastuzumab), with a positive troponin measurement prompting further cardiologic evaluation.[30] The ESMO and ASCO are also supportive of serial biomarker measurements to monitor for cardiac toxicity.[8,9] Current ESC guidelines note a lack of evidence in support of adjusting or holding cancer treatment in response to biomarker abnormalities.[5]

Evidence

Troponin in the detection of anthracycline and trastuzumab toxicity

There have been several observational studies that have demonstrated that TnI,[12–14,16,23,31] hs-TnI,[17] TnT,[32] and hsTnT[33] levels predicted subsequent onset of decrease in LVEF after anthracycline or trastuzumab therapy. The largest of these, in 703 patients receiving anthracyclines primarily for breast cancer and lymphoma demonstrated that

an increase in TnI within 72 hours of chemotherapy and 1 month after the completion of treatment course was associated with cardiac toxicity. The risk was greatest (84%) in patients with a persistent increase in TnI (>0.08 ng/mL), but still significantly increased (37%) in the subgroup with only an initially increased troponin.[31] Another study demonstrated that the rate of increase in troponin after anthracycline therapy correlated with the risk of clinical heart failure or decreased LVEF at 3 years.[17]

With regard to trastuzumab, Cardinale and colleagues[12] demonstrated an association between an increase in TnI and cardiotoxicity after trastuzumab therapy. As noted above, the cohort was notable for a high rate of previous anthracycline treatment.

The use of multiple biomarkers in an additive fashion may enhance prediction of cardiac toxicity from anthracyclines and trastuzumab. Ky and colleagues[29] measured 8 biomarkers (TnI, high-sensitivity CRP [hsCRP], NT-proBNP, GDF-15, MPO, PIGF, sFLT-1, and Gal-3) along with LVEF serially in 78 patients with breast cancer. Interval changes in TnI and MPO were associated with increased risk of a drop in LVEF when examined individually and also in a model combining biomarkers, with a risk of cardiac toxicity of 46.5% in the subset of patients with the largest increases in both biomarkers. MPO and GDF-15 were found to correlate with LVEF reduction in another analysis of this population.[34]

B-type natriuretic peptide in the detection of anthracycline toxicity

Increases in BNP and NT-proBNP seem to be more sensitive than LVEF in predicting the development of cardiac toxicity after anthracycline therapy. Lenihan and colleagues[18] found BNP levels to be significantly higher after every anthracycline cycle in subjects who experienced cardiac events, and every patient who experienced a cardiac event had at least 1 BNP measurement >100 pg/mL, whereas only 30% of subjects who experienced a cardiac event had a significant reduction in LVEF detected beforehand. Another study demonstrated an association between an increased BNP at 72 hours after chemotherapy and a decreased LVEF at 1 year.[35] Similar associations between BNP levels after treatment and cardiac endpoints have been seen in other studies.[36,37]

High-sensitivity C-reactive protein in the detection of anthracycline and trastuzumab toxicity

One study of 54 women undergoing trastuzumab treatment reported hsCRP >3 mg/L to be a sensitive marker of subsequent cardiotoxicity.[38] Studies by Ky and colleagues[29] and Lipshultz and colleagues,[21] however, did not find an association with increased hsCRP levels and cardiac outcomes after anthracycline and trastuzumab therapy. The low specificity of CRP to cardiovascular disease, especially in patients with underlying cancer, may hinder its clinical application to this population.

MicroRNAs and anthracycline toxicity

Two studies have found plasma miRNAs levels to be higher 24 hours after anthracycline therapy and trastuzumab.[39,40] With regard to outcomes, an ancillary study from the "Carvedilol Effect on Chemotherapy-induced Cardiotoxicity" (CECCY) trial, with 56 patients in the placebo arm, demonstrated that miR-1 was superior to TnI in prediction of cardiotoxicity at 12 months by area under the curve (AUC) analysis (AUC = 0.851 and 0.544, P = .0016). miR-208a, which has been found to be increased in acute myocardial infarction, was undetectable in the population.[27,41]

Limitations of the published studies of miRNA in detection of anthracycline toxicity include the limited number of miRNA studied, a lack of assessment for overt cardiac dysfunction, and a lack of normalization for quantification of miRNA expression by qRT-PCR.[42] Low concentration of miRNA in the peripheral blood and wide variation in levels in the general population are additional hurdles to the implementation of miRNA in clinical use.[43]

Peripheral blood mononuclear cell transcriptome and anthracycline toxicity

The peripheral blood mononuclear cell (PBMC) transcriptome has been found to have increased DNA-base oxidation after doxorubicin treatment, and demonstrates expression of common genes in oxidative stress pathways in heart tissue in a rat model.[44,45] A pilot study of PBMC gene expression after anthracycline therapy demonstrated a consistent PBMC gene profile in patients who subsequently developed cardiotoxicity.[46] Further studies are needed to determine if this product of translational research is of clinical use in cardio-oncology.

Arginine-nitric oxide metabolites

One recent study examined levels of multiple arginine-NO metabolites in 170 patients with breast cancer undergoing treatment with anthracyclines with or without trastuzumab, and found levels of asymmetric dimethylarginine and *N*-monomethylarginine at 2 months were associated with a 3-fold increase in the development of cardiac dysfunction at 5 years follow-up.[28] This is an intriguing finding because products of this pathway are thought to mediate generation of reactive oxygen species in anthracycline toxicity.[47]

Monitoring for tyrosine kinase inhibitor toxicity

Tyrosine kinase inhibitors, including sunitinib and sorafenib, have been associated with heart failure and cardiac ischemia.[4] Several studies have demonstrated increases in TnT and NT-proBNP after TKI treatment, however, they found no significant relationship between biomarker levels and other cardiovascular outcomes.[3,48,49]

Monitoring for radiation-induced cardiac disease

TnI has been found to be increased after left-sided chest radiation specifically.[50,51] However, the degree of increase does not necessarily correlate with radiation dose.[52] On the other hand, BNP levels appear to correlate with radiation dose to the heart, with levels greater than 125 pg/mL associated with higher radiation doses in 1 study.[52,53] PIGF and GDF-15 have been found also to be increased in the acute period after radiation therapy for breast, lung cancer, and lymphoma.[54] Studies with longer follow-up are necessary to determine if early increases of these biomarkers predict development of clinical disease.

MONITORING FOR LATE ADVERSE EFFECTS OF CANCER THERAPY
Current Guidelines

Almost 6 in 10 survivors of pediatric cancer have received treatment with anthracyclines or radiation, making the early identification of cardiovascular dysfunction after therapy a major concern. However, the optimal protocol for screening is unclear.[55] ESC guidelines recommend considering multimodality screening in cancer survivors treated with potentially cardiotoxic regimens using a combination of imaging and biomarkers, whereas the ASMO recommends consideration of biomarker measurement in symptomatic cancer survivors.[5,8] In the population of pediatric cancer survivors, the International Late Effects of Childhood Cancer Guideline Harmonization Group reports that the diagnostic value of troponins and natriuretic peptides for detecting asymptomatic survivors of childhood cancer is poor. However, they note it is reasonable to consider the use of biomarkers in symptomatic individuals with preserved LVEF or a history of borderline cardiac function.[55]

Evidence

Several studies have examined troponin in the detection of subsequent left ventricular (LV) dysfunction after anthracyclines and radiation therapy, with none showing a significant association.[52,56–59] BNP and NT-proBNP levels, however, correlate with cumulative anthracycline dose and have been associated with Doppler imaging showing abnormal tissue, LV end-diastolic dimension, and LV systolic dysfunction in survivors of anthracycline therapy.[56,58–61] In addition, NT-proBNP has been found to be increased late after radiation therapy and is highest in patients who have received anthracyclines and radiation.[52,60]

Other biomarkers have also been studied in cancer survivors. Levels of GDF-15 in 38 patients at an average 1.9 years after anthracycline chemotherapy were found to correlate with diastolic dysfunction.[57] Another study of patients during the 10 years after anthracycline therapy did not find an association with Gal-3 or ST2 and LV dysfunction.[58] A separate study that included tumor necrosis factor alpha, Gal-3, interleukin-6, ST2, and sFlt-1 found no association with these biomarkers and LVEF 1 year after therapy.[59]

Biomarker-Guided Prevention of Cardiovascular Toxicity

There is significant interest in the use of biomarker-guided intervention to prevent clinical cardiac disease in patients with cancer (**Table 3**). Some biomarker levels seem to be responsive to preventative therapies and may identify patients who stand to benefit from cardiovascular intervention during cancer therapy. Lipshultz and colleagues[62] demonstrated that increases of TnT in pediatric patients could be mitigated with the administration of dexrazoxane before chemotherapy treatment. Cardinale and colleagues[63] randomized 114 patients undergoing high-dose chemotherapy who had a posttreatment increase of TnI of greater than 0.08 ng/mL after either a course of enalapril therapy or placebo. At 1 year, the incidence of cardiotoxicity was null in patients who had received enalapril therapy (0% vs 43% risk, $P<.001$). The treatment group also had a significantly higher LVEF (62.4±3.5 vs 48.3±9.3, $P<.001$) and a lower risk of arrhythmias requiring treatment (2% vs 17%, $P = .01$) at 1 year.

Prophylactic treatment of heart failure with trastuzumab has also been studied. Two hundred and six patients with breast cancer and a history of anthracycline therapy were randomized to candesartan treatment or placebo, with serial biomarker measurements and echocardiography. Although there was no significant difference in LVEF decrease or biomarker levels after treatment, there was a nonsignificant trend toward less-frequent

symptomatic heart failure in the treatment group (7.8% vs 12.6%, $P = .36$).

Biomarker-guided prevention of cardiotoxicity in trastuzumab therapy requires further study. The ongoing CARE trial will assess if TnT-guided initiation of angiotensin receptor and β-blockers prevent cardiac injury arising from anthracycline and trastuzumab therapy.[64]

The value of biomarker-guided treatment of cardiac toxicity may not be limited to anthracyclines and trastuzumab. One report from phase I trials of an antivascular endothelial growth factor (anti-VEGF) monoclonal antibody, anti-VEGF receptor TKIs, and a kinesin inhibitor, in metastatic solid tumors identified 10 patients with asymptomatic TnI increases. Patients were initiated on β-blocker and aspirin therapy and eventually rechallenged with the study drugs, with no further increases in TnI or other cardiac toxicity seen.[65]

SUMMARY
Clinical Recommendations

Based on the available evidence as presented here and current clinical practice guidelines provided by the societies, we summarize recommendations regarding the use of cardiovascular biomarkers in assessment of patients with cancer in **Box 1**. Unfortunately, there are major limitations to the published studies.

Limitations of Current Studies

Primary among these is the small sample size of existing studies. Second, the most commonly studied outcome in cardio-oncology is echocardiographic LVEF, which is an insensitive and late marker of cardiac injury, with criteria that often encompass changes in ejection fraction that remain within normal limits. Third, there is significant heterogeneity in patient care among the studies.

In addition, the use of biomarkers in prediction of risk of arrhythmia, venous thromboembolism, pericardial disease, and severe hypertension due to cancer therapy remain understudied. The number of biomarkers studied continues to grow, many only published in small preliminary studies. It is difficult to determine which of these biomarkers to prioritize in research efforts. Whereas there is evidence of association between certain biomarkers and cardiovascular outcomes in some areas, such as anthracyclines and trastuzumab toxicities, evidence supporting a clinical benefit of routine biomarker use is lacking in most scenarios.

The available evidence suffers from significant heterogeneity, with differing definitions of

Table 3
Randomized trials in cardio-oncology that have incorporated biomarkers

Chemotherapy	Cancer Type	Biomarker	What Was Studied	Sample Size	Median Age,y	Sex	Primary Outcome	Result	Study
Anthracyclines	Acute lymphocytic leukemia	TnT	Randomized controlled trial (RCT) of dexrazoxane given before doxorubicin, TnT measured per study protocol	206	7	50% male	TnT increase >0.01 ng/mL	Rate of troponin increase lower in patients who received dexrazoxane (21% vs 50%, $P<.001$), no significant difference in survival or echocardiographic findings at 2.5 y	Lipshultz et al,[62] 2004
Mixed, largely anthracyclines	Mixed	TnI	RCT of enalapril vs placebo in patients with increased TnI detected after anthracycline therapy	114	45	37% male	Decrease in LVEF by >10 points to <50% at 1, 3, 6, and 12 mo after treatment	Patients treated with enalapril for 1 y had lower rate of primary outcome (0% vs 43%, $P<.001$)	Cardinale et al,[63] 2006
Anti-VEGF monoclonal antibody, anti-VEGF receptor tyrosine kinase inhibitors, and a kinesin inhibitor	Metastatic solid tumors	TnI	TnI measured in patients undergoing a clinical trial for cancer therapies	10	65	60% male		All patients given course of aspirin and β-blocker therapy, after which all tolerated retrial of study drug	Ederhy et al,[65] 2012
Anthracyclines and trastuzumab	Breast	Hs-TnT and NT-proBNP	RCT of candesartan in patients receiving trastuzumab who had previously received anthracycline therapy	206	50	0% male	Decline in LVEF by >15 points or to <45% at 40 wk after completion of therapy	Nonsignificant increase in primary outcome with candesartan treatment (19% vs 16%, absolute risk increase 3.8%, 95% CI −7 to 15, $P = .58$). No association with biomarker levels and treatment or changes in LVEF	Boekhout et al,[67] 2016

Box 1
Clinical recommendations regarding the use of cardiovascular biomarkers in patients with cancer

Assessment of cardiovascular risk before cancer therapy

- Consider pretreatment measurement of troponins in patients who are to receive trastuzumab therapy and have received anthracycline therapy in the past.
- The evidence of benefit in pretreatment risk stratification with troponin in anthracycline therapy is lacking, although baseline measurement may be considered as part of serial monitoring for cardiac toxicity during therapy.
- Consider BNP/NT-proBNP measurement before anthracycline therapy, increased levels may portend an increased risk of development of LV dysfunction or clinical heart failure during or after treatment.

Monitoring for cardiovascular toxicity during cancer therapy

- Consistent with ASCE/ESCI guidelines, serial measurements of troponin or BNP with cardiovascular imaging should be obtained to assess for subclinical cardiac dysfunction; biomarker increases should prompt further cardiac evaluation.
- Consider initiation of heart failure therapy in asymptomatic patients who develop increase of troponin during anthracycline therapy.
- Evidence for initiation of heart failure therapy in asymptomatic patients who develop increase in biomarkers during trastuzumab therapy is currently lacking.
- Symptomatic heart failure during treatment should be managed as per ACC/AHA guidelines.
- No evidence of use in routine biomarker monitoring in TKI therapy; however, clinical concern for cardiac ischemia during TKI and other therapies associated with cardiac ischemia should prompt further workup and treatment of acute coronary syndromes as per established ACC/AHA guidelines.
- No evidence of use of biomarker monitoring routinely after radiation therapy.

Surveillance for cardiovascular toxicity after completion of cancer therapy

- Consider regular posttreatment screening with BNP or NT-proBNP along with cardiac imaging after anthracycline therapy for detection of subclinical cardiac dysfunction.
- Increases in BNP and NT-proBNP in asymptomatic cancer survivors who have received anthracyclines should prompt further assessment of cardiac function with cardiac imaging.
- Symptomatic heart failure during treatment should be managed as per ACC/AHA guidelines.
- No evidence of use of serial troponin measurement for detection of subclinical cardiac dysfunction in asymptomatic cancer survivors who have received anthracyclines.

---

cardiotoxicity among studies. Biomarker assays are variable in their sensitivity and there is often a lack of clear distinction between normal and abnormal biomarker levels. Biomarker levels in the upper end of the normal range, as defined in other disease states, may confer increased risk of toxicity from cancer therapies.

Potential Solutions and Outlook

Potential solutions exist to address many of these limitations. Standardizing definitions of cardiovascular toxicities and biomarker cutoffs could be of significant benefit in homogenizing study results. This could help to clarify biomarker abnormalities that should trigger further assessment or treatment of the cardio-oncology patient. Future studies could incorporate multiple biomarkers to develop cardiac risk-prediction models. Studies of biomarker-guided interventions to prevent overt cardiovascular disease will be essential to translate promising biomarkers into clinical practice. Finally, trials that take a multimodal approach to cardiovascular risk mitigation combining assessment of both imaging and biomarkers would be of significant benefit in validating emerging practice guidelines.

Cardiovascular biomarkers have emerging use in the prediction and management of cardiovascular effects of cancer therapy. The rapidly growing list of biomarkers being studied demonstrates the significant interest in the field. Although further studies are needed to translate this promise into clinical practice, emerging evidence suggests that biomarkers have the potential to become effective tools central to the practice of cardio-oncology.

REFERENCES

1. Siegel RL, Miller KD, Jemal A. Cancer statistics, 2016. CA Cancer J Clin 2016;66(1):7–30.
2. Seidman A, Hudis C, Pierri MK, et al. Cardiac dysfunction in the trastuzumab clinical trials experience. J Clin Oncol 2002;20(5):1215–21.
3. Hall PS, Harshman LC, Srinivas S, et al. The frequency and severity of cardiovascular toxicity from targeted therapy in advanced renal cell carcinoma patients. JACC Hear Fail 2013;1(1):72–8.
4. Chang H-M, Moudgil R, Scarabelli T, et al. Cardiovascular complications of cancer therapy. J Am Coll Cardiol 2017;70(20):2536–51.
5. Lenihan DJ, Rodriguez Muñoz D, Lyon AR, et al. 2016 ESC position paper on cancer treatments and cardiovascular toxicity developed under the auspices of the ESC Committee for Practice Guidelines. Eur Heart J 2016;37(36):2768–801.
6. Morrow DA, de Lemos JA. Benchmarks for the assessment of novel cardiovascular biomarkers. Circulation 2007;115(8):949–52.
7. Tan LL, Lyon AR. Role of biomarkers in prediction of cardiotoxicity during cancer treatment. Curr Treat Options Cardiovasc Med 2018;20(7):55.
8. Armenian SH, Lacchetti C, Barac A, et al. Prevention and monitoring of cardiac dysfunction in survivors of adult cancers: American Society of Clinical Oncology clinical practice guideline. J Clin Oncol 2017;35(8):893–911.
9. Curigliano G, Cardinale D, Suter T, et al. Cardiovascular toxicity induced by chemotherapy, targeted agents and radiotherapy: ESMO clinical practice guidelines. Ann Oncol 2012;23(suppl 7):vii155–66.
10. Virani SA, Dent S, Brezden-Masley C, et al. Canadian Cardiovascular Society guidelines for evaluation and management of cardiovascular complications of cancer therapy. Can J Cardiol 2016;32(7):831–41.
11. Zardavas D, Suter TM, Van Veldhuisen DJ, et al. Role of troponins I and T and N-terminal prohormone of brain natriuretic peptide in monitoring cardiac safety of patients with early-stage human epidermal growth factor receptor 2-positive breast cancer receiving trastuzumab: a herceptin adjuvant study ca. J Clin Oncol 2017;35(8):878–84.
12. Cardinale D, Colombo A, Torrisi R, et al. Trastuzumab-induced cardiotoxicity: clinical and prognostic implications of troponin I evaluation. J Clin Oncol 2010;28(25):3910–6.
13. Cardinale D, Sandri MT, Martinoni A, et al. Left ventricular dysfunction predicted by early troponin I release after high-dose chemotherapy. J Am Coll Cardiol 2000;36(2):517–22.
14. Cardinale D, Sandri MT, Martinoni A, et al. Myocardial injury revealed by plasma troponin I in breast cancer treated with high-dose chemotherapy. Ann Oncol 2002;13(5):710–5.
15. Morandi P, Ruffini PA, Benvenuto GM, et al. Serum cardiac troponin I levels and ECG/echo monitoring in breast cancer patients undergoing high-dose (7 g/m2) cyclophosphamide. Bone Marrow Transplant 2001;28(3):277–82.
16. Sandri MT, Cardinale D, Zorzino L, et al. Minor increases in plasma troponin I predict decreased left ventricular ejection fraction after high-dose chemotherapy. Clin Chem 2003;49(2):248–52.
17. Garrone O, Crosetto N, Lo Nigro C, et al. Prediction of anthracycline cardiotoxicity after chemotherapy by biomarkers kinetic analysis. Cardiovasc Toxicol 2012;12(2):135–42.
18. Lenihan DJ, Stevens PL, Massey M, et al. The utility of point-of-care biomarkers to detect cardiotoxicity during anthracycline chemotherapy: a feasibility study. J Card Fail 2016;22(6):433–8.
19. Feola M, Garrone O, Occelli M, et al. Cardiotoxicity after anthracycline chemotherapy in breast carcinoma: effects on left ventricular ejection fraction, troponin I and brain natriuretic peptide. Int J Cardiol 2011;148(2):194–8.
20. Ruggiero A, De Rosa G, Rizzo D, et al. Myocardial performance index and biochemical markers for early detection of doxorubicin-induced cardiotoxicity in children with acute lymphoblastic leukaemia. Int J Clin Oncol 2013;18(5):927–33.
21. Lipshultz SE, Miller TL, Scully RE, et al. Changes in cardiac biomarkers during doxorubicin treatment of pediatric patients with high-risk acute lymphoblastic leukemia: associations with long-term echocardiographic outcomes. J Clin Oncol 2012;30(10):1042–9.
22. Dodos F, Halbsguth T, Erdmann E, et al. Usefulness of myocardial performance index and biochemical markers for early detection of anthracycline-induced cardiotoxicity in adults. Clin Res Cardiol 2008;97(5):318–26.
23. Sawaya H, Sebag IA, Plana JC, et al. Early detection and prediction of cardiotoxicity in chemotherapy-treated patients. Am J Cardiol 2011;107(9):1375–80.
24. De Iuliis F, Salerno G, Ludovica and T, et al. Serum biomarkers evaluation to predict chemotherapy-induced cardiotoxicity in breast cancer patients. Tumour Biol 2016;37(3):3379–87.
25. Nousiainen T, Jantunen E, Vanninen E, et al. Natriuretic peptides as markers of cardiotoxicity during doxorubicin treatment for non-Hodgkin's lymphoma. Eur J Haematol 1999;62(2):135–41.
26. Beer LA, Kossenkov AV, Liu Q, et al. Baseline immunoglobulin E levels as a marker of doxorubicin- and trastuzumab-associated cardiac dysfunction. Circ Res 2016. https://doi.org/10.1161/CIRCRESAHA.116.309004.

27. Rigaud VO-C, Ferreira LRP, Ayub-Ferreira SM, et al. Circulating miR-1 as a potential biomarker of doxorubicin-induced cardiotoxicity in breast cancer patients. Oncotarget 2016;8(4):6994–7002.

28. Finkelman BS, Putt M, Wang T, et al. Arginine-nitric oxide metabolites and cardiac dysfunction in patients with breast cancer. J Am Coll Cardiol 2017; 70(2):152–62.

29. Ky B, Putt M, Sawaya H, et al. Early increases in multiple biomarkers predict subsequent cardiotoxicity in patients with breast cancer treated with doxorubicin, taxanes, and trastuzumab. J Am Coll Cardiol 2014; 63(8):809–16.

30. Plana JC, Galderisi M, Barac A, et al. Expert consensus for multimodality imaging evaluation of adult patients during and after cancer therapy: a report from the American Society of Echocardiography and the European Association of Cardiovascular Imaging. Eur Hear J Cardiovasc Imaging 2014; 15(10):1063–93.

31. Cardinale D, Sandri MT, Colombo A, et al. Prognostic value of troponin I in cardiac risk stratification of cancer patients undergoing high-dose chemotherapy. Circulation 2004;109(22):2749–54.

32. Auner HW, Tinchon C, Linkesch W, et al. Prolonged monitoring of troponin T for the detection of anthracycline cardiotoxicity in adults with hematological malignancies. Ann Hematol 2003;82(4):218–22.

33. Katsurada K, Ichida M, Sakuragi M, et al. High-sensitivity troponin T as a marker to predict cardiotoxicity in breast cancer patients with adjuvant trastuzumab therapy. Springerplus 2014;3(1):1–7.

34. Putt M, Hahn VS, Januzzi JL, et al. Longitudinal changes in multiple biomarkers are associated with cardiotoxicity in breast cancer patients treated with doxorubicin, taxanes, and trastuzumab. Clin Chem 2015;61(9):1164–72.

35. Sandri MT, Salvatici M, Cardinale D, et al. N-Terminal pro-B-type natriuretic peptide after high-dose chemotherapy: a marker predictive of cardiac dysfunction? Clin Chem 2005;51(8):1405–10.

36. Okumura H, Iuchi K, Yoshida T, et al. Brain natriuretic peptide is a predictor of anthracycline-induced cardiotoxicity. Acta Haematol 2000;104(4): 158–63.

37. Hayakawa H, Komada Y, Hirayama M, et al. Plasma levels of natriuretic peptides in relation to doxorubicin-induced cardiotoxicity and cardiac function in children with cancer. Pediatr Blood Cancer 2001; 37(1):4–9.

38. Onitilo AA, Engel JM, Stankowski RV, et al. High-sensitivity C-reactive protein (hs-CRP) as a biomarker for trastuzumab-induced cardiotoxicity in HER2-positive early-stage breast cancer: a pilot study. Breast Cancer Res Treat 2012;134(1):291–8.

39. Leger KJ, Leonard D, Nielson D, et al. Circulating microRNAs: potential markers of cardiotoxicity in children and young adults treated with anthracycline chemotherapy. J Am Heart Assoc 2017;6(4) [pii: e004653].

40. Frères P, Bouznad N, Servais L, et al. Variations of circulating cardiac biomarkers during and after anthracycline-containing chemotherapy in breast cancer patients. BMC Cancer 2018;18(1):1–9.

41. Oliveira-Carvalho V, Ferreira LRP, Bocchi EA. Circulating mir-208a fails as a biomarker of doxorubicin-induced cardiotoxicity in breast cancer patients. J Appl Toxicol 2015;35(9):1071–2.

42. Ruggeri C, Gioffré S, Achilli F, et al. Role of microRNAs in doxorubicin-induced cardiotoxicity: an overview of preclinical models and cancer patients. Heart Fail Rev 2018;23(1):109–22.

43. Min PK, Chan SY. The biology of circulating microRNAs in cardiovascular disease. Eur J Clin Invest 2015;45(8):860–74.

44. Doroshow JH, Synold TW, Somlo G, et al. Oxidative DNA base modifications in peripheral blood mononuclear cells of patients treated with high-dose infusional doxorubicin. Blood 2001;97(9):2839.

45. Todorova VK, Beggs ML, Delongchamp RR, et al. Transcriptome profiling of peripheral blood cells identifies potential biomarkers for doxorubicin cardiotoxicity in a rat model. PLoS One 2012;7(11): e48398. Song Q, ed.

46. Todorova VK, Makhoul I, Siegel ER, et al. Biomarkers for presymptomatic doxorubicin-induced cardiotoxicity in breast cancer patients. PLoS One 2016; 11(8):e0160224. Coleman WB, ed.

47. Wolf MB, Baynes JW. The anti-cancer drug, doxorubicin, causes oxidant stress-induced endothelial dysfunction. Biochim Biophys Acta 2006;1760(2): 267–71.

48. Schmidinger M, Zielinski CC, Vogl UM, et al. Cardiac toxicity of sunitinib and sorafenib in patients with metastatic renal cell carcinoma. J Clin Oncol 2008; 26(32):5204–12.

49. Narayan V, Keefe S, Haas N, et al. Prospective evaluation of sunitinib-induced cardiotoxicity in patients with metastatic renal cell carcinoma. Clin Cancer Res 2017;23(14):3601–9.

50. Erven K, Florian A, Slagmolen P, et al. Subclinical cardiotoxicity detected by strain rate imaging up to 14 months after breast radiation therapy. Int J Radiat Oncol Biol Phys 2013;85(5):1172–8.

51. Nellessen U, Zingel M, Hecker H, et al. Effects of radiation therapy on myocardial cell integrity and pump function: which role for cardiac biomarkers? Chemotherapy 2010;56(2):147–52.

52. D'Errico MP, Grimaldi L, Petruzzelli MF, et al. N-Terminal pro-B-type natriuretic peptide plasma levels as a potential biomarker for cardiac damage after radiotherapy in patients with left-sided breast cancer. Int J Radiat Oncol Biol Phys 2012;82(2):e239-46.

53. D'Errico MP, Petruzzelli MF, Gianicolo EAL, et al. Kinetics of B-type natriuretic peptide plasma levels in patients with left-sided breast cancer treated with radiation therapy: results after one-year follow-up. Int J Radiat Biol 2015;91(10):804–9.

54. Demissei BG, Freedman G, Feigenberg SJ, et al. Early changes in cardiovascular biomarkers with contemporary thoracic radiation therapy for breast cancer, lung cancer, and lymphoma. Int J Radiat Oncol Biol Phys 2019;103(4):851–60.

55. Armenian SH, Hudson MM, Mulder RL, et al. Recommendations for cardiomyopathy surveillance for survivors of childhood cancer: a report from the International Late Effects of Childhood Cancer Guideline Harmonization group. Lancet Oncol 2015;16(3):e123–36.

56. Sherief LM, Kamal AG, Khalek EA, et al. Biomarkers and early detection of late onset anthracycline-induced cardiotoxicity in children. Hematology 2012;17(3):151–6.

57. Arslan D, Cihan T, Kose D, et al. Growth-differentiation factor-15 and tissue Doppler imaging in detection of asymptomatic anthracycline cardiomyopathy in childhood cancer survivors. Clin Biochem 2013;46(13–14):1239–43.

58. Armenian SH, Gelehrter SK, Vase T, et al. Screening for cardiac dysfunction in anthracycline-exposed childhood cancer survivors. Clin Cancer Res 2014; 20(24):6314–23.

59. van Boxtel W, Bulten BF, Mavinkurve-Groothuis AMC, et al. New biomarkers for early detection of cardiotoxicity after treatment with docetaxel, doxorubicin and cyclophosphamide. Biomarkers 2015;20(2):143–8.

60. Zidan A, Ahmad H, Saleh SH, et al. NT-proBNP as early marker of subclinical late cardiotoxicity after doxorubicin therapy and mediastinal irradiation in childhood cancer survivors. Dis Markers 2015; 2015:1–10.

61. Mavinkurve-Groothuis AMC, Groot-Loonen J, Bellersen L, et al. Abnormal NT-pro-BNP levels in asymptomatic long-term survivors of childhood cancer treated with anthracyclines. Pediatr Blood Cancer 2009;52(5):631–6.

62. Lipshultz SE, Rifai N, Dalton VM, et al. The effect of dexrazoxane on myocardial injury in doxorubicin-treated children with acute lymphoblastic leukemia. N Engl J Med 2004;351(2):145–53.

63. Cardinale D, Colombo A, Sandri MT, et al. Prevention of high-dose chemotherapy-induced cardiotoxicity in high-risk patients by angiotensin-converting enzyme inhibition. Circulation 2006; 114(23):2474–81.

64. MacLean M. ISRCTN24439460: The Cardiac CARE Trial – can heart muscle injury related to chemotherapy be prevented? 2017. https://doi.org/10.1186/ISRCTN24439460.

65. Ederhy S, Massard C, Dufaitre G, et al. Frequency and management of troponin I elevation in patients treated with molecular targeted therapies in phase i trials. Invest New Drugs 2012;30(2): 611–5.

66. Sawaya H, Sebag IA, Plana JC, et al. Assessment of echocardiography and biomarkers for the extended prediction of cardiotoxicity in patients treated with anthracyclines, taxanes, and trastuzumab. Circ Cardiovasc Imaging 2012;5(5):596–603.

67. Boekhout AH, Gietema JA, Milojkovic Kerklaan B, et al. Angiotensin II-receptor inhibition with candesartan to prevent trastuzumab-related cardiotoxic effects in patients with early breast cancer. JAMA Oncol 2016;2(8):1030–7.

Approach to Surgery for Cardiac Tumors
Primary Simple, Primary Complex, and Secondary

Bobby Yanagawa, MD, PhD[a], Edward Y. Chan, MD[b], Robert J. Cusimano, MD[c], Michael J. Reardon, MD[d],*

KEYWORDS

- Cardiac tumor • Malignant tumor • Sarcoma • Tumor team

KEY POINTS

- Cardiac tumors can be conceptualized as primary simple, primary complex, and secondary.
- Most simple primary and some complex primary cardiac tumors should be surgically resected.
- The prognosis for secondary tumors to the heart remains dismal. In select cases, surgical debulking may be indicated to improve quality of life.
- Patients with complex primary and secondary tumors to the heart should be managed by a multidisciplinary cardiac tumor team in a center of excellence.

INTRODUCTION

Cardiac tumors can be conceptualized as primary simple, primary complex, and secondary. Primary cardiac tumors are rare. The estimated incidence from autopsy studies ranges from 0.001% to 0.3%.[1] Approximately three-quarters of primary cardiac tumors are benign, and one-quarter are malignant.[2] Myxomas represent the most common benign primary cardiac tumors, accounting for nearly half of all benign tumors.[1] Other less common benign primary cardiac tumors include lipoma, hemangioma, fibroma, and paraganglioma. Most primary malignant cardiac tumors are sarcomas, with undifferentiated sarcomas and angiosarcomas being the most common, followed by leiomyosarcomas and rhabodmyosarcomas.[1] Secondary cardiac tumors are approximately 30 times more common than primary cardiac tumors.[3,4] The incidence ranges from 2% to 18% in patients with metastatic cancer, and almost every type of malignant tumor has been known to reach the heart.[3,4] The most common primary sites of metastatic cardiac tumors are lung adenocarcinoma, squamous cell carcinoma, leukemia, lymphoma, and breast carcinoma.[4] Overall survival ranges from several months to 2 years from the time of diagnosis, with worse prognosis once malignant pericardial effusions occur.[5]

Primary tumors of the heart can present with various nonspecific symptoms or can be asymptomatic and detected incidentally during

The authors have no disclosures for this article.
[a] Division of Cardiac Surgery, Department of Surgery, St Michael's Hospital, University of Toronto, 30 Bond St, Toronto, ON M5B 1W8, Canada; [b] Department of Surgery, Houston Methodist Hospital, 6550 Fannin Street, Suite 1401, Houston, TX 77030, USA; [c] Division of Cardiac Surgery, Peter Munk Cardiac Centre, Toronto General Hospital, University of Toronto, 200 Elizabeth St, Toronto, ON M5G 2C4, Canada; [d] Department of Cardiovascular Surgery, Houston Methodist DeBakey Heart & Vascular Center, Houston Methodist Hospital, 6550 Fannin Street, Suite 1401, Houston, TX 77030, USA
* Corresponding author.
E-mail address: mreardon@houstonmethodist.org

cardiovascular assessment or at autopsy.[1] Symptoms include:

- Constitutional or systemic manifestations such as weight loss, malaise, and fatigue
- Obstructive cardiac symptoms, including dyspnea, presyncope angina, and sudden cardiac death
- Other cardiac manifestation symptoms related to atrial or ventricular tachyarrhythmia, conduction abnormalities, pericardial effusion, and tamponade
- Embolic manifestations including stroke
- Manifestations caused by local invasion and metastases

Patients with cardiac metastases are often asymptomatic, as they present late in the course of malignancy.[5,6] Malignant tumors can spread to the heart by lymphatic, hematogenous, transvenous, and direct invasion, which ultimately determines the type of cardiac involvement.[3,4] Secondary cardiac tumors can be classified anatomically as pericardial, epicardial/myocardial, and endocardial/intracavitary. The pericardium is the most common site of cardiac metastases, representing approximately two-thirds of cases.[3] Most commonly, pericardial metastases result in serosanguineous malignant pericardial fluid. Patients may present with shortness of breath, pleuritic chest pain, and/or peripheral edema. Epicardial and myocardial metastases constitute about one-third of cardiac metastatic cases.[3] Palpitations from arrhythmias are the most common sign of metastatic myocardial disease. Although uncommon, myocardial metastases may cause left or right heart failure. Endocardial metastases are mostly asymptomatic, but intracavitary lesions may lead to obstruction and embolization. Finally, benign metastatic spread can occur with intravenous cardiac extension of pelvic leiomyomas, and benign metastasizing leiomyomas from the uterus, the latter being rare.[3,4]

The goals of diagnostic evaluation are to confirm the presence of a cardiac tumor; to describe its size, location, and extension; and to rule out malignancy. The main imaging modalities are echocardiography, MRI, and ultrafast computed tomography (CT). A multi-modality approach is often desirable. In select patients, adjunctive diagnostic modalities such as coronary angiography, positron emission tomography (PET), and transvenous biopsy may also be useful.

In 2002 at the Houston Methodist Hospital and MD Anderson Cancer Center, the authors began a multidisciplinary cardiac tumor team that included a cardiac surgeon, cardiologist, cardio-oncologist, oncologist, radiologist, and palliative care specialists. Since then, this cardiac tumor heart team has extended to an international effort. The authors believe that complex benign and all malignant cardiac tumors should be referred to an experienced, multidisciplinary team. Realistic goals and expectations are discussed with the patient. Although the patient is central, family support, care, and understanding are also important to the overall treatment plan and should not be forgotten.

This article presents the authors' surgical approach to primary simple, primary complex, and secondary cardiac tumors.

SURGERY FOR PRIMARY SIMPLE TUMORS

The first decision upon finding a new cardiac mass is to decide if it indeed represents a tissue mass versus nontissue such as clot, calcium, vegetation, or foreign body. If a tumor is suspected, then the next decision is to attempt to classify the tumor as benign or malignant. The misdiagnosis of malignant primary tumors as benign and lack of recognition for the complexity of benign tumors such as paraganglioma and large fibroma can lead to inappropriate decisions on care. The authors suggest that multidisciplinary cardiac tumor heart teams be considered for any suspected primary complex tumor cases.

Myxoma

Myxomas account for 50% of all benign cardiac tumors in adults.[1] Most cardiac myxomas are solitary (**Fig. 1**). They arise from the endocardium and protrude into a cardiac chamber. Cardiac myxomas show a predilection for the left atrium (75%), right atrium (15%), with the remaining cases equally distributed between the right and left ventricle. Surgical resection of myxomas is recommended because of the risk of embolization and complications. Outcomes in these cases are excellent. The authors' current experience at the Houston Methodist DeBakey Heart & Vascular Center is 135 myxomas with no deaths and 2 recurrences. At the Toronto General Hospital (1990–2016), the authors have operated on 139 myxomas with 2 deaths and 2 recurrences, both of whom had Carney syndrome.

Papillary Fibroelastoma

Papillary fibroelastomas (PFEs) are the second most common adult cardiac tumor occurring in about 10% of primary cardiac tumor cases.[7] They occur most commonly on the valvular endocardium, with the noncoronary cusp being the

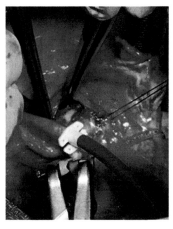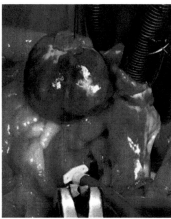

Fig. 1. Primary simple cardiac tumor. Uncomplicated resection of a left atrial myxoma from a superior left atrial approach in a 55-year-old man with symptoms of shortness of breath and fatigue.

most prevalent, but they can occur anywhere on the cardiac endocardium.[8] They are usually single but can be multiple, with as many as 40 PFEs reported in a single patient.[9] Surgery is recommended for left-sided lesions because of the risk of embolism. For right-sided lesions, the risk of embolization and surgical indication is unclear. Given the low operative risk, the authors resect most right-sided PFEs larger than 1 cm. The authors' previous experience with PFEs has shown 50% of the tumors arising from the left side and most (13 of 14) involving cardiac valves. There were no operative deaths, and no valves required resection or had insufficiency after tumor excision.[10]

Lipoma

Cardiac lipomas are well-encapsulated homogenous tumors composed of mature adipocytes.[11] They can occur anywhere in the heart, but the most typical locations are the endocardium of the right atrium or left ventricle.[12] A finding of a low-attenuation mass with density similar to fat on CT is pathognomonic.[13] Large, symptomatic tumors should be resected.[14]

Lipomatous Hypertrophy of the Interatrial Septum

Lipomatous hypertrophy is the nonencapsulated collection of mature adipocytes, with associated mature intervening islands of myocardial or nonlipomatous cells. It is commonly found between the right and left atria.[15] It is more common than lipomas and commonly occurs in the typical location in elderly, obese female patients and is often found incidentally on testing for other reasons. Although arrhythmia has been associated with this condition, it is usually asymptomatic. There

is no evidence that prognosis is improved by resection.

Hemangioma

Cardiac hemangiomas are rare, representing about 2% of primary cardiac tumors.[16] The diagnosis of cardiac hemangiomas is challenging. These benign tumors may can develop anywhere in the heart. Cardiac hemangiomas occur most frequently in children and adolescents.[17] Most cardiac hemangiomas are discovered incidentally, but complications can include heart failure, right ventricular outflow tract obstruction,[18] coronary obstruction,[19] pericardial effusion, arrhythmias,[20] and sudden death.[21] Patients with a resectable tumor usually have a good prognosis, and surgery is recommended.[16] When complete resection is not feasible, partial resections are thought to produce long-term benefits.[17] At the Houston Methodist DeBakey Heart & Vascular Center, the authors have successfully operated on 5 cardiac hemangiomas that were causing obstructive symptoms. They also have 3 patients with tumors that met the characteristics of hemangioma that are in anatomically difficult areas to resect safely. The authors have been following these with patients with no changes for over 3 years.

SURGERY FOR PRIMARY COMPLEX TUMORS

This section investigates select primary benign tumors such as fibromas and paragangliomas, as well as all primary malignant tumors with a focus on sarcomas.

Benign - Fibroma

Cardiac fibromas are rare benign tumors occurring predominantly in children and adolescents.[22] These tumors are solitary and occur almost exclusively within the ventricular myocardium, usually in the left ventricle free wall or septum.[23] Most cardiac fibromas produce symptoms through arrhythmia and conduction disturbances, intracardiac blood flow obstruction, or interference with normal valvular and/or ventricular function.[22,23] These tumors are generally well circumscribed and noninfiltrating.

Surgery should be considered and can involve extensive resection requiring ventricular reconstruction.[24] Even large left ventricular fibromas can generally be resected and the left ventricle reconstructed, as these tumors tend to displace the left ventricular muscle away rather than replacing it.[24] Occasionally, mitral valve repair or replacement is needed.[23,24] Successful complete resection of the tumor is curative. When the tumor cannot be removed completely, partial resection provides good palliation.[23] In selected patients with unresectable tumors, cardiac transplantation may be considered.[25] The largest published series of surgically treated cardiac fibromas includes 18 patients who underwent surgery over a 38-year period, and were followed for up to 34 years.[23] There was 1 operative death and no late deaths. There was no tumor recurrence or change in size of the residual tumor in the 1 patient who had subtotal resection.

Benign - Paraganglioma

Chromaffin tumors arising from the neural crest cells originating from the sympathetic or parasympathetic chains are classified as paragangliomas. Only about 1% to 2% occur in the chest, and most of these arise in the posterior mediastinum.[26] They occur most commonly in the roof of the left atrium or the base of the pulmonary artery and aorta. These tumors can be hormonally active. About 10% of cardiac paragangliomas are malignant.[27] Patients presenting with hypertension or suspicion of tumor hormonal activity require testing and blockade before surgery.

Complete surgical excision is the only effective treatment for paraganglioma. Surgery is complicated by the fact that these tumors do not have a capsule and require complete excision for success. This lack of encapsulation and proximity to anatomically important structure can make the surgical approach to these highly vascular tumors complex.[28]

Malignant - Cardiac Sarcoma

Primary cardiac sarcomas are rare. Survival without surgical resection is generally measured in months. The authors classify primary cardiac sarcoma by its location, rather than histologically,

because they find that this determines the presentation, urgency of intervention, and surgical options available.[2,29] Their classification divides primary cardiac sarcomas into right heart, left heart, and pulmonary artery sarcomas.

Cardiac sarcomas have a propensity for early metastatic dissemination, and systemic neoadjuvant therapy should be strongly considered in hemodynamically stable patients with localized disease as it allows for easier resection by reducing the tumor volume and reducing the risk of systemic relapse. These advantages exist only in cases where response to therapy is demonstrated. A combination of doxorubicin and ifosfamide is used in the neoadjuvant therapy of most sarcomas of the right and left heart. Other regimens include gemcitabine/docetaxel combination and single-agent paclitaxel (for patients with angiosarcoma). In patients with metastatic disease, systemic therapy forms the mainstay of treatment.

Right Heart Sarcoma

Most right heart sarcomas are angiosarcomas.[30] These tumors are 2 to 3 times more common in men than in women. They show a strong predilection for the right atrium. These tumors tend to aggressively invade adjacent structures, including the great veins, tricuspid valve, right ventricular free wall, interventricular septum, and right coronary artery. When feasible, complete surgical resection is the mainstay of therapy, and it is the only treatment modality that has been shown to improve survival.[31] The authors' approach is for neoadjuvant chemotherapy following biopsy diagnosis.[32] Doxorubicin and ifosfamide comprise the authors' standard chemotherapy regimen, which is continued until unresponsive. Then candidacy for surgical resection is evaluated. Patients with metastatic disease unresponsive to chemotherapy or those who developed new metastatic disease while on treatment are not considered candidates for surgery. Patients with widely metastatic disease are also not considered candidates, unless palliative surgery is undertaken to relieve severe symptoms.

In the authors' experience, the introduction of this standardized multimodality treatment protocol, largely centered on the use of neoadjuvant chemotherapy, led to a significant increase in the rate of microscopically complete resection (ie, with R0 margins) from 24% to 61% ($P = .03$). Neoadjuvant chemotherapy was also associated with a doubling of median survival (20 vs 9.5 months).[32] Because of their infiltrative nature, right heart sarcomas require extensive resection to achieve negative margins. This may involve resection of the right atrium, the right coronary artery, tricuspid valve and up to a third of the right ventricle, total cardiac replacement with biventricular assist device implantation,[33] or total artificial heart implantation.[34] The primary reason for local failure is incomplete resection.

Left Heart Sarcoma

Primary sarcomas of the left heart are usually found in the left atrium and are most commonly solid. They often present with acute-onset heart failure secondary to obstruction of forward flow, so neoadjuvant chemotherapy is rarely considered possible. The 1- and 2-year survival for primary cardiac sarcoma in this series was 46% and 28%, respectively.

Left heart sarcomas present a surgical challenge in terms of achieving complete resection and may require autotransplantation with ex vivo tumor resection, reconstruction, and reimplantation.[35,36] The authors have used cardiac autotransplantation for large intracavitary left ventricular tumors to avoid ventriculotomy[37] and for left atrial sarcomas.[38] Incomplete resection of primary cardiac sarcoma is universally associated with rapid recurrence and poor outcomes. For the cases requiring cardiac autotransplant and pneumonectomy, the authors' approach is to separate the surgery into 2 stages: cardiac resection first, then standard pneumonectomy after the metabolic disturbance of cardiopulmonary bypass has abated. The authors refer to this approach, which has been successful in addressing this problem, as the Texas Two Step.[39]

Pulmonary Artery Sarcoma

Pulmonary artery sarcoma is rare. Patients present with symptoms of dyspnea, cough, hemoptysis, or chest pain, often resulting in a misdiagnosis of pulmonary embolism.[29,40] Treatment approaches have included palliative pulmonary artery stenting, pneumonectomy, debulking, tumor endarterectomy, and wide surgical excision. The Mayo Clinic has reported a series of 9 patients having surgical resection collected over a 19-year period.[41] The authors' group reported a series of 8 pulmonary artery sarcoma resections with a mean survival of 24.7 months compared with 8.0 months found in the literature.[29] The authors have shown that wide excision that often includes the pulmonary trunk can be safely done and improve survival.[29]

SURGERY FOR SECONDARY TUMORS

The management of secondary cardiac tumors is variable and contingent on the comorbidities, clinical presentation, and overall prognosis, which is largely based on the extent of tumor spread and the type of cancer. Because cardiac metastases often represent one of many locations of metastatic deposits, the main goals of therapy are the general treatment of the patients' overall cancer, not the cardiac lesion alone. The treatment options for patients with secondary cardiac tumors are adjuvant or neo-adjuvant chemotherapy, radiation, surgical resection and palliation. Most often, a combination of the aforementioned strategies is employed.

For symptomatic or large pericardial effusions, pericardiocentesis for both diagnosis and treatment should be considered. Malignant recurrent effusions may require the use of a sclerosing agent or drainage with a subxiphisternal window or percutaneous approach for symptomatic palliation.

Surgical tumor resection may be considered in highly selected malignant cases (**Fig. 2**). The lesion should be resectable while preserving sufficient cardiac function to sustain life. Surgical resection should be given particular consideration in individuals with endocardial metastases to prevent or treat acute and complete obstruction. These resections are often larger than anticipated and should likely be undertaken in a center of excellence for cardiac tumors, both for the decision to operate and for optimal operative and postoperative care. It is unknown if resection of

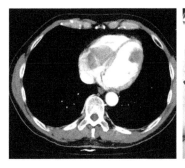 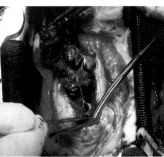

Fig. 2. Secondary cardiac tumor. Right atrial and left ventricular melanoma. Left: CT shows right atrial and left ventricular tumor masses. Right: the left ventriculotomy and ventricular apical tumor.

isolated cardiac metastatic deposits prolongs life or disease-free survival, although there are instances with prolonged survival.

Renal Tumors

For direct invasive renal carcinomas, radiation and chemotherapy are not effective in relieving the obstruction of blood flow, and surgical resection should be considered. If the kidney can be fully removed, as well as the tail of the tumor thrombus in the inferior vena cava (IVC), survival can approach 75% at 5 years.[42] The authors used to perform a concomitant median sternotomy and used cardiopulmonary bypass with hypothermic circulatory arrest. However, the authors have changed their approach and now work closely with liver transplant surgeons who have extensive experience in operating on the retro-hepatic vena cava. They expose the vena cava to the right atrium through an abdominal incision. With ligation of the arterial inflow, the tumor tail often shrinks below the diaphragm, and in almost all circumstances, this can be removed without the use of cardiopulmonary bypass (CPB). Occasionally venovenous bypass (as used in hepatic transplantation) may be necessary to occlude inflow through the IVC. If the tumor is too complex for this maneuver, then a median sternotomy is performed, and CPB with hypothermic circulatory arrest can be used to remove the tumor from the cardiac chambers down into the IVC.

Lung Tumors

The authors advocate for surgical treatment in selected patients with advanced carcinoma of the lung with intracardiac involvement. A partial atrial resection may be achieved by opening the pericardium and freeing the posterior left atrium from its pericardial attachments, a technique used routinely in lung transplantation. This approach makes it easy to apply an atrial vascular clamp. When the atrial clamping technique is not possible, cardiopulmonary bypass can be used to facilitate complete resection. Total cardiopulmonary bypass is used with either cardioplegia or fine ventricular fibrillation. These techniques may improve the chances of survival for patients in whom advanced carcinoma of the lung has spread to the pericardial or cardiac structures. The authors' group has also reported surgical resection of direct spread of advanced nonsmall cell lung carcinoma, which was incorporated into the inferior pulmonary vein and extended into the left atrium, right atrium, and the interatrial septum.[43] The tumor and the pulmonary specimen were excised successfully en bloc, the atrial margins were closed primarily, and

the pericardial defect was closed with a patch. Several groups have similarly described resection of lung carcinoma with direct atrial invasion with reasonable midterm success.[44]

SUMMARY

This article provided an overview of a surgical approach to cardiac tumors. Primary simple, tumors such as myxoma, fibroelastoma, lipoma, and hemangioma are generally safely resected with excellent outcomes. Primary complex benign tumors such as paraganglioma and fibroma and primary malignant cardiac tumors, commonly sarcomas, are less uncommon and more complex. Secondary cardiac tumors are more common but have poor overall outcomes. Surgical management may include percutaneous or open pericardial drainage for effusion and open surgical resection in highly select patients. Few surgeons or even institutions gain much experience with these complex cardiac tumor entities, and the authors recommend care by an established multidisciplinary cardiac tumor team in a highly experienced center of excellence. As always, individualized clinical assessment is of utmost importance for decision making.

REFERENCES

1. Butany J, Nair V, Naseemuddin A, et al. Cardiac tumours: diagnosis and management. Lancet Oncol 2005;6:219–28.
2. Bakaeen FG, Reardon MJ, Coselli JS, et al. Surgical outcome in 85 patients with primary cardiac tumors. Am J Surg 2003;186:641–7 [discussion: 647].
3. Bussani R, De-Giorgio F, Abbate A, et al. Cardiac metastases. J Clin Pathol 2007;60:27–34.
4. Goldberg AD, Blankstein R, Padera RF. Tumors metastatic to the heart. Circulation 2013;128:1790–4.
5. Hoffmeier A, Sindermann JR, Scheld HH, et al. Cardiac tumors–diagnosis and surgical treatment. Dtsch Arztebl Int 2014;111:205–11.
6. Reynen K, Kockeritz U, Strasser RH. Metastases to the heart. Ann Oncol 2004;15:375–81.
7. Bruckner BA, Reardon MJ. Benign cardiac tumors: a review. Methodist Debakey Cardiovasc J 2010;6:20–6.
8. Ngaage DL, Mullany CJ, Daly RC, et al. Surgical treatment of cardiac papillary fibroelastoma: a single center experience with eighty-eight patients. Ann Thorac Surg 2005;80:1712–8.
9. Kumar TK, Kuehl K, Reyes C, et al. Multiple papillary fibroelastomas of the heart. Ann Thorac Surg 2009; 88:e66–7.
10. Abu Saleh WK, Al Jabbari O, Ramlawi B, et al. Cardiac papillary fibroelastoma: single-institution

experience with 14 surgical patients. Tex Heart Inst J 2016;43:148–51.

11. Wijesurendra RS, Sheppard KA, Westaby S, et al. The many faces of cardiac lipoma-an egg in the heart! Eur Heart J Cardiovasc Imaging 2017; 18(7):821.

12. D'Souza J, Shah R, Abbass A, et al. Invasive cardiac lipoma: a case report and review of literature. BMC Cardiovasc Disord 2017;17:28.

13. Salanitri JC, Pereles FS. Cardiac lipoma and lipomatous hypertrophy of the interatrial septum: cardiac magnetic resonance imaging findings. J Comput Assist Tomogr 2004;28:852–6.

14. Zhu SB, Zhu J, Liu Y, et al. Surgical treatment of a giant symptomatic cardiac lipoma. J Thorac Oncol 2013;8:1341–2.

15. Cunningham KS, Veinot JP, Feindel CM, et al. Fatty lesions of the atria and interatrial septum. Hum Pathol 2006;37:1245–51.

16. Abu Saleh WK, Al Jabbari O, Bruckner BA, et al. Case report: a rare case of left atrial hemangioma: surgical resection and reconstruction. Methodist Debakey Cardiovasc J 2016;12:51–4.

17. Brizard C, Latremouille C, Jebara VA, et al. Cardiac hemangiomas. Ann Thorac Surg 1993;56:390–4.

18. Young AM, Danter MR, Lewis JS Jr, et al. Right ventricular hemangioma in the outflow tract: a rare cause of obstruction. Ann Thorac Surg 2017;103:e245–6.

19. Sulayman R, Cassels DE. Myocardial coronary hemangiomatous tumors in children. Chest 1975;68: 113–5.

20. Weston CF, Hayward MW, Seymour RM, et al. Cardiac haemangioma associated with a facial port-wine stain and recurrent atrial tachycardia. Eur Heart J 1988;9:668–71.

21. Abad C, Campo E, Estruch R, et al. Cardiac hemangioma with papillary endothelial hyperplasia: report of a resected case and review of the literature. Ann Thorac Surg 1990;49:305–8.

22. Burke AP, Rosado-de-Christenson M, Templeton PA, et al. Cardiac fibroma: clinicopathologic correlates and surgical treatment. J Thorac Cardiovasc Surg 1994;108:862–70.

23. Cho JM, Danielson GK, Puga FJ, et al. Surgical resection of ventricular cardiac fibromas: early and late results. Ann Thorac Surg 2003;76:1929–34.

24. Leja MJ, Perryman L, Reardon MJ. Resection of left ventricular fibroma with subacute papillary muscle rupture. Tex Heart Inst J 2011;38:279–81.

25. Valente M, Cocco P, Thiene G, et al. Cardiac fibroma and heart transplantation. J Thorac Cardiovasc Surg 1993;106:1208–12.

26. Aravot DJ, Banner NR, Cantor AM, et al. Location, localization and surgical treatment of cardiac pheochromocytoma. Am J Cardiol 1992;69:283–5.

27. Goldstein RE, O'Neill JA Jr, Holcomb GW 3rd, et al. Clinical experience over 48 years with pheochromocytoma. Ann Surg 1999;229:755–64 [discussion: 764–6].

28. Ramlawi B, David EA, Kim MP, et al. Contemporary surgical management of cardiac paragangliomas. Ann Thorac Surg 2012;93:1972–6.

29. Blackmon SH, Patel A, Reardon MJ. Management of primary cardiac sarcomas. Expert Rev Cardiovasc Ther 2008;6:1217–22.

30. Ramlawi B, Leja MJ, Abu Saleh WK, et al. Surgical treatment of primary cardiac sarcomas: review of a single-institution experience. Ann Thorac Surg 2016;101:698–702.

31. Look Hong NJ, Pandalai PK, Hornick JL, et al. Cardiac angiosarcoma management and outcomes: 20-year single-institution experience. Ann Surg Oncol 2012;19:2707–15.

32. Abu Saleh WK, Ramlawi B, Shapira OM, et al. Improved outcomes with the evolution of a neoadjuvant chemotherapy approach to right heart sarcoma. Ann Thorac Surg 2017;104:90–6.

33. Bruckner BA, Rodriguez LE, Bunge R, et al. Large cardiac tumor managed with resection and two ventricular assist devices. Ann Thorac Surg 2014;97:321–4.

34. Bruckner BA, Abu Saleh WK, Al Jabbari O, et al. Total artificial heart implantation after excision of right ventricular angiosarcoma. Tex Heart Inst J 2016; 43:252–4.

35. SH Blackmon RM. Cardiac autotransplanation. Oper Tech Thorac Cardiovasc Surg 2010;15:141–61.

36. Reardon MJ, DeFelice CA, Sheinbaum R, et al. Cardiac autotransplant for surgical treatment of a malignant neoplasm. Ann Thorac Surg 1999;67:1793–5.

37. Leja MJ, Kim M, Perryman L, et al. Metastatic melanoma to the intracavitary left ventricle treated using cardiac autotransplantation technique for resection. Methodist Debakey Cardiovasc J 2011;7:44–6.

38. Iskander SS, Nagueh SF, Ostrowski ML, et al. Growth of a left atrial sarcoma followed by resection and autotransplantation. Ann Thorac Surg 2005;79:1771–4.

39. Chan EY, Reul RM, Kim MP, et al. The "Texas Two-Step" procedure. J Thorac Cardiovasc Surg 2018; 155:285–7.

40. Srivali N, Yi ES, Ryu JH. Pulmonary artery sarcoma mimicking pulmonary embolism: a case series. QJM 2017;110:283–6.

41. Srivali N, Yi ES, Ryu J. Pulmonary artery sarcoma: 19-year cohort study. Int J Radiat Oncol Biol Phys 2017;98:226.

42. Prager RL, Dean R, Turner B. Surgical approach to intracardiac renal cell carcinoma. Ann Thorac Surg 1982;33:74–7.

43. Aburto J, Bruckner BA, Blackmon SH, et al. Renal cell carcinoma, metastatic to the left ventricle. Tex Heart Inst J 2009;36:48–9.

44. Shirakusa T, Kimura M. Partial atrial resection in advanced lung carcinoma with and without cardiopulmonary bypass. Thorax 1991;46:484–7.

Cardiovascular Toxicities in Pediatric Cancer Survivors

Thomas D. Ryan, MD, PhD[a],*, Rajaram Nagarajan, MD, MS[b],
Justin Godown, MD[c]

KEYWORDS

- Anthracycline • Cardiomyopathy • Cardio-oncology • Cardiotoxicity • Chemotherapy
- Heart failure • Oncocardiology • Pediatric cardiology

KEY POINTS

- Cardiovascular disease represents a significant cause of morbidity and mortality in survivors of childhood cancer.
- Cardiovascular screening represents an important component of current survivorship guidelines.
- The optimal treatment of established cardiac disease secondary to oncologic therapies remains unclear.
- Pediatric cardio-oncology is an evolving subspecialty that may play a crucial role in patient and family education and also help to facilitate earlier detection of cardiac disease.

INTRODUCTION

In the 1970s, Drs Meadows and D'Angio recognized the progress being made in the treatment of pediatric cancers and started the discussion of survivorship, including the idea that cure is not enough.[1,2] With greater than 15,000 cancers diagnosed each year in patients less than 19 years old,[3] this progress has resulted in approximately 450,000 survivors of pediatric cancer (**Table 1**).[4] Given this ever-increasing number of childhood cancer survivors, the long-term effects of cancer therapy have become increasingly important in this group.[5] Using this knowledge, researchers and clinicians have now developed surveillance recommendations for these late effects and have been able to adjust and modify current treatment strategies to maintain or improve overall survival, while decreasing associated morbidity and mortality.[6,7]

As the causes of morbidity and mortality are explored, it has been noted that, after recurrence and secondary malignancies, cardiovascular-related outcomes contribute most significantly to late effects of therapy.[6–9] Poor cardiac outcomes are related to cardiomyopathy, hypertension, diabetes, obesity, arrhythmias, structural abnormalities (eg, valvular disease), and coronary artery disease.[10,11] Therapies implicated included anthracyclines and radiation therapy. More recent has been the introduction of novel therapies, including tyrosine kinase inhibitors, monoclonal antibodies, immune checkpoint inhibitors, and chimeric antigen receptor T cell (CAR-T cell) therapy.[12,13] Some of these novel therapies are

Disclosure: The authors have nothing to disclose.
[a] Department of Pediatrics, Division of Pediatric Cardiology, Heart Institute, Cincinnati Children's Hospital Medical Center, University of Cincinnati College of Medicine, 3333 Burnet Avenue, MLC 2003, Cincinnati, OH 45229, USA; [b] Department of Pediatrics, Division of Oncology, Cancer and Blood Diseases Institute, Cincinnati Children's Hospital Medical Center, University of Cincinnati College of Medicine, 3333 Burnet Avenue, MLC 7018, Cincinnati, OH 45229, USA; [c] Department of Pediatrics, Division of Pediatric Cardiology, Monroe Carell Jr. Children's Hospital at Vanderbilt, 2200 Children's Way, Suite 5230 DOT, Nashville, TN 37232, USA
* Corresponding author.
E-mail address: thomas.ryan@cchmc.org

Table 1
Distribution of cases of childhood and adolescent cancers in the United States with common, potentially cardiotoxic treatment exposures

	Proportion of Cancers, Children 0–14 y (%)	Proportion of Cancers, Adolescents 15–19 y (%)	Cumulative Anthracycline Dose[c]	Potential Thoracic Radiation Exposure Scenarios
Leukemia				
Acute lymphocytic leukemia	26	8	Low[d]	Craniospinal photon radiation
Acute myeloid leukemia	5	4	High	—
Lymphoma				
Hodgkin lymphoma	4	15	Low or high[d]	Site dependent
Non-Hodgkin lymphoma	6	8	Low or high[d]	Site dependent
Central nervous system[a]	21	10	—	Craniospinal photon radiation
Neuroblastoma	7	—	Low[d]	Site dependent
Retinoblastoma	3	—	—	—
Wilms tumor	5	—	Low[d]	Select metastatic patients or abdominal radiation
Bone tumors[b]	4	7	High	Select metastatic patients
Soft tissue sarcoma	7	7	High[e]	Select metastatic patients
Germ cell tumors	3	12	—	—
Carcinoma and melanoma	4	20	—	Site dependent

Treatment is highly variable based on diagnosis, patient age, disease stage, site of disease, and several other factors. Represented in this table are general trends only.
[a] Includes ependymoma, astrocytoma, and medulloblastoma.
[b] Includes osteosarcoma and Ewing sarcoma.
[c] High (cumulative ≥ 250 mg/m^2) and low dose (<250 mg/m^2) applies to doxorubicin or doxorubicin equivalent of other anthracyclines.
[d] Anthracyclines included only in select high-risk and intermediate-risk regimens, not all treatment protocols.
[e] Anthracycline inclusion dependent on the specific tumor type and therapy treatment selected included only in select high-risk regimens, not all treatment protocols.
Adapted from Ward E, DeSantis C, Robbins A, *et al.* Childhood and adolescent cancer statistics, 2014. *CA: a cancer journal for clinicians.* 2014;64(2):83-103 and *data from* Howlader N, Noone AM, Krapcho M, *et al.* SEER cancer statistics review, 1975-2009 (vintage 2009 populations), national cancer institute. Available at: https://seer.cancer.gov/csr/1975_2009_pops09.

established in current treatment regimens for pediatric patients, whereas the use of others is still being established. Although the acute repercussions for these novel therapies are generally known, longer-term outcomes are not well described, particularly in patients treated during the pediatric and adolescent period of life.

MECHANISMS OF CARDIAC TOXICITY

The mechanisms of cancer treatment–related cardiotoxicity (CTRC) are covered in detail by other articles in this series. Herein is a brief review of both commonly used agents and novel therapies, with data in pediatric populations emphasized where available.

Anthracyclines

Most of the data pertaining to CTRC are related to anthracyclines. A number pathways are involved, including mitochondrial DNA damage, apoptosis from generation of reactive oxygen species, and damage to nuclear DNA through direct interaction of anthracyclines on topoisomerase 2β.[11,14] The presumed safe range for doses of chemotherapy has decreased steadily over time, with several studies in pediatric populations showing effects on echocardiographic parameters after administration of just a single dose (doxorubicin equivalent, 60 mg/m²).[15,16] The current generally accepted definition of low-dose versus high-dose anthracycline exposure is 250 mg/m² doxorubicin equivalent (see **Table 1**).

Radiation

Radiation therapy also increases the risk for development of CTRC, accounting for much of the reported injury to the pericardium, coronaries, conduction pathways, and myocardial diastolic function.[11] There is dose dependence related to extent of injury produced; however, it has not been established whether there is a limit below which injury does not occur.[17] Mechanisms of injury include induction of proinflammatory cascades, endothelial injury, generation of fibrosis, and initiation of oxidative stress.[11,17] Alternate therapeutic approaches, such as proton therapy, may spare the heart from radiation exposure and thus reduce cardiotoxicity, although this is not yet definitively proved.[18]

Targeted Cancer Therapies

An improved understanding of the molecular pathways important in cancer has led to the development of directed therapies,[12] as exemplified by the successful introduction of imatinib to treat chronic myeloid leukemia, which was US Food and Drug Administration (FDA) approved in 2001, and specifically for use in pediatric patients in 2003.[19–23] Presently, more than 20 small molecule tyrosine kinase inhibitors are available for clinical use.[24] Off-target binding with disruption of cellular signaling has been implicated in the CTRC associated with tyrosine kinase inhibitors, which vary considerably across therapeutic agents.[25] Kinase inhibitors have been associated with hypertension, thromboembolism, pulmonary hypertension, and ventricular dysfunction.[26–30] It is unclear whether the risk profiles of these agents differ between adults and children.

In pediatric patients specifically, antibody therapies have shown effectiveness in various cancers.[31–34] Similar to the cardiotoxic effects seen in small molecule inhibitors of kinases, monoclonal antibodies with a similar mechanism of action can also cause CTRC.[35] Clinical trials have shown the ability to offer protection against CTRC with these agents,[36] and other trials are underway to better understand this process.[37]

Cancer Immunotherapy

There are now multiple FDA-approved immune checkpoint inhibitors with applications in metastatic melanoma, lung cancer, and renal cancer.[38] Cardiac toxicity is rare, occurring in less than 0.1% of patients receiving these medications.[39,40] However, severe and potentially fatal myocarditis as well as arrhythmias have been reported with their use and represent important considerations as these therapies expand into the pediatric population.[40–45]

Chimeric Antigen Receptor T Cells

Patients with relapsed or refractory disease after anthracycline therapy show poor survival.[46] CAR-T cell therapy specifically targets cancer cells, and has achieved a nearly 90% overall remission rate in children with refractory or relapsed acute lymphocytic leukemia.[46–48] However, cytokine release syndrome can occur and may result in vasoplegic shock and/or ventricular dysfunction. Although tocilizumab has been shown to be beneficial in treating these side effects, hypotension necessitating the use of inotropic support is common, and ventricular dysfunction can persist.[49,50]

CURRENT SURVEILLANCE

For most cancer treatment modalities, there is a lag between clinical introduction of the therapy and the recognition of cardiotoxicity. In the case of anthracyclines, several decades passed from first use to such recommendations, and it was several more decades before statements were produced from the various cardiology and oncology professional societies. However, with time and experience, the gap between these steps has significantly narrowed for emerging therapies.[51] In the case of pediatric and adult survivors of pediatric cancers, although a wide variety of therapies are used in cancer treatment, almost all of the published data and recommendations for surveillance focus on anthracyclines and radiation. This focus is likely because of a combination of early data on anthracycline toxicity in this population, relative novelty of many newer therapies, and smaller patient numbers making identification of cardiotoxicity trends challenging.

Risk Stratification

An important component of any surveillance program is to determine risk for development of the disease or comorbidity in question. According to the National Comprehensive Cancer Network, those who have undergone treatment of cancer should be considered American College of Cardiology/American Heart Association stage A heart failure (no structural abnormality, but at risk to develop heart failure) at a minimum.[52] For survivors of pediatric cancers, the Childhood Cancer Survivor Study has been a wealth of information in this regard. This cohort study compared patients with sibling controls and showed an increased incidence of heart failure, valvular disease, pericardial disease, and coronary artery disease. For development of heart failure specifically, important risk factors included female gender, age less than 10 years at diagnosis, treatment era, and higher doses of anthracycline and/or radiation.[53] Data from this cohort have also shown the importance of modifiable risk factors, such as hypertension, obesity, and dyslipidemia, on cardiovascular outcomes.[54] Using these data, an online risk calculator (www.ccss.stjude.org) is available to predict risk of heart failure, ischemic heart disease, and stroke by age 50 years in survivors of childhood cancer.[55,56] This calculator focuses primarily on anthracycline and radiation therapies, and is

not used in making specific surveillance recommendations.

Available Guidelines

Several medical societies or organizations have produced guidelines, consensus statements, or position papers on the care of patients who have undergone therapy for cancer. Some resources are intended for all adult patients (**Table 2**),[52,57–60] whereas others have specifically focused on pediatric and/or adult survivors of pediatric cancers (**Box 1**).[11,61,62] Recent efforts have been made to consolidate the various guidelines for survivors of pediatric cancers, including specific direction on surveillance modality and strength of recommendation[61]; however, there are still limited resources regarding treatment once cardiovascular toxicity develops. All screening should include assessment by a physician, with additional testing dependent on the individual resource. For most cases, if abnormalities are detected, then referral to a

---

Table 2
Recommendations for care of adult patients after therapy for cancer based on leading resources

Discussion or Recommendations	ESMO[a]	ASE + EACVI[b]	ESC[c]	CCS[d]	ASCO[e]	NCCN[f]
Anthracycline/radiation exposure/risks	Yes	Yes	Yes	Yes	Yes	Yes
Other chemotherapy agents exposure/risks	Yes	Yes	Yes	Yes	No	Yes
LVEF assessment by imaging modalities	Yes	Yes	Yes	Yes	Yes	Yes
Use of circulating biomarkers	Yes	Yes	Yes	Yes	Yes	Yes
Assessment/diagnosis of other cardiovascular disease[g]	Yes	Yes	Yes	Yes	No	No
Treatment of ventricular dysfunction or heart failure	Yes	No	Yes	Yes	Yes	No
Treatment of other cardiovascular disease	Yes	No	Yes	Yes	No	No
Survivors of pediatric cancers	No	No	Per Harmonization[h]	Per COG[i]	No	Per COG[i]

Abbreviations: ASCO, American Society of Clinical Oncology; ASE, American Society of Echocardiography; CCS, Canadian Cardiovascular Society; COG, Children's Oncology Group; ESC, European Society of Cardiology; EACVI, European Association of Cardiovascular Imaging; ESMO, European Society for Medical Oncology; LVEF, left ventricular ejection fraction; NCCN, National Comprehensive Cancer Network.
  [a] European Society for Medical Oncology Clinical Practice Guidelines (2012).[57]
  [b] American Society of Echocardiography and European Association of Cardiovascular Imaging Expert Consensus for Multimodality Imaging (2014).[58]
  [c] European Society of Cardiology Position Paper (2016).[59]
  [d] Canadian Cardiovascular Society Guidelines (2016).[60]
  [e] American Society of Clinical Oncology Clinical Practice Guideline (2017).[62]
  [f] National Comprehensive Cancer Network (US) Clinical Practice Guidelines (2018).[52]
  [g] For example, hypertension, ischemia, QT-prolongation, thrombosis, valvular disease, pericardial disease.
  [h] International Late Effects of Childhood Cancer Guideline Harmonization Group.[61]
  [i] Children's Oncology Group (www.childrensoncologygroup.org).
Data from Refs.[52,57–62]

specialist in cardiovascular disease, preferably with expertise in cardio-oncology, is indicated.

Components of the Cardiac Evaluation

The specific evaluations performed as part of cardiovascular assessment in survivors of pediatric cancer depend, in large part, on the therapies used and thus the potential cardiotoxic effects.[10] For patients in whom only anthracycline chemotherapy was used, assessment of ventricular systolic function is the primary concern, whereas patients also exposed to radiation should be followed for valvular abnormalities, pericardial disease, and coronary artery disease as well. At a minimum, most protocols recommend assessment with physical examination by a primary provider, electrocardiogram (ECG), and echocardiogram. If additional specific concerns are realized, then further assessment of blood pressure, peripheral vascular disease, arrhythmia, valvular disorder, and pulmonary hypertension should be appropriately undertaken.[59] In general, most guidelines for survivors of pediatric cancer cover only ventricular function based on therapies used in the past; however, the field is rapidly expanding and recommended surveillance must be updated to keep pace.

Screening Modalities

Electrocardiography

Many chemotherapy protocols include serial assessment of the ECG, with emphasis on the corrected QT interval to track risk of the development of torsades de pointes.[59] Monitoring for prolongation of the QT interval and management of electrolytes are important when QT-prolonging medications are required for therapy (eg, arsenic trioxide) and/or the management of therapy-related and disease-related side effects (eg, 5-hydroxytryptamine antiemetics, methadone for pain). Most guidelines for surveillance of survivors of pediatric cancer include ECG monitoring.

Echocardiography, cardiac magnetic resonance, and multigated radionuclide angiography

Guidelines are available for the multimodality imaging assessment of adult patients throughout cancer therapy, and include recommendations for echocardiographic two-dimensional (2D) and three-dimensional (3D) assessments of function, strain imaging, and measures of right ventricular function.[58] Both 3D ejection fraction (EF) and parameters of tissue deformation (myocardial strain and tissue Doppler) have shown the ability to detect subclinical dysfunction in adult and pediatric studies.[63–65] Despite this, most current

screening efforts in pediatric patients focus on shortening fraction (SF) and EF, and only in long-term survivors.[61] One recent study detailed abnormal myocardial strain despite normal EF in a heterogeneous group of 25 pediatric patients immediately after their final treatment, but did not include time points during treatment.[66] As opposed to studies in adult patients, those in pediatric and adolescent populations have not yet proved the ability of decreases in myocardial strain to predict subsequent decreases in EF or development of symptomatic heart failure.[63] In considering the guidance from various organizing bodies, the International Late Effects of Childhood Cancer Guideline Harmonization Group (hereafter referred to as the Harmonization Group; **Box 1**) recommended echocardiography as the primary method of surveillance for assessment of left ventricular systolic function in patients previously treated with anthracyclines and/or chest radiation, no later than 2 years after completion of therapy, and repeated a maximum of every 5 years. More frequent and lifelong surveillance can be considered in high-risk survivors.[61] Echocardiography continues to have many advantages as an imaging modality, including portability and ease of use, availability at most centers, provider comfort with the information provided, and decades of published research using this modality.

Multigated radionuclide angiography (MUGA; also multigated blood pool imaging or multigated acquisition) provides quantification of left ventricular systolic function using first-pass or equilibrium radionuclide angiography, and has been used in CTRC since the late 1970s.[58] The technique is known to be reproducible and standardized for

---

Box 1
Resources providing information and/or guidance for cardiovascular care of survivors of pediatric cancers

Resource

American Heart Association Scientific Statement on Pediatric, Adolescent, and Young Adult Long-Term Survivors[11]

Children's Oncology Group (www.childrensoncologygroup.org)

Dutch Childhood Oncology Group[111]

Scottish Intercollegiate Guidelines Network (www.sign.ac.uk)

UK Children's Cancer and Leukemia Group (www.cclg.org.uk)

International Late Effects of Childhood Cancer Guideline Harmonization Group[61]

this patient population. However, several disadvantages exist. First, MUGA does not provide information on structure, chamber sizes, right ventricular systolic function, or diastolic function. Second, and more important, is radiation exposure to the patient. With improvements in echocardiography, and particularly cardiac magnetic resonance (CMR), the risk/benefit profile of MUGA is less attractive to many physicians. Further, although this is a common modality in adult centers, many pediatric providers have limited experience with its use in the current era.

CMR has utility in detecting CTRC, particularly in patients with limited imaging windows, and for assessment of the right ventricle, which is incompletely assessed by echocardiogram. One study of adult survivors of pediatric cancers found that nearly 15% had left ventricular EF less than 50% by CMR, with 75% of this group misclassified as left ventricular EF greater than 50% by 2D echocardiography.[64] As such, the investigators recommended consideration of CMR as further assessment for any patient with left ventricular EF less than 60% by echocardiography. In addition, CMR can assess for myocardial fibrosis and edema, which may have an important role in development of anthracycline cardiotoxicity.[67] The Harmonization Group determined that it is reasonable to use CMR for cardiomyopathy surveillance in at-risk survivors when echocardiography is technically suboptimal. When both CMR and MUGA are available, the preference is for CMR because of the lack of ionizing radiation exposure as well as additional information provided compared with MUGA.[61]

Serum biomarkers and other testing modalities

Troponins, brain natriuretic peptide (BNP), and n-terminal pro-BNP (NT-proBNP) levels are increased before initiation of therapy in pediatric patients, particularly anthracycline therapy, indicating a baseline state of cardiac stress or injury related to cancer with further increase in these biomarkers throughout the treatment course.[68–71] Patients in long-term follow-up may continue to show increases in levels of these biomarkers as evidence for ongoing or subclinical cardiotoxicity.[72,73] The Harmonization Group recommends that "assessment of cardiac blood biomarkers ... in conjunction with imaging studies may be reasonable in instances where symptomatic cardiomyopathy is strongly suspected or in individuals who have borderline cardiac function during primary surveillance."[61]

Additional testing modalities, such as cardiopulmonary exercise testing and ambulatory rhythm monitoring, are also included as potentially useful in adult-based guidelines; however, their utility depends on the clinical scenario.[59] Protocols still less than development, such as noninvasive measurement of arterial stiffness[74] or determination of left ventricular EF by collection of carotid arterial pulse waveform and phonocardiogram from a handheld device,[75] may have a place in surveillance if validated in larger studies.

Barriers to Follow-Up

Review of Childhood Cancer Survivor Study data shows that approximately 30% of adult survivors of pediatric cancer reported receiving care focused on their cancer history. Among those at increased risk for cardiomyopathy, fewer than 30% had undergone a recommended echocardiogram.[76] Several factors can negatively influence the transition from pediatric to adult care, including lack of knowledge about potential outcomes, lack of symptoms, the sense of cure after treatment, change in environment from pediatric to adult providers, prior dependence on parents/guardians to manage medical issues, and lack of a transition plan.[77] In addition, there is variability between centers regarding upper age limit at which patients may be seen, meaning some individuals who were previously well served by a pediatric center may find no equivalent if they "age out" of their institution.

MANAGEMENT STRATEGIES

There are studies addressing therapies for cardiotoxicity in adult survivors of childhood cancer; however, pediatric-specific data are lacking.[78,79] Therefore, management of CTRC in children is largely based on adult experience. Adult heart failure guidelines are enhanced by cardio-oncology–specific recommendations that include guidelines for management in response to changes in cardiovascular imaging and serum biomarkers and the presence of heart failure symptoms, and are directed by specific oncologic exposures. However, it should be acknowledged that because of the lack of robust data showing efficacy and the potential adverse effects of treatment, the use of standard heart failure therapies in children with CTRC remains controversial.[80,81]

Pharmacologic Therapies

Standard heart failure therapies have shown benefit in adults with CTRC, including angiotensin-converting enzyme inhibitors, β-blockers, and statins.[82–84] Comparable data in the pediatric population are limited. Angiotensin-converting enzyme inhibitors have been shown to improve markers of subclinical cardiac dysfunction in children and have also been shown to decrease left ventricular end-systolic wall stress.[85,86] A small retrospective study in survivors of pediatric cancer showed improvements in left ventricular dimensions, mass, afterload, and systolic function with angiotensin-converting enzyme inhibitor therapy. However, these benefits were not sustained, with subsequent deterioration after 6 years on therapy.[87] In one small single-center study, pretreatment with a β-blocker provided a potential protective effect for children with acute lymphoblastic leukemia, improving echocardiographic indices and inhibiting troponin leak following anthracycline administration.[88] In addition, there is an ongoing randomized controlled trial to assess the efficacy of carvedilol in preventing the development of left ventricular dysfunction in survivors of childhood cancer.[89] There are no data available on the cardioprotective effect of statins in children; however, in women with breast cancer receiving anthracycline chemotherapy, statin therapy was associated with a lower risk of heart failure.[84]

Timing of Therapy Initiation

The optimal timing and strategy for therapy initiation is unclear given the lack of available data. Although practitioners may not initiate heart failure therapies in the absence of objective changes in ventricular performance, there is increasing evidence to suggest that assessment of EF and/or SF are inadequate to detect subclinical myocardial dysfunction.[85] Up to 65% of children with acute lymphoblastic leukemia show progressive cardiac abnormalities 6 years following anthracycline completion.[90–92] Therefore, there may be some children with subclinical myocardial changes with normal ventricular function based on conventional measures. As cardiac imaging techniques evolve, including the increased use of myocardial strain and CMR, the threshold to detect and initiate heart failure therapies may change. However, the benefits of early therapy initiation remain unclear.

Risk Factor Mitigation and Modifiable Risk Factors

Cancer survivors may be at greater risk for the development of premature cardiovascular disease secondary to modifiable risk factors including hypertension, hyperlipidemia, diabetes, obesity, and sedentary lifestyle.[93–96] Addressing modifiable risk factors is of paramount importance in this population, which has a baseline risk of cardiovascular disease that is greater than the general population. Survivors of childhood cancer are more likely to have an inactive lifestyle compared with age-matched and sex-matched peers without cancer.[97,98] Aerobic exercise can mitigate certain aspects of CTRC; however, the specific mechanism of this benefit remains unclear.[99] The benefits of exercise also include improvement in cardiovascular function, body composition, immune function, chemotherapy completion rates, muscle strength and flexibility, and mood, as well as a reduction in medication side effects, stress, and anxiety.[59] A recent scientific statement from the American Heart Association proposes use of cardio-oncology rehabilitation to manage cardiovascular outcomes in survivors, including those of pediatric cancers.[100]

Advanced Heart Failure Therapies

Patients who fail maximal medical therapy for heart failure may require more advanced therapies, which could include the need for continuous inotropic support, mechanical circulatory support, or even consideration of heart transplant. Active malignancy is considered a contraindication to heart transplant at most pediatric heart transplant centers. However, in the absence of ongoing malignancy following completion of therapy and if the risk of recurrence of the tumor is deemed to be low, transplant may be considered. For appropriately selected patients, recent data suggest that posttransplant graft survival in patients with CTRC is comparable with that of children with dilated cardiomyopathy of other causes.[101] For patients with progressive cardiac dysfunction or for whom it is not currently appropriate to consider transplant, mechanical circulatory support may be considered as a bridge to transplant, a bridge to decision, or as destination therapy.[102]

The Role of Cardiology/Cardio-Oncology in the Care of Survivors of Pediatric Cancers

Cardiac-related mortality in cancer survivors has decreased in association with the use of more contemporary heart failure therapies.[6,103] Despite this improvement, the incidence of severe heart failure in this population has increased.[103] This increase has led to the evolution of cardio-oncology, aiming to provide cardiovascular care to patients throughout cancer therapy and during long-term follow-up.[104] Although there are currently several well-established adult cardio-oncology programs, establishment of similar practices in the pediatric population is equally important. Given the potential for cardiac dysfunction to remain subclinical,[104–107] early cardiology involvement may help to improve recognition of disease, leading to earlier initiation of appropriate therapies with the potential to affect patient outcomes.

Earlier cardiology involvement may also aid in addressing modifiable risk factors for cardiovascular disease. Risk factors present in childhood predict cardiovascular disease in adults.[108] Addressing risk factors in childhood and establishing healthy lifestyle choices early on is important for all children, but likely even more important in cancer survivors, who have a significantly increased risk of future cardiovascular disease. Childhood obesity is increasing, present in approximately 20% of children aged 2 to 19 years.[109] In conjunction with this, hypertension, dyslipidemia, and impaired glucose tolerance are becoming more prevalent.[110]

Communication is also enhanced by involving a cardiologist in the care of children with cancer. A formal pediatric cardio-oncology program could improve the consistency of cardiology involvement in the care of this population. An identified cardio-oncology provider can be a resource for the oncology team, helping to improve communication and collaboration. Families also benefit from cardiology involvement through education regarding the spectrum of cardiac disease seen in cancer survivors, the signs and symptoms of cardiac disease, and education surrounding modifiable cardiac risk factors.

SUMMARY

Cardio-oncology, both pediatric and adult, will continue to evolve as novel pediatric cancer therapies emerge and the population of childhood cancer survivors who require cardiology involvement increases. As this occurs, standardizing the approach to cardiology involvement in the care of this complex group of patients will be critically important. A coordinated effort among pediatric and adult cardio-oncology programs will help to advance multicenter research efforts, better define best practices, and help to further define the role of cardiologists in the care of survivors of childhood cancer.

REFERENCES

1. D'Angio GJ. Pediatric cancer in perspective: cure is not enough. Cancer 1975;35:866–70.
2. Meadows AT, D'Angio GJ. Late effects of cancer treatment: methods and techniques for detection. Semin Oncol 1974;1:87–90.
3. American Cancer Society. Cancer facts & figures 2019. Atlanta (GA): American Cancer Society; 2019.
4. Ward E, DeSantis C, Robbins A, et al. Childhood and adolescent cancer statistics, 2014. CA Cancer J Clin 2014;64:83–103.
5. Robison LL, Hudson MM. Survivors of childhood and adolescent cancer: life-long risks and responsibilities. Nat Rev Cancer 2014;14:61–70.
6. Armstrong GT, Chen Y, Yasui Y, et al. Reduction in late mortality among 5-Year survivors of childhood cancer. N Engl J Med 2016;374:833–42.
7. Gibson TM, Mostoufi-Moab S, Stratton KL, et al. Temporal patterns in the risk of chronic health conditions in survivors of childhood cancer diagnosed 1970-99: a report from the Childhood Cancer Survivor Study cohort. Lancet Oncol 2018;19:1590–601.
8. Armstrong GT, Pan Z, Ness KK, et al. Temporal trends in cause-specific late mortality among 5-year survivors of childhood cancer. J Clin Oncol 2010;28:1224–31.
9. Bhakta N, Liu Q, Ness KK, et al. The cumulative burden of surviving childhood cancer: an initial report from the St Jude Lifetime Cohort Study (SJLIFE). Lancet 2017;390:2569–82.
10. Babiker HM, McBride A, Newton M, et al. Cardiotoxic effects of chemotherapy: a review of both cytotoxic and molecular targeted oncology therapies and their effect on the cardiovascular system. Crit Rev Oncol Hematol 2018;126:186–200.
11. Lipshultz SE, Adams MJ, Colan SD, et al. Long-term cardiovascular toxicity in children, adolescents, and young adults who receive cancer therapy: pathophysiology, course, monitoring, management, prevention, and research directions: a scientific statement from the American Heart Association. Circulation 2013;128:1927–95.
12. Moslehi JJ. Cardiovascular toxic effects of targeted cancer therapies. N Engl J Med 2016;375:1457–67.
13. Neilan TG, Rothenberg ML, Amiri-Kordestani L, et al. Myocarditis associated with immune checkpoint inhibitors: an expert consensus on data gaps and a call to action. Oncologist 2018;23:874–8.
14. Vejpongsa P, Yeh ET. Prevention of anthracycline-induced cardiotoxicity: challenges and opportunities. J Am Coll Cardiol 2014;64:938–45.
15. Ganame J, Claus P, Uyttebroeck A, et al. Myocardial dysfunction late after low-dose anthracycline treatment in asymptomatic pediatric patients. J Am Soc Echocardiography 2007;20:1351–8.
16. Ganame J, Claus P, Eyskens B, et al. Acute cardiac functional and morphological changes after Anthracycline infusions in children. Am J Cardiol 2007;99:974–7.
17. Darby SC, Cutter DJ, Boerma M, et al. Radiation-related heart disease: current knowledge and future prospects. Int J Radiat Oncol Biol Phys 2010;76:656–65.
18. Menezes KM, Wang H, Hada M, et al. Radiation matters of the heart: a mini review. Front Cardiovasc Med 2018;5:83.

19. Krause DS, Van Etten RA. Tyrosine kinases as targets for cancer therapy. N Engl J Med 2005;353:172–87.

20. Kantarjian H, Sawyers C, Hochhaus A, et al. Hematologic and cytogenetic responses to imatinib mesylate in chronic myelogenous leukemia. N Engl J Med 2002;346:645–52.

21. FDA approves Gleevec for pediatric leukemia. FDA Consum 2003;37:6.

22. Druker BJ, Talpaz M, Resta DJ, et al. Efficacy and safety of a specific inhibitor of the BCR-ABL tyrosine kinase in chronic myeloid leukemia. N Engl J Med 2001;344:1031–7.

23. Druker BJ, Guilhot F, O'Brien SG, et al. Five-year follow-up of patients receiving imatinib for chronic myeloid leukemia. N Engl J Med 2006;355:2408–17.

24. Jiao Q, Bi L, Ren Y, et al. Advances in studies of tyrosine kinase inhibitors and their acquired resistance. Mol Cancer 2018;17:36.

25. Chaar M, Kamta J, Ait-Oudhia S. Mechanisms, monitoring, and management of tyrosine kinase inhibitors-associated cardiovascular toxicities. Onco Targets Ther 2018;11:6227–37.

26. Jain D, Russell RR, Schwartz RG, et al. Cardiac complications of cancer therapy: pathophysiology, identification, prevention, treatment, and future directions. Curr Cardiol Rep 2017;19:36.

27. Chu TF, Rupnick MA, Kerkela R, et al. Cardiotoxicity associated with tyrosine kinase inhibitor sunitinib. Lancet 2007;370:2011–9.

28. Ewer MS, Suter TM, Lenihan DJ, et al. Cardiovascular events among 1090 cancer patients treated with sunitinib, interferon, or placebo: a comprehensive adjudicated database analysis demonstrating clinically meaningful reversibility of cardiac events. Eur J Cancer 2014;50:2162–70.

29. Ewer SM, Ewer MS. Cardiotoxicity profile of trastuzumab. Drug Saf 2008;31:459–67.

30. Schmidinger M, Zielinski CC, Vogl UM, et al. Cardiac toxicity of sunitinib and sorafenib in patients with metastatic renal cell carcinoma. J Clin Oncol 2008;26:5204–12.

31. Ladenstein R, Potschger U, Valteau-Couanet D, et al. Interleukin 2 with anti-GD2 antibody ch14.18/CHO (dinutuximab beta) in patients with high-risk neuroblastoma (HR-NBL1/SIOPEN): a multicentre, randomised, phase 3 trial. Lancet Oncol 2018;19:1617–29.

32. Grill J, Massimino M, Bouffet E, et al. Phase II, open-label, randomized, multicenter trial (HERBY) of bevacizumab in pediatric patients with newly diagnosed high-grade glioma. J Clin Oncol 2018;36:951–8.

33. Chisholm JC, Merks JHM, Casanova M, et al. Open-label, multicentre, randomised, phase II study of the EpSSG and the ITCC evaluating the addition of bevacizumab to chemotherapy in childhood and adolescent patients with metastatic soft tissue sarcoma (the BERNIE study). Eur J Cancer 2017;83:177–84.

34. Zhukova N, Rajagopal R, Lam A, et al. Use of bevacizumab as a single agent or in adjunct with traditional chemotherapy regimens in children with unresectable or progressive low-grade glioma. Cancer Med 2019;8:40–50.

35. Chen ZI, Ai DI. Cardiotoxicity associated with targeted cancer therapies. Mol Clin Oncol 2016;4:675–81.

36. Gulati G, Heck SL, Ree AH, et al. Prevention of cardiac dysfunction during adjuvant breast cancer therapy (PRADA): a 2 x 2 factorial, randomized, placebo-controlled, double-blind clinical trial of candesartan and metoprolol. Eur Heart J 2016;37:1671–80.

37. Guglin M, Munster P, Fink A, et al. Lisinopril or Coreg CR in reducing cardiotoxicity in women with breast cancer receiving trastuzumab: a rationale and design of a randomized clinical trial. Am Heart J 2017;188:87–92.

38. Kerr WG, Chisholm JD. The next generation of immunotherapy for cancer: small molecules could make big waves. J Immunol 2019;202:11–9.

39. Jain V, Bahia J, Mohebtash M, et al. Cardiovascular complications associated with novel cancer immunotherapies. Curr Treat Options Cardiovasc Med 2017;19:36.

40. Johnson DB, Balko JM, Compton ML, et al. Fulminant myocarditis with combination immune checkpoint blockade. N Engl J Med 2016;375:1749–55.

41. Heinzerling L, Ott PA, Hodi FS, et al. Cardiotoxicity associated with CTLA4 and PD1 blocking immunotherapy. J Immunother Cancer 2016;4:50.

42. Behling J, Kaes J, Munzel T, et al. New-onset third-degree atrioventricular block because of autoimmune-induced myositis under treatment with anti-programmed cell death-1 (nivolumab) for metastatic melanoma. Melanoma Res 2017;27:155–8.

43. Laubli H, Balmelli C, Bossard M, et al. Acute heart failure due to autoimmune myocarditis under pembrolizumab treatment for metastatic melanoma. J Immunother Cancer 2015;3:11.

44. Semper H, Muehlberg F, Schulz-Menger J, et al. Drug-induced myocarditis after nivolumab treatment in a patient with PDL1- negative squamous cell carcinoma of the lung. Lung Cancer 2016;99:117–9.

45. Mahmood SS, Fradley MG, Cohen JV, et al. Myocarditis in patients treated with immune checkpoint inhibitors. J Am Coll Cardiol 2018;71:1755–64.

46. Mahadeo KM, Khazal SJ, Abdel-Azim H, et al. Management guidelines for paediatric patients receiving chimeric antigen receptor T cell therapy. Nat Rev Clin Oncol 2019;16:45–63.

47. Grupp SA, Kalos M, Barrett D, et al. Chimeric antigen receptor-modified T cells for acute lymphoid leukemia. N Engl J Med 2013;368:1509–18.

48. Maude SL, Frey N, Shaw PA, et al. Chimeric antigen receptor T cells for sustained remissions in leukemia. N Engl J Med 2014;371:1507–17.

49. Burstein DS, Maude S, Grupp S, et al. Cardiac profile of Chimeric antigen receptor T Cell therapy in children: a single-institution experience. Biol Blood Marrow Transplant 2018;24:1590–5.

50. Fitzgerald JC, Weiss SL, Maude SL, et al. Cytokine release syndrome after Chimeric antigen receptor T cell therapy for acute lymphoblastic leukemia. Crit Care Med 2017;45:e124–31.

51. Kenigsberg B, Wellstein A, Barac A. Left ventricular dysfunction in cancer treatment: is it relevant? JACC Heart Fail 2018;6:87–95.

52. Denlinger CS, Sanft T, Baker KS, et al. Survivorship, version 2.2018, NCCN clinical practice guidelines in oncology. J Natl Compr Canc Netw 2018;16: 1216–47.

53. Mulrooney DA, Yeazel MW, Kawashima T, et al. Cardiac outcomes in a cohort of adult survivors of childhood and adolescent cancer: retrospective analysis of the Childhood Cancer Survivor Study cohort. BMJ 2009;339:b4606.

54. Armstrong GT, Oeffinger KC, Chen Y, et al. Modifiable risk factors and major cardiac events among adult survivors of childhood cancer. J Clin Oncol 2013;31:3673–80.

55. Chow EJ, Chen Y, Kremer LC, et al. Individual prediction of heart failure among childhood cancer survivors. J Clin Oncol 2015;33:394–402.

56. Chow EJ, Chen Y, Hudson MM, et al. Prediction of ischemic heart disease and stroke in survivors of childhood cancer. J Clin Oncol 2018;36:44–52.

57. Curigliano G, Cardinale D, Suter T, et al. Cardiovascular toxicity induced by chemotherapy, targeted agents and radiotherapy: ESMO clinical practice guidelines. Ann Oncol 2012;23(Suppl 7):vii155–66.

58. Plana JC, Galderisi M, Barac A, et al. Expert consensus for multimodality imaging evaluation of adult patients during and after cancer therapy: a report from the American Society of Echocardiography and the European Association of Cardiovascular Imaging. J Am Soc Echocardiogr 2014;27: 911–39.

59. Zamorano JL, Lancellotti P, Rodriguez Munoz D, et al. 2016 ESC Position Paper on cancer treatments and cardiovascular toxicity developed under the auspices of the ESC Committee for Practice Guidelines: the Task Force for cancer treatments and cardiovascular toxicity of the European Society of Cardiology (ESC). Eur Heart J 2016;37:2768–801.

60. Virani SA, Dent S, Brezden-Masley C, et al. Canadian cardiovascular society guidelines for evaluation and management of cardiovascular complications of cancer therapy. Can J Cardiol 2016;32:831–41.

61. Armenian SH, Hudson MM, Mulder RL, et al. Recommendations for cardiomyopathy surveillance for survivors of childhood cancer: a report from the International late effects of childhood cancer guideline Harmonization group. Lancet Oncol 2015;16:e123–36.

62. Armenian SH, Lacchetti C, Barac A, et al. Prevention and monitoring of cardiac dysfunction in survivors of adult cancers: American Society of Clinical Oncology clinical practice guideline. J Clin Oncol 2017;35:893–911.

63. Thavendiranathan P, Poulin F, Lim KD, et al. Use of myocardial strain imaging by echocardiography for the early detection of cardiotoxicity in patients during and after cancer chemotherapy: a systematic review. J Am Coll Cardiol 2014;63:2751–68.

64. Armstrong GT, Plana JC, Zhang N, et al. Screening adult survivors of childhood cancer for cardiomyopathy: comparison of echocardiography and cardiac magnetic resonance imaging. J Clin Oncol 2012;30:2876–84.

65. Yu AF, Raikhelkar J, Zabor EC, et al. Two-dimensional speckle tracking echocardiography detects subclinical left ventricular systolic dysfunction among adult survivors of childhood, adolescent, and young adult cancer. Biomed Res Int 2016; 2016:9363951.

66. Pignatelli RH, Ghazi P, Reddy SC, et al. Abnormal myocardial strain indices in children receiving anthracycline chemotherapy. Pediatr Cardiol 2015; 36:1610–6.

67. Galan-Arriola C, Lobo M, Vilchez-Tschischke JP, et al. Serial magnetic resonance imaging to identify early stages of anthracycline-induced cardiotoxicity. J Am Coll Cardiol 2019;73:779–91.

68. Lipshultz SE, Rifai N, Dalton VM, et al. The effect of dexrazoxane on myocardial injury in doxorubicin-treated children with acute lymphoblastic leukemia. N Engl J Med 2004;351:145–53.

69. Mavinkurve-Groothuis AM, Kapusta L, Nir A, et al. The role of biomarkers in the early detection of anthracycline-induced cardiotoxicity in children: a review of the literature. Pediatr Hematol Oncol 2008; 25:655–64.

70. Lipshultz SE, Scully RE, Lipsitz SR, et al. Assessment of dexrazoxane as a cardioprotectant in doxorubicin-treated children with high-risk acute lymphoblastic leukaemia: long-term follow-up of a prospective, randomised, multicentre trial. Lancet Oncol 2010;11:950–61.

71. Lipshultz SE, Miller TL, Scully RE, et al. Changes in cardiac biomarkers during doxorubicin treatment of pediatric patients with high-risk acute lymphoblastic leukemia: associations with long-term echocardiographic outcomes. J Clin Oncol 2012;30:1042–9.

72. Mavinkurve-Groothuis AM, Groot-Loonen J, Bellersen L, et al. Abnormal NT-pro-BNP levels in

asymptomatic long-term survivors of childhood cancer treated with anthracyclines. Pediatr Blood Cancer 2009;52:631–6.

73. Sherief LM, Kamal AG, Khalek EA, et al. Biomarkers and early detection of late onset anthracycline-induced cardiotoxicity in children. Hematology 2012;17:151–6.

74. Krystal JI, Reppucci M, Mayr T, et al. Arterial stiffness in childhood cancer survivors. Pediatr Blood Cancer 2015;62:1832–7.

75. Armenian SH, Rinderknecht D, Au K, et al. Accuracy of a novel handheld wireless platform for detection of cardiac dysfunction in anthracycline-exposed survivors of childhood cancer. Clin Cancer Res 2018;24:3119–25.

76. Nathan PC, Greenberg ML, Ness KK, et al. Medical care in long-term survivors of childhood cancer: a report from the childhood cancer survivor study. J Clin Oncol 2008;26:4401–9.

77. Rosenberg-Yunger ZR, Klassen AF, Amin L, et al. Barriers and facilitators of transition from pediatric to adult long-term follow-up care in childhood cancer survivors. J Adolesc Young Adult Oncol 2013;2:104–11.

78. Sieswerda E, van Dalen EC, Postma A, et al. Medical interventions for treating anthracycline-induced symptomatic and asymptomatic cardiotoxicity during and after treatment for childhood cancer. Cochrane Database Syst Rev 2011;(9):CD008011.

79. Conway A, McCarthy AL, Lawrence P, et al. The prevention, detection and management of cancer treatment-induced cardiotoxicity: a meta-review. BMC Cancer 2015;15:366.

80. Lipshultz SE, Colan SD. Cardiovascular trials in long-term survivors of childhood cancer. J Clin Oncol 2004;22:769–73.

81. Bansal N, Amdani SM, Hutchins KK, et al. Cardiovascular disease in survivors of childhood cancer. Curr Opin Pediatr 2018;30:628–38.

82. Cardinale D, Colombo A, Bacchiani G, et al. Early detection of anthracycline cardiotoxicity and improvement with heart failure therapy. Circulation 2015;131:1981–8.

83. Kalay N, Basar E, Ozdogru I, et al. Protective effects of carvedilol against anthracycline-induced cardiomyopathy. J Am Coll Cardiol 2006;48:2258–62.

84. Seicean S, Seicean A, Plana JC, et al. Effect of statin therapy on the risk for incident heart failure in patients with breast cancer receiving anthracycline chemotherapy: an observational clinical cohort study. J Am Coll Cardiol 2012;60:2384–90.

85. Harrington JK, Richmond ME, Fein AW, et al. Two-dimensional speckle tracking echocardiography-derived strain measurements in survivors of childhood cancer on angiotensin converting enzyme inhibition or receptor blockade. Pediatr Cardiol 2018;39:1404–12.

86. Silber JH, Cnaan A, Clark BJ, et al. Enalapril to prevent cardiac function decline in long-term survivors of pediatric cancer exposed to anthracyclines. J Clin Oncol 2004;22:820–8.

87. Lipshultz SE, Lipsitz SR, Sallan SE, et al. Long-term enalapril therapy for left ventricular dysfunction in doxorubicin-treated survivors of childhood cancer. J Clin Oncol 2002;20:4517–22.

88. El-Shitany NA, Tolba OA, El-Shanshory MR, et al. Protective effect of carvedilol on adriamycin-induced left ventricular dysfunction in children with acute lymphoblastic leukemia. J Card Fail 2012;18:607–13.

89. Armenian SH, Hudson MM, Chen MH, et al. Rationale and design of the Children's Oncology Group (COG) study ALTE1621: a randomized, placebo-controlled trial to determine if low-dose carvedilol can prevent anthracycline-related left ventricular remodeling in childhood cancer survivors at high risk for developing heart failure. BMC Cardiovasc Disord 2016;16:187.

90. Lipshultz SE, Colan SD, Gelber RD, et al. Late cardiac effects of doxorubicin therapy for acute lymphoblastic leukemia in childhood. N Engl J Med 1991;324:808–15.

91. Lipshultz SE, Lipsitz SR, Mone SM, et al. Female sex and drug dose as risk factors for late cardiotoxic effects of doxorubicin therapy for childhood cancer. N Engl J Med 1995;332:1738–43.

92. Harake D, Franco VI, Henkel JM, et al. Cardiotoxicity in childhood cancer survivors: strategies for prevention and management. Future Cardiol 2012;8:647–70.

93. Hutchins KK, Siddeek H, Franco VI, et al. Prevention of cardiotoxicity among survivors of childhood cancer. Br J Clin Pharmacol 2017;83:455–65.

94. Meacham LR, Sklar CA, Li S, et al. Diabetes mellitus in long-term survivors of childhood cancer. Increased risk associated with radiation therapy: a report for the childhood cancer survivor study. Arch Intern Med 2009;169:1381–8.

95. Neville KA, Cohn RJ, Steinbeck KS, et al. Hyperinsulinemia, impaired glucose tolerance, and diabetes mellitus in survivors of childhood cancer: prevalence and risk factors. J Clin Endocrinol Metab 2006;91:4401–7.

96. Armenian SH, Sun CL, Vase T, et al. Cardiovascular risk factors in hematopoietic cell transplantation survivors: role in development of subsequent cardiovascular disease. Blood 2012;120:4505–12.

97. Ness KK, Leisenring WM, Huang S, et al. Predictors of inactive lifestyle among adult survivors of childhood cancer: a report from the Childhood Cancer Survivor Study. Cancer 2009;115:1984–94.

98. Miller TL, Lipsitz SR, Lopez-Mitnik G, et al. Characteristics and determinants of adiposity in pediatric cancer survivors. Cancer Epidemiol Biomarkers Prev 2010;19:2013–22.

99. Chen JJ, Wu PT, Middlekauff HR, et al. Aerobic exercise in anthracycline-induced cardiotoxicity: a systematic review of current evidence and future directions. Am J Physiol Heart Circ Physiol 2017; 312:H213–22.

100. Gilchrist SC, Barac A, Ades PA, et al. Cardio-Oncology Rehabilitation to manage cardiovascular outcomes in cancer patients and survivors: a scientific statement from the American Heart Association. Circulation 2019;139(21):e997–1012.

101. Bock MJ, Pahl E, Rusconi PG, et al. Cancer recurrence and mortality after pediatric heart transplantation for anthracycline cardiomyopathy: a report from the Pediatric Heart Transplant Study (PHTS) group. Pediatr Transplant 2017;21. https://doi.org/10.1111/petr.12923.

102. Cavigelli-Brunner A, Schweiger M, Knirsch W, et al. VAD as bridge to recovery in anthracycline-induced cardiomyopathy and HHV6 myocarditis. Pediatrics 2014;134:e894–9.

103. Feijen E, Font-Gonzalez A, Van der Pal HJH, et al. Risk and temporal changes of heart failure among 5-year childhood cancer survivors: a DCOG-LATER study. J Am Heart Assoc 2019;8:e009122.

104. Kostakou PM, Kouris NT, Kostopoulos VS, et al. Cardio-oncology: a new and developing sector of research and therapy in the field of cardiology. Heart Fail Rev 2019;24:91–100.

105. Mavinkurve-Groothuis AM, Groot-Loonen J, Marcus KA, et al. Myocardial strain and strain rate in monitoring subclinical heart failure in asymptomatic long-term survivors of childhood cancer. Ultrasound Med Biol 2010;36:1783–91.

106. Cetin S, Babaoglu K, Basar EZ, et al. Subclinical anthracycline-induced cardiotoxicity in long-term follow-up of asymptomatic childhood cancer survivors: assessment by speckle tracking echocardiography. Echocardiography 2018;35:234–40.

107. Corella Aznar EG, Ayerza Casas A, Jimenez Montanes L, et al. Use of speckle tracking in the evaluation of late subclinical myocardial damage in survivors of childhood acute leukaemia. Int J Cardiovasc Imaging 2018;34:1373–81.

108. Morrison JA, Friedman LA, Gray-McGuire C. Metabolic syndrome in childhood predicts adult cardiovascular disease 25 years later: the Princeton lipid research clinics follow-up study. Pediatrics 2007; 120:340–5.

109. Skinner AC, Ravanbakht SN, Skelton JA, et al. Prevalence of obesity and severe obesity in US children, 1999-2016. Pediatrics 2018;141(3) [pii: e20173459].

110. Wittcopp C, Conroy R. Metabolic syndrome in children and adolescents. Pediatr Rev 2016;37: 193–202.

111. Sieswerda E, Postma A, van Dalen EC, et al. The Dutch Childhood Oncology Group guideline for follow-up of asymptomatic cardiac dysfunction in childhood cancer survivors. Ann Oncol 2012;23: 2191–8.

Implementing a Cardio-oncology Center of Excellence
Nuts and Bolts, Including Coding and Billing

Anita M. Arnold, DO, MBA[a],*, Cathleen Biga, MSN[b]

KEYWORDS

- Cardio-oncology service line • Financial • Coding • Billing

KEY POINTS

Developing and sustaining a cardio-oncology program has 3 key components:

- Establishing the need: would the oncology and cardiology communities support a program; is there competition that would have a negative impact on the program; and is there administrative support for a dedicated cardio-oncology program?
- Developing the program: it must address community needs and the organizational strategy for service line development. The strategy should consist of an early phase with limited components, followed by expansion as a center of excellence.
- Financing the program: establishing the up-front clinical needs, payor mix, and services required as well as attention to billing and coding to maximize sustainability and growth of the program is paramount.

INTRODUCTION: WHAT IS CARDIO-ONCOLOGY AND WHY IS IT NEEDED?

Cardio-oncology is an evolving subspecialty of cardiology that deals with the acute and long-term care of cancer patients as well as cancer survivors. It has developed in concordance with the advances in oncology that have vastly increased the armamentarium of therapies for cancer patients and the subsequent cardiac toxicities that have emerged, both during therapy and sometimes decades later as cancer-related cardiac dysfunction.[1] The enormous complexity of the cancer treatments, with the myriad cardiac issues that can arise during therapy, mandate a collaboration that is diverse, knowledgeable, streamlined, cost efficient, and, most of all, able to navigate patients through an increasingly complicated health care system in a timely fashion.[2] Although the prototype for cardiotoxicity is the anthracyclines, initial reports were of their cancer benefit[3,4] and it was not until later that cardiotoxicity was reported. It was usually the oncologist who managed screening with periodic multigated acquisition scanning and referred to cardiology at later stages.[5] Eventually, increasing cardiac toxicities were seen, not only from older agents like anthracyclines but also with contemporary agents as well. This was most notable in childhood cancer survivors, where the rate of

Disclosures: C. Biga is the owner of Cardiovascular Management of Illinois. A.M. Arnold has nothing to disclose.
[a] Florida State University School of Medicine, Cardio-Oncology, Lee Health, 9800 South Health Park Drive #320, Ft Myers, FL 33908, USA; [b] Cardiovascular Management of Illinois, 900 South Frontage Road, Suite 325, Woodridge, IL 60517, USA
* Corresponding author.
E-mail address: Anita.Arnold@leehealth.org

0733-8651/19/© 2019 Elsevier Inc. All rights reserved.

subsequent cardiac death was more common than recurrent cancer.[6] This sparked an interest in cancer-related cardiac dysfunction as a consequence of cancer cure or transformation to a chronic disease, leading some to advocate for a cardio-oncology specialty.[7,8]

The American College of Cardiology (ACC) has supported the creation of a Council of Cardio-Oncology with multiple working groups to advance the field with evidence-based recommendations. Training programs are being developed,[9] and the council has begun educating lawmakers and health policy advisors about the specialty and advocating for cardio-oncology patients. A 2014 needs assessment of cardiology program directors about cardio-oncology reported 27% of centers had dedicated cardio-oncology programs, but only 12% were developing service lines. More than 70%, however, agreed that cardiac complications were increasingly common in cancer patients, and felt a cardio-oncology program would improve overall patient care.[10,11] A more contemporary survey of practicing cardiologists in Florida noted half had no cardio-oncology program at their institutions and only 18% were comfortable treating cardiac complications due to cancer therapy, which speaks to the need for further education of practitioners as well as development of formal cardio-oncology training programs.[12] As a testament to the need, there has been a huge increase in cardio-oncology publications, conferences with dedicated cardio-oncology lectures, and whole conferences devoted to the emerging field and its needs (imaging, training, research, coding, and billing as well as funding), to name a few.

SHOULD A CARDIO-ONCOLOGY PROGRAM BE STARTED?

Similar to deciding on the development of any service line, the decision to develop a cardio-oncology program for an institution takes some research and planning. There is no question that some of the drivers for cardio-oncology programs are unique. The shifting paradigm of cancer becoming a chronic disease, with therapies lasting years, requires long-term follow-up for ongoing cardiac toxicity. As more cancer patients are cured and enter the survivorship phase, there needs to be identification of those at risk and strategies for how best to monitor long-term cancer therapy–related cardiac disease. It has been estimated that by 2040, the number of cancer survivors in the United States will increase by approximately 11 million: from 15.5 million in 2016 to 26.1 million in 2040. The proportion of

survivors older than age 65 will increase from 61 years to 73 years. By 2040, only 18% of cancer survivors will be between ages 50 and 64, and 8% will be less than age 50. This represents a very elderly population of patients who have suffered cardiotoxic therapy and also are susceptible to cardiovascular disease due to aging alone. This is the so-called silver tsunami population that will undoubtedly benefit from cardio-oncology while undergoing treatment and follow-up in the years to come (D. Sadler, personal communication, 2019). This aging of the cancer population will add to the cost of health care along with struggles with with physician shortages, burnout, and health care funding.[13] Providing cardio-oncology services early in the treatment plan would mitigate early toxicity and allow for proactive treatment as well as surveillance protocols for survivors. This should result in better outcomes at lesser cost for these patients.

Cancer and heart disease traditionally have been the 2 leading causes of death in the United States,[14] and it stands to reason that many patients suffer both diseases. For those with advanced heart disease who develop cancer, there are unique challenges for which cardio-oncology would be most beneficial. This will require multiple types of providers, some of whom may be shared with the oncology service line to benefit the patients and providers on multiple levels (such as social work, pharmacy, and rehabilitation services).

Cardio-oncology is a fast-growing field and the questions are whether or not an institution should commit to a dedicated program to develop a center of excellence and how that would be structured to best serve the community.[15] Similar to many other advances in cardiology (electrophysiology [EP] and ablation; structural heart disease with transcatheter aortic value replacement; and MitraClip, Human Cells, Tissues and Organs, or transplantation services), it first needs to be decided if this service line can be supported or if it is even needed at a particular institution. The benefits of such a program would first be to the cancer and cardiac patients cared for as well as the providers who need expertise in problems that can arise during cancer treatment and survivorship. The complexity of caring for cancer patients has grown to the point that a dedicated program in most institutions would greatly benefit the streamlined, collaborative care of these patients as well as allow them to remain locally for their care. It is estimated that 30% of all patients undergoing cancer therapy have some cardiovascular issues associated with their care, with cardiovascular disease as the leading cause of morbidity and mortality in the years after cancer treatment.[16]

The structure of an organization is a critical first step in deciding if it should have a stand-alone cardio-oncology program, or perhaps, if an organization has already started down the path of having a cardiovascular service line, it may be the best option to develop a cardio-oncology center of excellence. As cardiology continues to be subspecialized (structural heart, athletic heart, EP, vascular, and so forth), it is paramount to design the clinical, financial, operational, and quality aspects of this broad spectrum of care across a continuum. Starting with the overall strategy of a cardiovascular service line allows for the creation of subspecialties as they evolve.

WHICH PATIENTS WOULD BE EXPECTED TO BENEFIT FROM THE SERVICE LINE?

It is anticipated that 3 types of patients would benefit from a cardio-oncology program:

1. Cancer patients who are undergoing treatment with potentially cardiotoxic therapy (chemotherapy or radiation therapy) or surgery for cancer treatment, to have a risk assessment prior to undergoing any therapy and optimize their cardiovascular status.
2. Patients with known cardiac disease who develop cancer: to insure they can withstand the rigors of treatment and avoid worsening of their cardiac status as well as work with the oncology team in unique patient circumstances: patients needing dual anti-platelet therapy for coronary stenting who may develop pancytopenia; patients needing anticoagulation for atrial fibrillation, with arrhythmias and ischemic heart disease; and patients with limited life expectancy, cardiomyopathy, and possible device therapy.
3. Survivor of cancer need surveillance, especially childhood cancers with treatment usually involving anthracyclines and radiation and where there is an 80% 5-year survival; with 50% of subsequent deaths due to cardiac disease. The longer a childhood cancer survivor lives, the more likely the patient is to develop cardiac disease but at a much earlier age than siblings or aged-matched cohorts.[17] These patients require follow-up for years and may develop any number of cardiac comorbidities as a result of their childhood therapies.

WHAT SHOULD BE THE GOALS OF A PROGRAM?

Within the mission statement of an organization, the vision of the service line (the goals of a cardio-oncology program) should focus on providing services that

- Ensure better outcomes (early and late) for patients with heart disease and cancer
- Recognize early cardiotoxicity of cancer therapy and how best to prevent and manage
- Prevent, reduce, and, if possible, reverse cardiac damage that has occurred
- Develop collaborative research with others in the community and nationally
- Remove cardiac disease as a barrier to effective cancer therapy and prevent delays in cancer treatment
- Participate in establishing survival standards for cardiac surveillance

It is anticipated that by providing cardio-oncology services within the cancer community, earlier toxicities can be better managed and possibly subsequent future outcomes improved.[18]

GETTING STARTED; WHICH BASELINE DATA ARE NEEDED?

Although it seems intuitive from the previous discussion, it is imperative to do some background research for an organization before embarking on program development. The administrative staff will expect the following issues to be addressed:

1. What are the demographics—the age, socio-economics, mobility, and education—of the service area? What is the geographic referral area? How many patients are served and what is the payor mix? Studies show that patients are more likely to participate in clinical studies and engage in health care if delivered locally, which is important for program development.[19]
2. What is the incidence of cancer within the community; are there specific types and do they differ by gender, ethnicity, or age? These data are available from a cancer registry or from the American Cancer Society.[20]
3. Are there already robust oncology and cardiology service lines to support the care for these complex patients? Do they perceive that this center of excellence within their existing service line is needed (if the initial response is "no," that may be the perfect place to start, with education of the medical community as to the services of cardio-oncology and how it would

benefit patients and providers; try to identify gaps in knowledge and start to bridge them)?

4. Is there a nearby a university/academic/cancer program that already meets the cardio-oncology needs of the community? Are patients more likely to go out of the area to those programs? These data may be able to be extrapolated from other types of cancer programs within the institution.

5. Who regionally has or could easily develop a cardio-oncology program, and how likely is it that patients would go there for their cardio-oncology care (classic SWOT analysis, looking realistically at institutional strengths, weaknesses, opportunities, and threats)?

6. While working within the team, the creation of a 5-year, financial forecast often is required. This focused approach to new program development pulls together all those elements needed for a successful program and allows for the setting of realistic expectations in the financial component of the program development.

   a. The key elements of a successful development of an accurate financial forecast should include payor mix (what insurances are in the market area), patient volume, services that are needed (*Current Procedural Terminology* [*CPT*] codes), average reimbursement/*CPT* code/payor, what staff are required, how much space is needed, and what staff are required to perform these services. A critical but often overlooked element of the financial forecast is what hospital administrators refer to as down-stream revenue. What services are anticipated that this subset of patients will require—imaging, procedures, and laboratories are just a few of the considerations that should be incorporated into this 5-year, financial forecast. This will give the administration the needed information—in addition to the clinical component—necessary to make these decisions.

   b. The most successful programs have a dyad/triad relationship—the cardiologist, the oncologist, and the administrator—all are required to ensure the appropriate resources are planned for and the execution of the plan seamless.

Once it has been ascertained that a cardio-oncology program is needed in an area, the needed financial resources identified, and there are clinicians to support the program, the help of key stakeholders crucial for supporting the program must be engaged. A great place to start is with the oncology providers (medical, radiation,

and surgical) as well as the cardiology groups in the area. It is important to address 2 key concepts:

1. A cardio-oncologist can provide an expertise for cancer patients that would be helpful during therapy and survivorship time frames (in other words, How is this program different from the cardiology already available, and why should resources be devoted to this program?). A mini-survey of providers regarding their understanding and use (if subsequently available) of cardio-oncology services may help understand not only the needs but also the potential referral patterns of the institution.

2. Cardiology colleagues can be reassured that the cardio-oncologist will be the liaison for events during the cancer therapy and assist in long-term follow-up as needed. It would be inconceivable to care for all the needs of the cardio-oncology population, and, over time, most programs have expanded so certain members of the cardiac team (interventional and EP) have developed expertise in caring for these patients as well. It serves to elevate the entire spectrum of cardiac and oncologic care for the community.

Once a collegiality is established for the program's existence, buy-in from the hospital's administration is needed; explain the vision so that they see the potential of such a program and are willing to support the service line. One word of caution is to not go too far with the clinical set up without bringing in the administrator dyad—and if there is not one in cardio-oncology, it is good to find a nurse, advanced practice provider, or administrator who understands hospital politics/financials/process to help take this project from design through implementation. Likely there will be questions about how the service line will grow, what is needed to get started, if it will support itself with downstream revenue, how long would that take, and so forth. These issues are a bit harder to get at, but several programs have benchmarked early successes.[21]

WHO IS ACTUALLY PART OF THE CARDIO-ONCOLOGY TEAM?

Initially, it is expected the team would be small and then expanded as a program develops. At minimum, a team should be 3 dedicated persons who are the base of the cardio-oncology program; this can easily evolve from an existing cardiology practice:

1. Cardio-oncologist: in most cases the cardio-oncologist is not formally trained but has a

passion for providing care for the cancer patient. Working with an oncologist who will assist in building the program and help identify the needs of the oncology community is vital.

2. Nurse: helps navigate referrals, coordinate testing and visits, facilitate communication among the various providers, and helps triage patients and procedures and be the link between other service lines. The nurse also is instrumental in teaching cancer nurse navigators about cardio-oncology and is available for early and quick consultation.

3. Dedicated cardiac sonographer who images most, if not all the cardio-oncology patients, with an expertise in strain or 3-D imaging. Ideally this service should be offered same day and on site if possible.

BUT SPECIFICALLY, HOW TO BEGIN?

Most cardio-oncology programs started by having a dedicated cardiologist start to detail the vision and dream to others. Begin at a place that feels comfortable, for example, start attending tumor boards or a multidisciplinary breast clinic, with an introduction as cardio-oncology, and join the discussions. Offering to help staff manage their high-risk cardiac patients or being a resource is beneficial and helps to grow the program. If possible, have office space (even 1–2 days a week) physically located near the oncology team, making it easier for oncology (and their staff) to think of cardio-oncology and send patients for evaluation. Many of the most successful multidisciplinary clinics start with a simple time share agreement—take 4 hours 2 times a month in an oncology office. Alternatively, depending on the specific situation, perhaps a clinic in the hospital would offer more of a Switzerland-like approach—one where several oncologists feel comfortable referring. There will be hurdles to plan for—such as electronic health records (EHRs), billing, and staffing; but those are all resolvable elements that an administrative team can help plan for and execute a solid implementation strategy for. In some practices, offering same-day cardio-oncology consultations, or 24-hour to 48-hour turnaround for preoperative clearance for oncologic surgery, for example, has provided great value to the oncology teams. Several PowerPoint presentations should be prepared for the general public, especially cancer support groups with patients and family members (let them help drive the discussion of need for the program) as well as targeted to physician groups at the hospital, local medical society, nurses, and training programs in the area.

If possible, get the hospital to publish blogs on its Web site (or on the cancer Web site) about available cardio-oncology services and printed brochures about how to get in touch and why the services are important; call local media outlets describing the new program and its benefit for the community. The hospital may help with many of the media concerns because they are usually looking for ways to celebrate their services to the community. Do not underestimate the power of word of mouth; patients usually are involved in many community groups (Rotary, Knights of Columbus, Shriners, and so forth) as well as church groups (with parish nurses). Try to get as much exposure as possible to these community resources to help grow the program and spread awareness of cardio-oncology.

Considering a cardio-oncologist is probably practicing general cardiology as well, it becomes important to identify the cardio-oncology population of a practice. The receptionist and scheduler, as well as triage nurse, need to ask patients if they are cardio-oncology, because they may have special concerns, and triage them appropriately. Our staff has reacted with the utmost empathy and compassion and gone to great lengths to accommodate the needs of cardio-oncology patients. They understand the urgency of doing an "add-on echocardiogram with strain" to allow the next dose of chemotherapy, they facilitate communication for cardio-oncology patients, and they have at numerous times adjusted schedules to accommodate the needs of the patients. There is a sense of double urgency to help these patients with 2 of the most devastating illnesses a person can have, cancer and heart disease. The authors are blessed for having such a wonderful staff, and as a program develops, I trust it will have a similar experience. Staff also will make a program a success and help grow the service line.

Considering most cardio-oncology programs initially are not physically located in or near the oncology offices, there may be a degree of disconnect that does not allow for early patient referral or dialogue. This needs to be addressed by having cardio-oncology as part of the initial treatment team similar to palliative care. Studies have shown integrating palliative care services early in cancer care provided better outcomes for patients,[11] Cardio-oncology should be integrated into the cancer care program and be delivered through interdisciplinary cardio-oncology teams, with consultation available early in the course of therapy.

USE ELECTRONIC RECORDS

It is helpful to have information technology (IT) involved early, because tracking cardio-oncology patients and being able to prove service line growth and downstream revenue are important. A few simple ideas from IT have proved helpful, and, as the program expands, other ways to utilize IT to provide better care for patients may be found:

1. Some EHRs have imbedded registries that can pull patient information that may be found helpful. In particular, the authors chose to merge some fields from the cancer registry as well as from certain of the cardiovascular registries (heart failure, arrhythmia, coronary artery disease, device implantation, hypertension, and hyperlipidemia) and add specific fields to track, such as assessment of left ventricular function. This eliminated having to duplicate all the demographics and, if the fields already exist, a separate cardio-oncology registry can be created at a fairly low cost.

2. Best practice alerts can identify patients with cancer (the authors excluded nonmelanoma skin cancers) AND certain high-risk features for heart disease, OR known heart disease by a pop-up that asks if a patient may benefit from a cardio-oncology consult. Keep in mind there are a lot of best practice alerts and they may get ignored. The field may be limited to a specific cancer initially and to see if it drives referrals. If, after a period of time, it is more of an annoyance to the providers, that strategy may be rethought.

3. The authors recently developed a strategy to have the cancer intake nurses use a brief chart, adapted from a Mayo Clinic strategy that identifies high-risk patients and generates a referral to cardio-oncology for a cardiac risk assessment and ongoing follow-up if indicated. After discussion and evaluating the evidence of cardio-oncology data, leadership felt best practices dictated an automatic referral for high-risk patients.

4. Other cardio-oncology programs have used a pharmacy database, such that when an order is written for a cardiotoxic agent, a cardio-oncology consult is suggested to the prescribing oncologist. This may be difficult in situations with multiple EHRs or providers not integrated in the same health system.

5. An efficient way to help with differing EHRs is to obtain permission for a read-only status. Cardio-oncology can access real-time records without having to do a formal record release and wait for the data. Within the authors' program, only the cardio-oncologist and nurse have that access.

6. A simple way to identify and track a patient as cardio-oncology is to have scheduling identify the visit type as cardio-oncology. The authors have created 4 visit types that can subsequently be tracked and analyzed:
   a. Cardio-oncology consult
   b. Cardio-oncology follow-up
   c. Cardio-oncology preoperative clearance
   d. Cardio-oncology survivorship

ORGANIZATION OF THE CARDIO-ONCOLOGY PROGRAM

As a program grows, there are several suggested team members[22,23] but, ultimately, it will be the needs of the community and referring oncology providers that help drive the direction of the program. Many cardio-oncology programs have evolved based on the needs of their patients and particular champions for the program.[24]

The authors' program has evolved to include other team members believed needed to care for cardio-oncology patients (**Fig. 1**). They have proved to be an integral part of the cardio-oncology team and add greatly to the patient experience and satisfaction. As a team continues with needs assessments for the community, it may be found that other services should be added. For example, in rural areas or socioeconomically disadvantaged communities, help may be needed with transportation or child care for patients to benefit from the services. Paying for prescription therapies is challenging enough with both cancer and heart disease; patients may need help navigating the financial programs available for them. Language services are important, and not all of these services need to be provided by high-cost employees. A 2017 study from the University of Alabama used a novel approach using lay navigators to assist patients throughout their cancer experience and noted a significant decrease in overall cancer costs, with increased patient satisfaction.[25] Dieticians, social workers, and exercise physiologists may all need to become part of this new team. Looking past normal treatment modalities will expand a center of excellence and treat the whole patient. There is a movement to try to include cardio-oncology patients into a cardiac/oncology rehabilitation–like environment—all of these dedicated specialties should be evaluated as potential team members. This speaks to

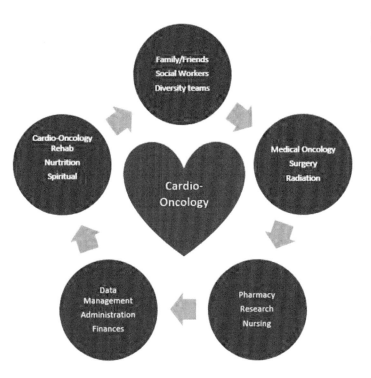

Fig. 1. Components of the cardio-oncology program, Lee Health.

WHICH ANCILLARY CARDIO-ONCOLOGY SERVICES SHOULD BE PROVIDED?

Cardio-oncology patients present unique challenges and require collaboration with other cardiovascular specialists to provide care that does not compromise the oncologic treatment of the patient. Unique situations, such as treatment of ischemia with antiplatelets, need to be discussed with oncology due to pancytopenia with chemotherapy, or, if there is a need for urgent oncologic surgery, then revascularization with a bare metal stent or even balloon angioplasty may be more appropriate for this type of patient, rather than a drug-eluting stent, or maximization of medical therapy without stenting to get the patient through a critical point in the oncologic care. Arrhythmia is common both in the cardiac and oncologic patient but especially with certain anticancer therapies. Anticoagulation and antiarrhythmic strategies (long corrected QT interval [QTc] frequently is seen in many cancer patients) can significantly compromise the oncology treatment plan if not discussed in advance with EP and oncology colleagues. This also is important with device therapy and pacemaker placement with respect to radiation fields and life expectancy. The multidisciplinary heart failure team often is involved when there is acute cardiac decompensation as with myocarditis but can help as a resource for chronic failure as well. Expertise in cardiovascular imaging in an institution to assess left ventricular function is critical to follow oncology patients exposed to cardiotoxic agents. Although many institutions are using echocardiography particularly with strain or 3-D imaging, the cardiac sonographers should be trained and comfortable with the technology before the team makes treatment decisions based on strain or 3-D. Many programs (the authors' included) try to keep the bulk of the strain work with 1 or 2 technicians and reporting cardiologists. Cardiac magnetic resonance is still the gold standard for left ventricular assessment but for any number of reasons is not as accessible, although indications are expanding, especially in survivorship programs.[26,27] The most important part of cardio-oncology is to monitor for possible early cardiac complications that may require interruptions in oncologic therapy[28] and to minimize the impact on the cancer therapy. It involves a true collaboration of cardiovascular and oncologic teams, and the cardio-oncologist is the bridge for those interactions.

TAKE ADVANTAGE OF NETWORKING

As the specialty of cardio-oncology grows, local networking with other cardiologists interested in the field is helpful. Some groups have created monthly meetings to discuss interesting or challenging cases, others a yearly cardio-oncology update at ACC chapter meetings. The national ACC, Council of Cardio-Oncology, and CardioSource Web sites are excellent places to take advantage of national and international expertise in the field. The number of outstanding cardio-oncology meetings nationally and internationally grows yearly and provides an excellent venue for networking.

MAKING A PROGRAM FINANCIALLY VIABLE

A cardio-oncology program can be a valuable asset to a system, providers, and patients who are affected by cancer. But the reality is that in the current health care environment, a program must be financially solvent. Initially, a program may be an extension of a particular cardiology group or a cardiology department but eventually will need a separate cost center to support its work. In order to truly organize and implement a successful cardio-oncology center of excellence, a solid financial footing is mandatory. In addition to that initial financial forecast discussed previously, a solid understanding of the socioeconomic infrastructure is critical to developing a successful program. Some of these topics have been outlined in recent publications,[29] but the following section may help to build on that foundation.

START WITH THE BASICS

It might be best to start with a basic outline of health care economics—how do healthcare providers get paid for what they do? Health care economics often is referred to as the allocation of scarce health care resources.[30] Understanding the elements that are critical in the payment of services will help create a successful program that is viable and sustainable. It also is important to identify where health care economics is today—moving from a fee-for-service model to a value world.

Health care in the Unites States has dominated the social, political, and financial arena in the past decade. Although it is assumed that the United States having some of the best medical care is the explanation for higher costs, facts do not bear that out. In the United States, health care costs are indeed the highest in the world, yet the overall health of the population lags far behind other countries that spend much less. An analysis comparing health care spending, supply, utilization, prices, and health outcomes across 13 high-income countries shows the United States in 2013 spent far more on health care than these other countries. Despite this, Americans had poor health outcomes, including shorter life expectancy and higher rates of chronic conditions.[31] As a comparison, the United States spends 17.1% of the gross national product on health care whereas the United Kingdom spends less than that at 8.8% with better outcomes.[32] That model of increased spending with worse outcomes is not sustainable.

Although the debate as to why the United States spends so much and has worse outcomes is ongoing, the government has been trying not only to change the way it is practices (focusing more on evidence-based guidelines) but also to restructure the payment system that was spiraling out of control. Each year the government relied on the sustainable growth rate to hold down costs. The sustainable growth rate was part of the budget act of 1997 and proposed that if spending exceeded the expected target, then the payments to physicians would be cut to keep spending in check.[33] Year after year, as spending increased, the House of Medicine would descend on Capitol Hill and lobby for a real fix for the problem.

The paradigm shift that was thought to have been occurring rapidly has accelerated 10-fold in the past 24 months (2017–2019). In the past, health care focused largely on fee-for-service care, with providers paid by the number of visits, services, and tests ordered. The Institute for Healthcare Improvement launched the Triple Aim in October of 2007, which was designed to help health care organizations and providers redesign health care delivery. The belief was that new processes must be redesigned and adopted that would simultaneously pursue 3 dimensions:

1. Improve the patient experience of care (quality AND satisfaction).
2. Improve the health of populations.
3. Reduce the per capita cost of health care.

This compass of health care slowly but surely became widely accepted and yet there was an unexpected and unintended consequence—provider burn out. This has now evolved to what is commonly referred to as the Quadruple Aim—adding the prevention of provider burnout to the dimensions of the Triple Aim. The passage of the Affordable Care Act and the Health Care and Education Reconciliation Act in 2010 continued the comprehensive health care reform whose impact has been felt for the past 5 years and continues today in 2019 and will for years to come.[34] This act set the stage for rapid changes in health care delivery. It became imperative for every provider to look at how, when, where, and why health care is delivered.

With the advent of the Department of Health and Human Services (HHS) mandate released on January 26, 2015, and the passage of Medicare Access and Children's Health Insurance Program (CHIP) Reauthorization Act (MACRA) on April 20, 2015, the transition to payment based on the value of care delivered truly ramped up. The HHS mandate set the stage for payment reform—30% of all Medicare payments by the end of 2016 to be paid via alternative payment models (and not fee for service); and by the end of 2018, 90% of all payments would be tied to quality or value—with 50% paid via alternative payment models (Medicare Shares Savings, Next Generation Accountable Care Organizations, and so forth).

The result is MACRA—now referred to as Quality Payment Program—will continue to move the focus from fee-for-service to value-based payments. This has proponents and detractors on both sides, but it makes sense to be the best custodian of health care dollars and focus on providing the best care for patients at the same time. The value of work is publicly reported, accessible by consumers as well as payors. In 2019, one of the issues that providers are facing is that because the data collected are assessing outcomes as value, they ultimately will reflect financially on physician's compensation, both as bonuses and penalties. Many physicians in the United States are integrated and now work for a health care system. Some of those physicians have deluded themselves into thinking they are no longer responsible for data, coding, or documentation that supports a level of service, that it has become the system's problem. That may seem correct, but if the physicians do not code properly or document appropriately, billing is suboptimal, and patients cannot be cared for as cuts are made in staff and services. Providers need to understand how much of the data are reported and how personal data can be viewed, to see where there may be gaps in documentation. This becomes the infrastructure on the economic base for a successful cardio-oncology program.

REIMBURSEMENT IS EASY

In order to build a program, a few basics are critical, starting with how providers are paid. There are several fee schedules that are critical to understand in the realm of cardio-oncology:

1. The physician fee schedule—this is the mechanism whereby most Medicare Part B services are paid. It also is the followed (eventually) by most of the private payors—but it is critical to review and analyze how private payors interpret the rules.
   a. The physician fee schedule is a complete list of fees used by Medicare to pay doctors and other providers (advanced practice practitioners and suppliers). This is the base of the current fee-for-service model of payment.
   b. *CPT* codes (there are 3 levels of *CPT* codes—this article concentrates on Level 1). Level 1 CPT codes are divided into 6 categories that include work done in evaluation and management (E/M) (office/hospital visits, surgery, radiology, anesthesiology, pathology, and laboratory).
   c. ICD 10 is mechanism used to document the current medical classification of codes for diseases, signs and symptoms, abnormal findings, complaints, and so forth. This is referred to the diagnosis used for what is done (the *CPT* code) and results in payment.
2. The hospital outpatient prospective payment system (HOPPS) also referred to as hospital outpatient department (HOPD) is how Medicare pays for outpatient care—based on where the care was rendered. A hospital outpatient department may be physically located on the hospital campus, or it may be off-campus but following specific/complex rules.
   a. In use since 2000, HOPPS pays based on ambulatory payment classifications, which are designed for payment for services that have similar clinical characteristics and costs.

Cardio-oncology programs will use both these systems for payment. In addition, it is critical to understand that the Medicare payments are determined by local entities, called Medicare Administrative Contractors (MACs). The MACs are awarded geographic jurisdiction to process Medicare Part A and Part B claims for beneficiaries. There currently are 12 MACs that provide these services across the United States. It is critical to know who the carriers are because they are the ones that interpret the Medicare rules. Without getting too complicated, there are 2 main ways MACs adjudicate the bills submitted—local coverage determinations (LCDs) and national coverage determinations. If national coverage determinations are thought of as the basement—the minimal elements that must be met for being paid—these must be followed by every MAC. The LCDs, on the other hand are determined by the local MAC and often are where physicians go for help in adding *ICD-10* codes to a specific test (such as echocardiogram with strain) in order to get paid. THIS IS THE MOST CRITICAL THING TO UNDERSTAND IN DESIGNING A PROGRAM. If a cardio-oncologist is not getting paid for the diagnoses they use in this subset of patients, the cardio-oncologist needs to find the local MAC medical director, meet with that person, present data and rationale, and request a change in the LCD. It is possible that the state ACC advocacy section may be able to assist.

The national team of cardio-oncologists must band together and work on solutions to this crucial issue—how to get paid for what they do. This is one of the most frustrating elements of a fee for service payment model; imagine if a bundled payment or a payment could be designed for an episode of care that would not be as dependent on ICD-10 codes, CPT codes, and sites of service but just concentrate on providing the best care, in the right environment, and at the right time—what a world that would be for providers and their patients. The discussion on networking is critical and where national ACC health advocacy, in particular, cardio-oncology advocacy, can help.

THE NEXT WORK RELATIVE VALUE UNIT

It is often said that risk scores will become a provider's next benchmark—much like the work relative value unit is today. Yet most providers today pay little to no attention to this critical component of coding and documentation. What is a risk score? And why would providers care?

Risk scores have become foundational for any population health program. It may be asked, what does population health have to do with our cardio-oncology patients? "Everything" is the correct answer! By using big data and large sample sizes to better understand patterns of what is likely to happen to individuals, organizations can develop insights into how each unique patient is progressing along common disease trajectories and plan interventions accordingly. Fundamentally, a risk score is a metric used to determine the likelihood that an individual will experience a particular outcome. Initially used in Medicare Advantage Plans, risk scores are now calculated for every Medicare beneficiary on an annual basis. Although this topic might be found complex, and not one a physician chooses to concentrate on—beware! Oncologists and cardiologists are operating in a whole new world. The new mechanism to account for sick cardio-oncology patients is called hierarchical condition category (HCC) and is a mechanism to account for the additional care and subsequent added costs often associated with these complex patients.[35] A risk adjustment factor that predicts a patient's cost of care

based on both the ICD-10 codes used and how those cross-walk to the HCC codes. It may be asked, Why care? The answer is simple: insurance companies and Medicare see a high-risk adjustment factor and expect the cost of care for the patient will be higher than the benchmark for the primary condition. Patients with chronic conditions, such as cancer and coronary heart disease, need to have all their comorbidities—with as specific a diagnosis as possible—billed for in order for the insurance companies to give weight (value) to these complex patients.

Every provider must begin to understand this topic and ensure that coding and documentation embrace the core concepts. Those critical concepts include

1. Using THE most specific ICD-10 code that describes the reason for a patient's visit. Avoid at all costs unspecified codes. Although all ICD-10 codes do not qualify for HCC codes, all ICD-10 codes are cross-walked.
2. Documenting and billing as many ICD-10 codes as appropriate. If physicians fail to document the comorbidities that are core to the medical decision making in caring for these complex patients, they could be viewed as providing expensive care in a low value manner.
3. Many alternate payment models relying on risk adjustment factors
4. Merit-based incentive payment system (MIPS)—a pathway in Quality Payment Program—uses risk-adjusted scores to determine MIPS scores
5. Many physicians mistakenly thinking that they do not have to code for congestive heart failure, diabetes, hypertension, or other comorbidities, because they are not the principal or primary care physician who is managing those conditions. If a comorbidity influences the cancer or cardiac treatment decision or is assessed during a visit in any way, it should be coded, with a comment that a primary care provider or specialist is managing.[36]

In summary, on this critical element of coding and documentation, ensure the billing system can handle up to 12 ICD-10 codes, remembering that comorbidities need to be documented in the medical record annually, and document all conditions a patient may have that have an impact on the medical decision making.

TYING IT ALL TOGETHER

Although it is impossible to distill coding advice into a single comprehensive article, here are a few key tips—although it is imperative to understand the nuances of each code and use it compliantly. Make sure to be aware of the following codes and use them where appropriate with appropriate documentation:

- Use of communication codes: keep in mind that both telehealth and the new communication codes use technology to communicate, but they are separate and distinct services. Telehealth is meant to be a substitute for an in-person visit and has significant rules that must be followed. The new communication codes (G2012 and G2010) require patient consent and 5 minutes to 10 minutes; the G0071 code is reserved for rural health clinics and federally qualified health centers. They facilitate that needed post–clinic visit touch base and carry some reimbursement.
- Use of telehealth—as noted, telehealth encompasses a broad variety of technologies and methods to deliver health and educational services under specific rules and guidelines.[37]
- Use of non–face-to-face prolonged service codes: these 2 codes (99358 and 99359) are time-based codes that reimburse for providers' non–face-to-face prolonged services. The key to the successful use of these add-on codes is ensuring to document the specific time the physician used to review records (not the providers' own) and speak with referring physicians, consultants, family, and so forth. These services may or may not be provided on the same day as the face-to-face E/M code—but an E/M code MUST be billed. In addition, the time does not have to be continuous, but the time must be documented, including the lapsed time.[38]
- Use of chronic care codes: these codes are a bit complex but often critical for oncologic patients. One of the best references is the frequently asked questions from Centers for Medicare and Medicaid Services.[39]
- Use of advanced care planning codes: talking with all patients regarding their unique wishes for quality of life is never more critical than with cardio-oncology patients. Additionally, these codes are used as quality metrics for many of the bundled initiatives, such as Bundled Payments for Care Improvement Advanced. There are codes that are reimbursed[40]—based on time spent with the patients—as well as F codes that, although they carry no reimbursement, do leave a record in the EMR regarding a patient's wishes.[41]
- Use of transitional care codes: cardio-oncology patients transition through many different settings in their journey. Physicians and advanced practice practitioners utilize these codes to ensure continuity of care that may begin 30 days from discharge and include (1) interactive contact within 2 business days; (2) providing a non–face-to-face service, such as review of medications or upcoming tests/treatments; and (3) ensuring there is a face-face visit within 7 days or 14 days.[42]
- Use of echocardiogram, 3-D echocardiogram, and strain codes: echocardiography often is the first choice of imaging modality for diagnosing cardiac dysfunction in cancer patients. Traditionally, an echocardiogram determination of left ventricular ejection fraction is requested by the oncologists in all cancer patients at baseline, in any situation in which the suspicion of heart failure is plausible, and both during and after completion of the anticancer therapy.[43] These add-on codes to an echocardiogram facilitate care of cardio-oncology patients. The use of strain imaging has demonstrated its value in cardio-oncology patients.[44,45] The payment for 3-D and strain is *ICD-10*–dependent—and an area where working with MAC carriers often is needed to ensure inclusion of the critical oncology codes.

These are just a few of the codes that should be in a toolkit as a cardio-oncology program is begun. It is imperative to work closely with payors and medical societies to remain current in their application and to remain ever vigilant for new codes as they are released.

SUMMARY

With the current status of cancer care in the United States, it stands to reason that many, if not all, hospitals would benefit from a dedicated cardio-oncology service line, with some expanding to a true center of excellence. There is background work that needs to be done, with respect to planning and garnering support of colleagues and administration, as well at attention to keeping the program financially viable to continue to provide the services that patients need. In the end, the value and commitment to providing the best care for cancer patients will be the sustaining force for a program.

REFERENCES

1. Zamorano JL, Lancellotti P, Rodriguez Muñoz D, et al, Authors/Task Force Members, ESC Committee for Practice Guidelines (CPG). 2016 ESC Position Paper on cancer treatments and cardiovascular toxicity developed under the auspices of the ESC Committee for Practice Guidelines: the Task Force

for cancer treatments and cardiovascular toxicity of the European Society of Cardiology (ESC). Eur Heart J 2016;37(36):2768–801.

2. Herrmann J, Lerman A, Sandhu NP, et al. Evaluation and management of patients with heart disease and cancer: cardio-oncology. Mayo Clin Proc 2014; 89(9):1287–306.

3. Dimarco A, Gaetani M, Orezzi P, et al. 'Daunomycin', a new antibiotic of the rhodomycin group. Nature 1964;201(4920):706–7.

4. Adamson RH. Letter: daunomycin (NSC-82151) and adriamycin (NSC-123127): a hypothesis concerning antitumor activity and cardiotoxicity. Cancer Chemother Rep 1974;58(3):293.

5. Gilladoga AC, Manuel C, Tan CT, et al. The cardiotoxicity of adriamycin and daunomycin in children. Cancer 1976;37(2 Suppl):1070–8.

6. Alexander J, Dainiak N, Berger HJ, et al. Serial assessment of doxorubicin cardiotoxicity with quantitative radionuclide angiocardiography. N Engl J Med 1979;300:278–83.

7. Armstrong T, Liu Q, Yasui Y, et al. Late mortality among 5-year survivors of childhood cancer: a summary from the childhood cancer survivor study. J Clin Oncol 2009;27(14):2328–38.

8. Yoon GJ, Telli ML, Kao DP, et al. Left ventricular dysfunction in patients receiving cardiotoxic cancer therapies are clinicians responding optimally? J Am Coll Cardiol 2010;56:1644–50.

9. Albini A, Pennesi G, Donatelli F, et al. Cardiotoxicity of anticancer drugs: the need for cardio-oncology and cardio-oncological prevention. J Natl Cancer Inst 2010;102:14–25.

10. Lenihan DJ, Hartlage G, Decara J. Cardio-oncology training: a proposal from the International Cardioncology Society and Canadian Cardiac Oncology Network for a new multidisciplinary specialty. J Card Fail 2016;22(6):465–71.

11. Fradley MG, Brown AC, Shields B, et al. Developing a comprehensive cardio-oncology program at a Cancer Institute: the Moffitt Cancer Center Experience. Oncol Rev 2017;11(2):340, 65-73.

12. Barac A, Murtagh G, Carver JR, et al. Cardiovascular health of patients with cancer and cancer survivors: a roadmap to the next level. J Am Coll Cardiol 2015;65:2739–46.

13. Bluethmann SM, Mariotto AB, Rowland JH. Anticipating the "Silver Tsunami" prevalence trajectories and comorbidity burden among older cancer survivors in the United States. Cancer Epidemiol Biomarkers Prev 2016;25(7):1029–36.

14. Centers for Medicare and Medicaid Services. National health expenditure data. Available at: CMS. gov https://www.cms.gov/resaech-statistics-data-and-systems/statistics-trends-and-reports/national healthexpenddata/index.html. Accessed April 5, 2019.

15. Gonzales S, Cox C. Kaiser Family Foundation: what are recent trends in cancer spending and outcomes? Peterson-Kaiser: health system tracker. Available at: https://www.healthsystemtracker.org. Accessed April 5, 2019.

16. Baghai R, Levine EH, Sataria SS. Service line strategies for US hospitals. The McKinsey Quarterly. Health Care; 2008. Available at: http://healthcare.mckinsey.com/sites/default/files/737801_Serviceline_strategies_for_US_hospitals__.pdf. Accessed April 7, 2019.

17. Tan C, Denlinger C. Cardiovascular toxicity in cancer survivors: current guidelines and future directions. 2018. Available at: https://www.acc.org/latest-in-cardiology/articles/2018/06/29/12/57/cv-toxicity-in-cancer-survivors. Accessed April 7, 2019.

18. Henson KE, Reulen RC, Winter DL, et al. Cardiac mortality among 200 000 five-year survivors of cancer diagnosed at 15 to 39 years of age: the teenage and young adult cancer survivor study. Circulation 2016;134(20):1519–31.

19. Gujral DM, Lloyd G, Bhattacharyya S. Provision and clinical utility of cardio-oncology services for the detection of cardiotoxicity in cancer patients. J Am Coll Cardiol 2016;67:1499–500.

20. Wallington SF, Dash C, Sheppard VB, et al. Enrolling minority and underserved populations in cancer clinical research. Am J Prev Med 2016;50(1):111–7.

21. Available at: https://www.cancer.org/research/cancer-facts-figure/cancer-facts-figures-2019.html. Accessed April 2, 2019.

22. Ferrell BR, Temel JS, Temin S, et al. Integration of palliative care into standard oncology care: American Society of Clinical Oncology Clinical Practice Guidelines. J Clin Oncol 2017;35(1):96–112.

23. Fitzgerald W, Neilson P. Development of an outpatient cardio-oncology program. 2018. Available at: accccancer.org. Accessed April 2, 2019.

24. Ghosh AK. How to build a cardio-oncology service. 2017. Available at: https://www.acc.org/latest-in-cardiology/articles/2017/10/24/08/43/how-to-build-a-cardio-oncology-service. Accessed April 2, 2019.

25. Okwuosa TM, Yeh ETH, Barac A. Burgeoning cardio-oncology programs. J Am Coll Cardiol 2015;66(10):1193–7.

26. Rocque GB, Pisu M, Jackson BE, et al. Resource use and medicare costs during lay navigation for geriatric patients with cancer. JAMA Oncol 2017; 3(6):817–25.

27. Armenian SH, Lacchetti C, Barac A, et al. Prevention and monitoring of cardiac dysfunction in survivors of adult cancers: American Society of Clinical Oncology Clinical Practice Guideline. J Clin Oncol 2017;35:893–911.

28. Plana JC, Galderisi M, Barac A, et al. Expert Consensus for Multimodality imaging evaluation of adult patients during and after cancer therapy:

a report from the American Society of Echocardiography and the European Association of Cardiovascular Imaging. Eur Heart J Cardiovasc Imaging 2014;15:1063–93.

29. Arnold A, Biga C, Mariani D. How to code and bill for cardio-oncology. 2018. Available at: https://www.acc.org/latest-in-cardiology/articles/2018/05/07/08/34/how-to-code-and-bill-for-cardio-oncology. Accessed April 2, 2019.

30. Available at: https://pmj.bmj.com/content/79/929/147.

31. U.S. Health care from a global perspective: spending, use of services, prices, and health in 13 countries (the commonwealth fund website). 2015. Available at: http://www.commonwealthfund.org/publications/issue-briefs/2015/oct/us-health-care-from-a-global-perspective.

32. Health care spending in the United States & selected OECD countries (Henry J. Kaiser Family Foundation website). Available at: http://kff.org/health-costs/issue-brief/snapshots-health-care-spending-in-the-united-states-selected-oecd-countries/.

33. Available at: https://healthpayerintelligence.com/news/how-macra-solves-challenges-of-sustainable-growth-rate-formula.

34. Available at: https://www.healthcare.gov/glossary/affordable-care-act/.

35. Available at: https://healthitanalytics.com/features/using-risk-scores-stratification-for-population-health-management.

36. Available at: http://oncpracticemanagement.com/issue-archive/2018/september-2018-vol-8-no-9/dispelling-misconceptions-about-hcc-coding/.

37. Available at: https://www.cchpca.org/about/about-telehealth.

38. Available at: https://www.aappublications.org/news/2018/01/10/Coding010518.

39. Available at: https://www.cms.gov/Medicare/Medicare-Fee-for-Service-Payment/HospitalOutpatientPPS/Downloads/Payment-Chronic-Care-Management-Services-FAQs.pdf.

40. Available at: https://www.cms.gov/Medicare/Medicare-Fee-for-Service-Payment/PhysicianFeeSched/Downloads/FAQ-Advance-Care-Planning.pdf.

41. Available at: https://www.cms.gov/outreach-and-education/medicare-learning-network-mln/mlnproducts/downloads/advancecareplanning.pdf.

42. Available at: https://www.cms.gov/outreach-and-education/medicare-learning-network-mln/mlnproducts/downloads/transitional-care-management-services-fact-sheet-icn908628.pdf.

43. Neilan TG, Jassal DS, Perez-Sanz TM, et al. Tissue Doppler imaging predicts left ventricular dysfunction and mortality in a murine model of cardiac injury. Eur Heart J 2006;27:1868–75.

44. Available at: https://www.acc.org/latest-in-cardiology/articles/2017/06/26/08/15/echocardiographic-strain-has-clinical-use.

45. Available at: https://www.escardio.org/Journals/E-Journal-of-Cardiology-Practice/Volume-16/What-is-the-best-imaging-tool-in-cardio-oncology.

UNITED STATES POSTAL SERVICE ®

Statement of Ownership, Management, and Circulation
(All Periodicals Publications Except Requester Publications)

1. Publication Title	2. Publication Number	3. Filing Date
CARDIOLOGY CLINICS	000 – 701	9/18/2019

4. Issue Frequency	5. Number of Issues Published Annually	6. Annual Subscription Price
FEB, MAY, AUG, NOV	4	$349.00

7. Complete Mailing Address of Known Office of Publication (Not printer) (Street, city, county, state, and ZIP+4®)

ELSEVIER INC.
230 Park Avenue, Suite 800
New York, NY 10169

Contact Person
STEPHEN R. BUSHING

Telephone (Include area code)
215-239-3688

8. Complete Mailing Address of Headquarters or General Business Office of Publisher (Not printer)

ELSEVIER INC.
230 Park Avenue, Suite 800
New York, NY 10169

9. Full Names and Complete Mailing Addresses of Publisher, Editor, and Managing Editor (Do not leave blank)

Publisher (Name and complete mailing address)

TAYLOR BALL, ELSEVIER INC.
1600 JOHN F KENNEDY BLVD. SUITE 1800
PHILADELPHIA, PA 19103-2899

Editor (Name and complete mailing address)

STACY EASTMAN, ELSEVIER INC.
1600 JOHN F KENNEDY BLVD. SUITE 1800
PHILADELPHIA, PA 19103-2899

Managing Editor (Name and complete mailing address)

PATRICK MANLEY, ELSEVIER INC.
1600 JOHN F KENNEDY BLVD. SUITE 1800
PHILADELPHIA, PA 19103-2899

10. Owner (Do not leave blank. If the publication is owned by a corporation, give the name and address of the corporation immediately followed by the names and addresses of all stockholders owning or holding 1 percent or more of the total amount of stock. If not owned by a corporation, give the names and addresses of the individual owners. If owned by a partnership or other unincorporated firm, give its name and address as well as those of each individual owner. If the publication is published by a nonprofit organization, give its name and address.)

Full Name	Complete Mailing Address
WHOLLY OWNED SUBSIDIARY OF REED/ELSEVIER, US HOLDINGS	1600 JOHN F KENNEDY BLVD. SUITE 1800 PHILADELPHIA, PA 19103-2899

11. Known Bondholders, Mortgagees, and Other Security Holders Owning or Holding 1 Percent or More of Total Amount of Bonds, Mortgages, or Other Securities. If none, check box ► ☐ None

Full Name	Complete Mailing Address
N/A	

12. Tax Status (For completion by nonprofit organizations authorized to mail at nonprofit rates) (Check one)
The purpose, function, and nonprofit status of this organization and the exempt status for federal income tax purposes:
☒ Has Not Changed During Preceding 12 Months
☐ Has Changed During Preceding 12 Months (Publisher must submit explanation of change with this statement)

PS Form **3526**, July 2014 [Page 1 of 4 (see instructions page 4)] PSN: 7530-01-000-9931 PRIVACY NOTICE: See our privacy policy on www.usps.com.

13. Publication Title	14. Issue Date for Circulation Data Below
CARDIOLOGY CLINICS	MAY 2019

15. Extent and Nature of Circulation			Average No. Copies Each Issue During Preceding 12 Months	No. Copies of Single Issue Published Nearest to Filing Date
a. Total Number of Copies (Net press run)			149	183
b. Paid Circulation (By Mail and Outside the Mail)	(1)	Mailed Outside-County Paid Subscriptions Stated on PS Form 3541 (Include paid distribution above nominal rate, advertiser's proof copies, and exchange copies)	66	90
	(2)	Mailed In-County Paid Subscriptions Stated on PS Form 3541 (Include paid distribution above nominal rate, advertiser's proof copies, and exchange copies)	0	0
	(3)	Paid Distribution Outside the Mails Including Sales Through Dealers and Carriers, Street Vendors, Counter Sales, and Other Paid Distribution Outside USPS®	36	51
	(4)	Paid Distribution by Other Classes of Mail Through the USPS (e.g., First-Class Mail®)	0	0
c. Total Paid Distribution (Sum of 15b (1), (2), (3), and (4))		►	102	141
d. Free or Nominal Rate Distribution (By Mail and Outside the Mail)	(1)	Free or Nominal Rate Outside-County Copies included on PS Form 3541	35	26
	(2)	Free or Nominal Rate In-County Copies Included on PS Form 3541	0	0
	(3)	Free or Nominal Rate Copies Mailed at Other Classes Through the USPS (e.g., First-Class Mail)	0	0
	(4)	Free or Nominal Rate Distribution Outside the Mail (Carriers or other means)	0	0
e. Total Free or Nominal Rate Distribution (Sum of 15d (1), (2), (3) and (4))		►	35	26
f. Total Distribution (Sum of 15c and 15e)		►	137	167
g. Copies not Distributed (See Instructions to Publishers #4 (page #3))		►	12	16
h. Total (Sum of 15f and g)		►	149	183
i. Percent Paid (15c divided by 15f times 100)		►	74.45%	84.43%

* If you are claiming electronic copies, go to line 16 on page 3. If you are not claiming electronic copies, skip to line 17 on page 3.

16. Electronic Copy Circulation		Average No. Copies Each Issue During Preceding 12 Months	No. Copies of Single Issue Published Nearest to Filing Date
a. Paid Electronic Copies	►		
b. Total Paid Print Copies (Line 15c) + Paid Electronic Copies (Line 16a)	►		
c. Total Print Distribution (Line 15f) + Paid Electronic Copies (Line 16a)	►		
d. Percent Paid (Both Print & Electronic Copies) (16b divided by 16c x 100)	►		

☒ I certify that 50% of all my distributed copies (electronic and print) are paid above a nominal price.

17. Publication of Statement of Ownership

☒ If the publication is a general publication, publication of this statement is required. Will be printed in the NOVEMBER 2019 issue of this publication. ☐ Publication not required.

18. Signature and Title of Editor, Publisher, Business Manager, or Owner

STEPHEN R. BUSHING - INVENTORY DISTRIBUTION CONTROL MANAGER

Stephen R. Bushing   Date 9/18/2019

I certify that all information furnished on this form is true and complete. I understand that anyone who furnishes false or misleading information on this form or who omits material or information requested on the form may be subject to criminal sanctions (including fines and imprisonment) and/or civil sanctions (including civil penalties).

PS Form **3526**, July 2014 (Page 3 of 4) PRIVACY NOTICE: See our privacy policy on www.usps.com.